D1446296

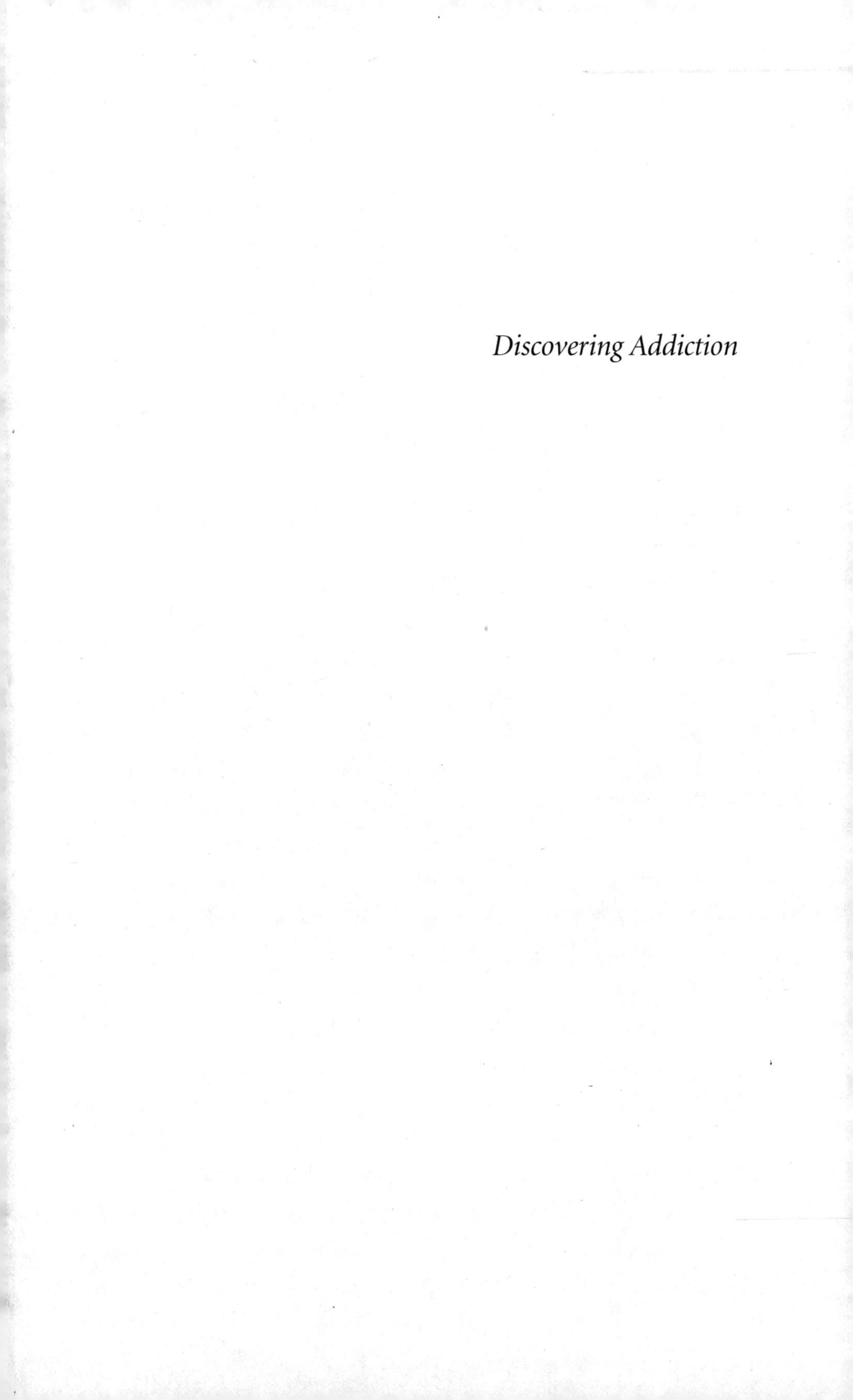

Discovering Addiction

Discovering Addiction

The Science and Politics of Substance Abuse Research

NANCY D. CAMPBELL

The University of Michigan Press
Ann Arbor

Published in the United States of America by
The University of Michigan Press
Manufactured in the United States of America
⊗ Printed on acid-free paper

2010 2009 2008 2007 4 3 2 1

A CIP catalog record for this book is available from the British Library.

Library of Congress Cataloging-in-Publication Data

Campbell, Nancy Dianne.
Discovering addiction : the science and politics of substance abuse research / Nancy D. Campbell.
p. ; cm.
Includes bibliographical references and index.
ISBN-13: 978-0-472-11610-2 (cloth : alk. paper)
ISBN-10: 0-472-11610-X (cloth : alk. paper)
1. Substance abuse. I. Title.
[DNLM: 1. Substance-Related Disorders. 2. Health Policy.
WM 270 C189d 2007]

RC564.C33 2007
362.29—dc22 2007023393

Against amnesia,
this book is dedicated to the researchers at Lexington
and the postaddicts who served as human subjects
in the obscurity of long-dead laboratories

Acknowledgments

The social worlds of drug policy historians and substance abuse researchers are convivial thought collectives. I would particularly like to thank Joseph Spillane, who forged a relationship with the University of Michigan Substance Abuse Research Center (UMSARC). Carol Boyd and Sean MacCabe facilitated our relationship with the College on Problems of Drug Dependence (CPDD), the modern-day incarnation of the original National Research Council committee described (under its various names) in this book. CPDD remains the premier professional association in the field but is now a large membership organization. The CPDD Board of Directors granted over twelve thousand dollars for the interviews on which this book is based. I am grateful to Martin and Toby Adler, Bob Schuster and Chris-Ellyn Johanson, Conan Kornetsky, Wallace Pickworth, and the dozens of CPDD members who allowed us to interview them. The University of Michigan Department of Pharmacology was especially hospitable, and I would like to thank Jim Woods and Gail Winger, Jonathan Maybaum, Ed Domino, and Graham Florry, who graciously volunteered time and insight without which this project would have been impossible. Of course, the author alone is responsible for all errors of omission and commission, as well as differences of interpretation. The interviews were transcribed by Elaine Farris with great generosity, good humor, and accuracy.

At a crucial point, the National Science Foundation funded the oral history project (grant #SES-0620320) so that we could create a digital archive for the interviews, which will be housed on the UMSARC Web site and in the Bentley Historical Library at the University of Michigan. Joseph Spillane joined me on some of the interviews, and a veritable cavalcade of stars agreed to serve on our advisory board. I would like to thank UMSARC's current director, Peggy Ngegy, for the initial inspiration for the advisory board; Carol Boyd for agreeing to head it; and Caroline Acker, David Courtwright, Eloise Dunlap, Sheigla Murphy, and David Musto for joining us. These people comprise a substantial part of the small but committed research community in drug policy history and drug ethnography. Jonathan Maybaum, creator of the SiteMaker software, skillfully guided us through the design of the Web site over the course of several wintry weekends. The process of writing and submitting the grant itself would have been far more difficult and less pleasant without the work of Dean Button of Rensselaer Polytechnic Institute.

During the writing process, I was surprised to encounter independent filmmakers J. P. Olsen and Luke Walden, who were as fascinated by Lexington as I was. Their film *The Narcotics Farm* tells the story of "Narco" from the perspective of those who experienced another side of that Lexington institution. My own archival work was ably assisted at the National Archives Southeast in Morrow, Georgia, by archivist Guy Hall and staple-puller extraordinaire Aaron Pevey and at College Park by Bureau of Prisons archivist John W. Roberts. Benefiting from the gifts of a fortuitous environment, I also enjoyed a shipment from the basement of Jon M. Harkness that illuminated the darker corners of the prison research enterprise. Basements served as my archives more than once: I am grateful to Chuck and Barbara Gorodetzky for allowing me to spend hours in theirs despite my advanced stages of pregnancy. I thank Andrea Tone for directing me to the American College of Neuropsychopharmacology (ACNP); Oakley Ray, longtime secretary of that organization, for supporting travel to the archives housed at the Eskind Biomedical Library at Vanderbilt University; and archivist Jeremy Nordmoe. The Rensselaer Polytechnic Institute Office of Research supported the first round of interviews with an internal seed grant to myself, Kim Fortun, and Mike Fortun titled "Pharmacogenomics, Toxicogenomics, and the Ethical Implications of Scientific Research on Complex Conditions: A Research Program to Study Emergent Decision Domains at the Intersection of Biotechnology and Information Technology."

I owe a great debt to Bill Eppridge and his wife, Adrienne Aurichio, whose generosity in the final days of this project led to Bill's extraordinary photographs appearing in this book. As a Time-Life photojournalist working on the first story about middle-class white heroin use to appear in the mainstream press, Bill was dispatched to the monkey laboratory at Michigan and the clinical research facility at Lexington late in the fall of 1964, after spending three months the previous summer photographing "John and Karen, Two Lives Lost to Heroin" (a *Life* magazine story and photo essay published on February 26, 1965 and March 5, 1965). Given the paucity of visual images of Lexington available in the National Archives, these photographs were extremely valuable for evoking the feel of the place.

Writing the acknowledgments to a book five years in the making feels like bringing together multiple lives. The feminist community sustains me despite the fact that gender, social policy, and the politics of reproductive rights are underplayed in this book. Michele Berger, Giovanna Di Chiro, Mary Margaret Fonow, Donna Haraway, Sally Kitch, Patti Lather, Nancy Naples, Lynn Paltrow, Sandy Schram, Susan Shaw, and Rickie Solinger remain important to everything that I do. Carol Bohmer and Amy Shuman graciously extended speaking invitations during this time. I am indebted to my doctoral students, Maral Erol, Virginia Eubanks, Jenrose Fitzgerald, and Lorna Ronald, as well as colleagues elsewhere, including Alexine Fleck, Kim Hewitt, Marcia Meldrum, and Noemi Tousignant. I thank the graduate students central to the Rensselaer science and technology studies community, especially Colin Beech, Jon Cluck, Ayala Cnaan, Camar Diaz-Torres, Rachel Dowty, Jill Fisher, Ken Fleischman, Allison Kenner, Eun-sung Kim, Natasha Lettis, Torin Monahan, Dean Nieusma, Casey O'Donnell, Marie Rarieya, Erich Schienke, Jeannette Simmonds, Peg Woodell, Shailaja Valdiya, and Bo Xie, as well as undergraduates Dalibel Bravo, Amrit Mohanran, Adam Marcus, Hasan Abdul-Mutakalli, Brandon Reiss, and Dane Dell and Jason Williams, who helped me with research in the last year of this book's writing. Members of my more local community who have helped me work through parts of this book include Steve Breyman, Linnda Caporael, Scott Christianson, Tamar Gordon, Kim Fortun, Mike Fortun, Rayvon Fouche, David Hess, Linda Layne, Sal Restivo, Sharra Vostral, Langdon Winner, and Edward J. Woodhouse. For collegiality and camaraderie at Rensselaer, I thank Sharon Anderson-Gold, Anne Borrea, Igor Broos, Dean Button, Lisa D'Angelo, John Harrington, Kathy High, Branda Miller, Don Moore, Pam Murarka, Barb Nelson, Allison Newman, Lee Odell, and Kathie Vumbacco. The intellectual hospitality of Kim, Mike, Kora, and Lena Fortun knows no peer. Finally, I would like to thank my family—my parents, Sandra Campbell and David R. Campbell, MD; Connie Campbell, MD, and Tony Diehl; Dave and Amanda Campbell; Gary Campbell; and my partner in all things, Ned Woodhouse, who, along with our children, Isaac Campbell Eglash and Grace Campbell Woodhouse, graciously and grudgingly tolerated my sporadic absences, increasingly insomniac work habits, and obscure enthusiasms. Getting me to play rather than work is their prime objective, and for that I am most grateful.

Contents

A Note on Sources

Travel and transcription were supported by the College on Problems of Drug Dependence, the University of Michigan Substance Abuse Research Center, the Center for Substance Abuse Research at Wayne State University, and the Office of Research at Rensselaer Polytechnic Institute.

Between 2003 and 2006, the following individuals were interviewed by me alone or with Joseph F. Spillane, at the places and times indicated in parentheses: Howard S. Becker, PhD, professor emeritus, Department of Sociology, University of California at Santa Barbara (January 2005); Edward Domino, professor of pharmacology, University of Michigan (Ann Arbor, Michigan, November 2006); Charles W. Gorodetzky, MD, PhD, retired vice president, deputy department head, and department head, Neurology Team Medical and Scientific Services, Quintiles Transnational (Kansas City, Missouri, July 2003); Donald Jasinski, PhD, chief, Center for Chemical Dependency, and professor, Department of Medicine, Johns Hopkins Bayview Medical Center (Baltimore, Maryland, May 2003); Herman Joseph, PhD, (Troy, New York, August 2005); Conan Kornetsky, PhD, professor, Departments of Psychiatry and Pharmacology, Boston University School of Medicine (Boston, Massachusetts, May 2003); Peter Mansky, MD, executive director, Nevada Health Professionals Assistance Foundation (December 2005, January 2006); Lucinda L. Miner, PhD, deputy director, Office of Science Policy and Communications, National Institute on Drug Abuse (May 2003); Sheigla Murphy, PhD, director, Center for Substance Abuse Studies, Institute for Scientific Analysis (New Orleans, Louisiana, June 2003); Oakley Ray, PhD, Vanderbilt University (Nashville, Tennessee, February 2006); Mark A. Rothstein, JD, Institute for Bioethics, Health Policy, and Law, University of Louisville School of Medicine (Louisville, Kentucky, March 2003); Marjorie Senechal, PhD, Louise Wolff Kahn professor in mathematics and the history of science, Smith College (Northampton, Massachusetts, September 2005); George R. Uhl, MD, PhD, chief, Molecular Neurobiology Branch, NIDA, Intramural Research Program (Baltimore, Maryland, 2003); Daniel Wikler, PhD, Mary B. Saltenstall professor of population ethics and professor of ethics and population health, Department of Population and International Health, Harvard University (2005); and James Woods, PhD, professor of pharmacology, University of Michigan (San Juan, Puerto Rico, June 2003; Ann Arbor, Michigan, March 2005).

The following individuals were interviewed at the annual meeting of the Conference on Problems of Drug Dependence in Phoenix, Arizona, in June 2006: Anna Rose Childress, PhD, research associate professor of psychology in psychiatry, Treatment Research Center, University of Pennsylvania; Theodore Cicero, PhD, professor of neuropharmacology in psychiatry, Washington University in St. Louis; James Inciardi, PhD, director, Center for Drug and Alcohol Studies, University of Miami; Bruce D. Johnson, PhD, director, Institute for Special Populations Research, National Development and Research Institute, New York; Beny Primm, MD, executive director, Addiction Research and Treatment Corporation, Brooklyn, New York; and Edward G. Singleton, National Institute on Drug Abuse.

The following individuals were interviewed by me alone or with Joseph F. Spillane at the annual meeting of the Conference on Problems of Drug Dependence in Orlando, Florida, in June 2005: George Bigelow, PhD, professor of behavioral pharmacology, Johns Hopkins University; Thomas Crowley, PhD, professor, University of Colorado; William Dewey, PhD, professor of pharmacology, Virginia Commonwealth University; Loretta Finnegan, MD; Roland Griffiths, PhD, professor of behavioral pharmacology, Johns Hopkins University; Rolley E. Johnson, PharmD, Reckitt-Benkhiser, Richmond, Virginia; Michael Kuhar, PhD, chief, Division of Neuroscience, Yerkes National Primate Research Center, and Candler professor of pharmacology, Emory University; Catherine A. Martin, PhD, professor, Department of Psychiatry, University of Kentucky, Lexington, Kentucky; Jane Maxwell, PhD, research professor, School of Social Work, University of Texas at Austin; Charles P. O'Brien, MD, PhD, director, Treatment Research Center, University of Pennsylvania; Charles O'Keefe, Virginia Commonwealth University, Richmond, Virginia; Richard Spence, PhD, research professor, School of Social Work, University of Texas at Austin; and Frank Vocci, PhD, director, Division of Treatment Research and Development, NIDA.

The following individuals were interviewed by me at the annual meeting of the Conference on Problems of Drug Dependence in San Juan, Puerto Rico, in June 2004: Robert Balster, PhD, professor of pharmacology and toxicology and director, Virginia Commonwealth University Institute for Drug and Alcohol Studies; Louis Harris, PhD, professor of pharmacology, Medical College of Virginia, Virginia Commonwealth University; Jack Henningfield, PhD, NIDA,

Intramural Research Program; Arthur Jacobsen, PhD, National Institute of Diabetes and Digestive and Kidney Diseases (NIDDK), National Institutes of Health (NIH); Chris-Ellyn Johanson, PhD, director, Wayne State University Center for Substance Abuse Research; Herb Kleber, MD, PhD, professor of psychiatry and director, Division on Substance Abuse, College of Physicians and Surgeons, Columbia University; Mary Jeanne Kreek, PhD, Laboratory of the Biology of Addictive Diseases, Rockefeller University; Wallace B. Pickworth, PhD, retired, NIDA, Intramural Research Program; Kenner Rice, PhD, NIDDK, NIH; Charles R. (Bob) Schuster, PhD, Wayne State University Center for Substance Abuse Research; Tsung-Ping Su, PhD, NIDA, Intramural Research Program; and Eddie Leong Way, PhD, professor emeritus, Department of Pharmacology, University of California at San Francisco.

The American College of Neuropsychopharmacology archives enabled me to look at the papers of Leo Hollister and Heinz Lehmann and to read transcripts or view videotaped interviews from the Oral History Collection for the following people: Martin Adler (1996), Julius Axelrod (1997), William Bunney (2001), Jonathan Cole (1994, 1999), Leonard Cook (n.d.), Peter B. Dews (n.d.), Edward Domino (n.d.), Fred Goodwin (1996), Leo Hollister (1996, 1999), Jerome Jaffe (1998), Murray Jarvik (n.d.), Donald Jasinski (1997), Seymour Kety (n.d.), Eva Killam (1994), Keith Killam (1994), Herb Kleber (n.d.), Conan Kornetsky (n.d.), Louis Lasagna (n.d.), Charles P. O'Brien (1998), Candace Pert (n.d.), Roy Pickens (1997), Solomon Snyder (n.d.), and Larry Stein (1995). David Healy's published interviews from this series were also a valuable data set. Finally, I am grateful to Jon M. Harkness, Jackie Orr, J. P. Olsen, and Luke Walden, all of whom generously shared interviews they conducted with researchers who did time at Lexington.

A Note on Interviews

Charles Gorodetzky was hired at the Addiction Research Center (ARC) in 1963, became deputy director in 1977 and scientific director of the ARC preclinical program that remained at Lexington in 1981, left public service for the pharmaceutical industry in 1984, and retired in 2005. Harris Isbell retired from the Public Health Service in 1963 to chair the Department of Medicine at the University of Kentucky and died in 1994. He was survived by his daughters. Donald Jasinski was hired at the ARC in 1965, became director in 1977 and scientific director of the ARC Baltimore in 1981, and was still working at Johns Hopkins University at the time of this writing. His pharmacist assistant, Rolley E. (Ed) Johnson, PharmD, spent several years on the Hopkins faculty before moving to Reckitt Benkhiser, the company that brought buprenorphine to the U.S. market. Herb Kleber, who was at the Lexington Hospital as a "two-year wonder" in 1963, was still directing the Division of Substance Abuse at the College of Physicians and Surgeons of Columbia University at the time of this writing. Conan Kornetsky was hired at the ARC as a University of Kentucky graduate student in 1948, departed in the early 1950s, and was still working at Boston University at the time of this writing. Isbell's successor, William R. Martin, was hired at the ARC in 1957 and appointed ARC director in 1963, retired in 1977 to become chair of pharmacology at the University of Kentucky School of Medicine, and died in 1992. He was survived by his wife, sons, and daughter. Charles R. (Bob) Schuster, former director of NIDA, was still working at Wayne State University at the time of this writing. Abraham Wikler retired in 1963, went to the University of Kentucky, and died in 1983. He was survived by his wife, Ada Wikler, and his children, Marjorie Senechal, now a professor at Smith College; Jeanne Wikler; Norma Wikler (now deceased); and Daniel Wikler, now a bioethicist at Harvard University.

Introduction

Popular beliefs about drugs and drug addiction are increasingly pitched in the language of science, which has become part of the stew of assumptions and stories we serve each other in everyday life. Drug users speak of being overtaken by cravings or uncontrollable urges, a way of speaking drawn from notions of appetite, habit, and craving that come not from unmediated drug experiences but from psychoanalysis. When relapse is attributed to "cues" or "triggers," patients and providers draw on a vocabulary of operant conditioning introduced by experimental psychologists and behavioral analysts. When drug users speak of feeling "chemically imbalanced," they rely on a late twentieth-century vocabulary of endorphins, neurotransmitters, opiate receptors, and brain chemistry drawn from neuroscience. Science offers specialized vocabularies that fuse with popular vernaculars—"the fix," "the rush," "getting high," "hitting bottom," or "kicking the habit"—through which people describe their innermost sensations. Expressive argots recursively feed into science: scientific theories affect how people interpret drug experiences, and users' reports in turn become research material. The frames used in science are consequential, for the production of scientific knowledge is a social privilege inextricably bound to questions of social justice.

Scientific knowledge about drug addiction is believed to reveal the inner workings of brains, minds, and bodies.[1] Addiction knows none of the social distinctions imposed by policy regimes that have repeatedly constructed drug use as a crime or as a disease in the United States.[2] Calling something a "disease" appeals to scientific conventions and clinical vocabularies but generates a cascade of questions: Is it curable or incurable? Does it mark its victims? Is it a metabolic disease, an infectious disease, a brain disease, a social contagion, a biochemical imbalance, a disease of the will, a disease of desire, a disease of stress? Is it chronic, lifelong, or episodic? Is it more like diabetes or allergy? Is it genetic? Addiction researchers have taken up all these possibilities at one time or another as they struggle to explain individual variation in vulnerability to addiction and relapse.

Discovering Addiction reveals that scientific efforts to explicate addiction have each answered the preceding questions differently and that none have stabilized any one set of answers for long. Scientific categories are also social distinctions, for habits of mind and body promote psychoactive drugs to positions of social and cultural significance. Access to drugs deemed problematic is restricted through formal laws, informal policies, and social norms; access to drugs deemed useful or medicinal is not only encouraged but prescribed. Some drugs are taken to cause problems; others to solve them. "Bad" drugs are shunned; "good" ones are promoted. Whether legal or illegal, recreation or medication, lubricant or barrier, drugs structure identities and relationships, social routines of work and play, and local and global economies.

BRINGING TO LIFE THE HISTORY OF ADDICTION RESEARCH

Scientific inquiry has substantially influenced the shifting lexicons and logics through which drug use is understood. This book is about the scientific communities that contribute to the confluence of scientific research, clinical practice, and social policy through which addiction has been addressed. Substance abuse researchers have grappled with what "addiction" means in the human and animal laboratories through which they have brought their science to life. *Discovering Addiction* reenacts the technical and ethical dilemmas that pervade the political, ethical, economic, and policy contexts in which this branch of science originated and is situated today.

Addiction researchers comprised one of the first multidisciplinary collaborative clinical research teams assembled expressly to mount a collective assault on a scientific frontier that was simultaneously considered a social problem (Walsh 1973a, 1229). The historical origins of addiction research lie in the Addiction Research Center (ARC), a laboratory that was once part of a federal prison-hospital in Lexington, Kentucky, and in the "monkey colony" at the University of Michigan at Ann Arbor. Characterizing addiction research as an "extraordinarily closed world," a *Science* magazine reporter described dominant personalities who exerted a "virtual monopoly" over knowledge production at the time (Walsh 1973a).[3] I analyze the making and unmaking of that closed world, mapping how the field morphed into a bewildering array of intersecting social worlds, each with its own vocabularies, hierarchies of credibility, and laboratory logics.[4] In writing the history of substance abuse research, I have struggled to come to terms with the scruples of those who conducted experiments on animals and human beings in these two sites. How did they construct, maintain, preserve, and defend their self-identity as ethical scientists, as physicians who were taught the precept, "first do no harm," and as scientific authorities who worked within an "illegitimate" or "stigmatized" research enterprise?

Despite attempts to clear the air, a whiff of stigma surrounds not only the objects and subjects of drug research but researchers themselves (Becker 1963; Clarke 1998; Goffman 1963). They differ on how to define and pose the problems they study. Many eschew the term *addiction,* already a dirty word in "drug dependence" research by the early 1950s. Since then, an array of substitutes has been offered—from "drug abuse" research in the 1970s, "substance abuse" or "chemical dependency" research in the 1980s, and research on "chronic, relapsing brain disorders" in the 1990s (White 2004). Today the phenomena under study have mutated into matters of "disrupted volition" (Volkow 2006) and "neurobiology gone awry" (Volkow and Li 2004), and the term *addiction* is in the process of returning to vogue (O'Brien, Volkow, and Li 2006). Each generation reconfigures the lexicon. Semantic shifts signal conceptual and technological changes in how science is done, as well as the changing social contexts, material conditions, and institutions within which scientific knowledge is made.

Discovering Addiction provides a history of the changing status of drug users as objects and subjects of knowledge. Terms like *paradigm shift* or *zeitgeist* are somewhat mystical explanations for how change happens in scientific communities. Instead of using such terminology, this book is organized around the focal concept of "laboratory logics," the pattern of beliefs that shape practical reasoning in science. Practitioners within epistemic communities trade in relatively narrow and coherent structures of belief that enable and constrain the lexicons, techniques, technologies, and practices that are considered legitimate ways to speak authoritatively about drugs in a given domain. Laboratory logics connect cultural beliefs and prior commitments to the actual practices enacted in the lab. Some laboratory logics incite research subjects to speak; others require their silence. Despite my emphasis on the laboratory, I believe that drug users themselves know quite a bit about how drugs work. This book tells the story of how they have come to play a lesser role in producing scientific and clinical knowledge than they once did.

In the 1950s, scientific researchers argued that drug addiction should be treated as a public health problem. They won few adherents beyond a handful of lawyers and sociologists opposed to framing addiction as either a crime or a disease (Becker 1963; Lindesmith 1946, 1947). No alliance formed between those who sought to reframe addiction as a public health matter. When I first encountered the scientific voices of the mid-twentieth century, I wondered who these "science guys" were, where they came from, and what authority led them to stand up to resist a law enforcement apparatus that was bent on prosecuting physicians and scorned scientific knowledge. Where did their knowledge come from? What were their relationships with addicted persons? Did they exploit the bodies and minds of their subjects—human or animal—in the name of science? Their research subjects, too, testified that addicts should be treated as if they were sick persons rather than criminals (Campbell 2000). What did these drug users think about those who put them under a microscope? Did they feel used, like the "human guinea pigs" the popular press made them out to be? Archives are largely silent on such questions. Interrogating the ethos that the addiction research culture carried into its work required bringing back to life long-dead laboratories where conversations arose about the ethics of experimental work with human and animal subjects. Long before clinical researchers confronted today's compulsory ethical questions, addiction researchers debated whether "treatment-naive populations" were preferable to "knowledgeable subjects" who had experiences with drugs behind them. Taking a fresh look at how addiction researchers coped with their predicaments casts today's unresolved dilemmas into sharper relief and puts historical flesh on bioethical bones.

LOOKING INSIDE THE SOCIAL WORLDS OF ADDICTION RESEARCH

While no science speaks with a unified voice, substance abuse researchers comprise a remarkably disunified chorus. Listening closely to substance abuse researchers can tax even the most scientifically literate scholars and the most well-informed policy makers. Although this cauldron of conceptual confusion can be a barrier to understanding, multiplicity in the sciences can also be a source of strength rather than a failing (Mol 2002). Multiple literacies are less a problem to manage than valuable tools for mapping boundaries between different communities of practice and attending to what it means to cross them. Doing oral history interviews forced me to cross boundaries between science and policy that I would once have left intact. I have become accustomed to being scolded about using terminology that issues from a social domain, scientific approach, or historical moment different from those of my interviewee. Thus my favorite definition of a drug has become the most prosaic one: "a substance that, when injected into a rat, produces a scientific paper" (Leake 1975, 30).

Given the centrality of drugs in social life, it is surprising that the history of scientific research on addiction has not yet been mapped in the social studies of scientific knowledge. Though *Science* magazine decades ago cast narcotics research as ripe for the sociology of science (Walsh 1973a), addiction research has yet to attract its share of sociologists, historians, or cultural theorists of science, medicine, and technology.[5] Griffith Edwards, longtime editor of *Addictions,* has observed, "Despite the growing interest in building a cadre of specialists devoted to the study, management, and prevention of addiction, there is still virtually no systematic information, much less an organized body of knowledge, about the individual and social factors that contribute to the evolution of a specialist field like addiction studies" (2002, 383). Historian Virginia Berridge has lamented the lack of analytic history of addiction despite increased availability of primary source materials such as oral histories and visual material (2006). *Discovering Addiction* replies to these lacunae by providing a historical account of the social organization of scientific knowledge production about drug addiction, a history of the ethics of human and animal experimentation, and a historical sociological account of the structure of a public science that was organized in the face of a proprietary pharmaceutical industry.

Listening to insider accounts by lifelong inhabitants of the addiction research enterprise is instructive for discerning the social structure of the scientific communities involved in "discovering" or constructing addiction. My work is indebted to "participant-historians" who have written accounts of their scientific careers or conducted interviews with one another. These sources informed my own interviews with key figures. I am grateful as well to scientists and surviving family members who granted me access to primary materials moldering in basements and filing cabinets. I have used all of these materials as well as the sparse scholarly literature to understand the social structures and material conditions that shaped the beliefs, commitments, and practices I here describe.[6] The chapters of this book cohere around the figures of prominent scientists not because of their individual genius or acumen but because they were what Ludwik Fleck called "standard-bearers in discovery" (1979, 42), voicing new laboratory logics and embodying emerging configurations in ways that have periodically remade the social worlds of substance abuse research.

Participant-historians were invaluable in distinguishing scientific subgroups, establishing patterns of interaction within social networks, and documenting accelerations in the pace of innovation or geographic mobility, formation of institutional infrastructures, and growth of coherent identity and shared history. For example, behavioral pharmacologist Joseph V. Brady's (2004) "revisionist" history of the field argues that the conceptual interplay between behavioral analysis and pharmacology came about not because of individual genius but from the "gifts of a fortuitous environment"—a widening pharmacopeia, increased federal support, and growth of in-house pharmaceutical industry testing. He attributed research pharmacologists' interest in drug abuse to regulatory efforts to assess the abuse liability of compounds not yet on the market, a point that insiders consider obvious but that an outsider might miss by emphasizing another facet of the addiction research enterprise, such as the search for less addictive painkillers or more effective addiction treatments. No one facet should be conflated with the others; no one facet is sufficient to understand the whole. No one definition of addiction has integrated enough levels of analysis to achieve universal acceptance or even to survive very long.

Insider accounts also offer invaluable clues to the thought styles at play in a scientific collective (Fleck 1979), but they are of course always political reconstructions of events (Clarke 1998, 5). Thus "internal history" must be handled with care so as to avoid overreliance on major figures at the expense of social-structural factors. Griffith Edwards has acknowledged: "The heroic view of history as something constructed by the deeds of great men and women is today not too fashionable. The historian in this case will rightly insist that what has happened over these decades in the drug and alcohol field must be understood in terms of technical innovations, the larger background social processes, and the great play of ideas" (1991, xiv). My focus on the conceptual interplay between the social organization of science and the discoveries of individual laboratories spurred the turn to oral history, which offers data on the shifting repertoire of lexicons and logics through which addiction has been theorized. Oral history plays a contested role in the history of science and medicine because it is often identified with internalist history. Pharmacologist David Healy, who has published interviews with his colleagues, has been taken to task for basing his analysis on "reminiscences, oral histories, and interviews made by the author with his fellow psychopharmacologists" (Rasmussen 2003). Yet interview transcripts tap into a reservoir of material on the social organization of the research enterprise and reveal how scientists perform their everyday ethical subjectivity.

Oral history interviews offer empirical pointers toward what begs for analysis. Research ethics were typically broached by those whose careers began at the Addiction Research Center in Lexington, Kentucky, many of whom assumed my interests lay primarily in the treatment of human subjects rather than the sociology of knowledge. Jerome H. Jaffe has explained that the ARC "stood virtually alone as [an] island of scholarship in a sea of general indifference to questions about the nature and treatment of alcohol and drug problems" and that "the few scholars who did become interested in these backwaters of science were either affiliated with th[is] center or dutifully made voyages to [it]" (2002, 101). Today's addiction research enterprise can be traced to these "backwaters," from which an impressive number of key figures sailed into prominent roles in government, academia, or industry.

UNSETTLING ASSUMPTIONS: EXPERIMENTATION ON HUMAN BEINGS

Bringing to life the hidden history of how clinical trials of analgesics were once conducted raises unsettling questions about governance. Regulatory requirements set in place by the Food and Drug Administration (FDA) in 1962 caused growing demand for human subjects, so pharmaceutical companies turned to prisons to find them (Adams and Cowan 1971). Certain events (recounted in chapter 6 in this book) forced them toward alternative populations in the mid-1970s. Thirty years later, prison research is being reconsidered due to a shortage of willing participants eligible for clinical trials (Urbina 2006). Because the U.S. population is "treatment saturated," private clinical research organizations now seek "treatment-naive" subjects the world over or turn to poor communities within the United States (Fisher 2005; Petryna 2006; Shah 2006). Clinical trials remain class- and race-stratified exercises that unevenly distribute risk and benefit.

What would it take to achieve socially responsible clinical trials? Research typically involves interaction between two classes of individuals. One group, who is usually white, middle-class, possessed of advanced degrees, and enfranchised within the social worlds of U.S. biomedicine, experiments on individuals from another group, who are usually less educated, less enfranchised, and living in poorer communities. The latter group is racially and ethnically more diverse and less experienced with the technoscientific aspects of biomedicine but is more experienced with directly adverse social impacts of science and extractive technologies. The increasing social distance between researchers and subjects forecloses public participation and leads to clashes between scientists and nonscientists.[7] Although these conflicts are often attributed to lack of scientific literacy or to inadequate public understanding of science, American publics have proved willing to bear some of the burdens and costs of scientific research (Lederer 1995, 137). Acceptable risk, however, is "in the eye of the beholder," according to a study by Ubel et al. (2006) showing that "the more distant the patient, the more likely people were to recommend [taking perceived risks]" (Bakalar 2006). Such results indicate how social distance enters into the human calculus of risk and benefit: the more distant the decision maker is, the more likely it is that there will be a recommendation to engage in risky practices.

The postaddicts described in this book were human subjects who were in far closer social proximity to the scientists who studied them than are many subjects of clinical trials today. Although postaddicts had their own reasons to submit their minds and bodies to science, they did so knowingly and without false hopes that participating in a study would somehow cure their personal dependency on addictive substances. Today, the political and economic climate of pharmaceutical research and promotion works against realizing the ideal of socially responsible clinical trials—by increasing social distance between the researcher and the researched and holding out hopes that cures will come about because of individual participation. Compounding these problems is the fact that "unbought scientific opinion is increasingly hard to find" (Le Carre 2001, 267). As *Discovering Addiction* reveals, research environments can and should be structured to guard against commercial interests colonizing the research agenda. Restraining commercial entities takes more than token representation or stepped-up attention to informed consent. Looking back to a time when researchers were in closer social proximity to their research subjects, this book tells the story of a committee of the National Research Council that directed the addiction research trajectory while buffering researchers from commercial interests. Centralized coordination by the National Academy of Sciences had great advantages but also created a "closed world" that relied on a mode of expertise that prevailed in a small enclave and was not readily translated beyond it. One might have expected misunderstandings between science and its publics to result from the practice of walling off scientific venues from public scrutiny.

By revealing how the social organization of the addiction research enterprise has worked since the 1920s, I hope to stimulate more-informed responses not only to drug problems but to pharmaceutical research. By showing how scientific lexicons, logics, and commitments move between the microsocial worlds of addicts, scientists, clinicians, and policy makers, I hope to offer fresh insight into the beliefs and assumptions that underlie concepts of drug addiction and dependence, as well as the ethics of drug research. Both research and drug policy would look different if advocacy from the perspectives of the communities most affected by the War on Drugs were taken into account. Science is not a very effective weapon in the War on Drugs, but it could be an enterprise that effectively calls wars on drugs into question and reduces the toll they take on the most vulnerable among us.

STUDYING UP: SITUATED KNOWLEDGES, UNSEEN AUDIENCES, AND IMPLICATED ACTORS

Anyone studying the rapid multiplication of the conceptual and experimental approaches through which science is made encounters challenges when navigating the incestuous social networks thick with unseen kinships that comprise scientific social worlds. External scrutiny enables outsiders to discern connections not apparent to those who inhabit scientific networks. Some of my connections, lexicons, and conclusions are counterintuitive for inhabitants of the social worlds I study. My work takes place in a different "universe of mutual discourse"—the social studies of science and technology. The historical sociology of scientific knowledge offers conceptual resources—hierarchies of credibility, epistemic cultures, and enunciative communities—suited for making sense of the social networks and practical discourses that form in "fortuitous environments" and for studying the political economy that structures such environments and shapes the cultures within them.

Multiple cognitive and interpretive resources are necessary to characterize shared beliefs, commitments, logics, material conditions, and institutional arrangements in which a research enterprise is situated (Haraway 1988; Harding 1991; Longino 1990, 2002). This book draws on the feminist sociology of knowledge despite the fact that I do not focus on women or gender. Drug-using women did not participate in the research related here. Nevertheless, all scientific work takes place through forms of expertise that are grounded in specific social situations and institutions that are gendered in ways that affect the research culture of laboratories just as surely as they pattern the microsocial dynamics of hospitals and prisons. Instead of centering explicit gender dynamics as I did in my previous book *Using Women: Gender, Drug Policy, and Social Justice* (Campbell 2000), here I am using feminist situational analysis to attend to power differentials and map connections between social worlds (Clarke 1998, 2000, 2005).

Each chapter of this book shows how "drugs" and "drug users" are constituted as objects and subjects of knowledge in a given domain; which techniques, technologies, and material practices are obligatory in that space; and which conceptual and practical logics are considered legitimate for making knowledge in that social world. Situating knowledge within the material constraints of its production also requires paying attention to the subjects whose lives, brains, and bodies are under study. Whether called "addicts," "patients," "users," "IVDUs" (intravenous drug users), "research subjects," "informants," "inmates," "participants," or "clients," they are "implicated actors" whose behavior and beliefs are targeted for change in all of the social worlds of substance abuse research (Clarke 1998, 16–17; Clarke and Montini 1993; Clarke 2005, 46–48). They are largely silent subjects who are often "only discursively present—constructed by others for their own purposes" (Clarke 2005, 46). In most addiction studies, addicts were not actively involved in negotiating their identities or the meanings of addiction but were instead acted on, "neither invited by those in greater power to participate nor to represent themselves on their own terms" (Clarke 2005, 46). Although users' voices appear rarely, they haunted the pages of this book just as they haunted the corridors of the laboratories that depended on them in the process of making science.

Addiction is a complex social phenomenon that exceeds the grasp of every explanatory account. Social questions have been largely foreclosed by the laboratory logics of most laboratory-based substance abuse research, which repeatedly disqualifies or "controls for" the social. Yet the meanings attributed to drugs differ among social contexts, which partly shape the experience of drug effects and the interpretation of seemingly physiological sensations. Although scientific lexicons are incorporated into the vernaculars through which people narrate their inner sensations, drug experiences obviously are not simply the stuff of science, nor do they occur entirely within the brain. Current neuroimaging studies attempt to visualize craving by invoking social cues, such as paraphernalia or ritualistic aspects of preparation to which addicts are conditioned. These return to the perennial question of how individual desire and experience is shaped by social setting and cultural context and to the puzzling variations in how individuals respond to drugs.

Yet the substance abuse research enterprise has become fully and even forcefully differentiated from social settings where drug use actually occurs. Even preclinical and clinical research programs now take place at considerable distance from each other. Pathways into the field have changed radically as neurobiological and molecular pharmacological routes supersede all others to focus at the cellular and subcellular level. Widening gaps between "science" and "service," "research" and "treatment," and "basic" and "applied" research have developed alongside an increasingly specialized vocabulary for naming, lamenting, closing, or bridging these gaps. The research effort coordinated by the U.S. government centered on addiction as an object of inquiry that required multiple approaches, but it never yielded completely to their integration.

Dynamic shifts in institutional structures and laboratory logics have required inhabitants of this research arena to retool often to keep pace with the evolving techniques used to study substance abuse. The ongoing quest to identify markers of addiction has been refracted through many different concepts, logics, and techniques, each linked to different political stances, ethical interpretations, and policy regimes. This book chronicles what scientific researchers from myriad disciplinary cultures have said and done to bring scientific knowledge about drug addiction into being. Its purpose is to show how researchers' commitments to particular beliefs and ways of speaking are predicated on a set of laboratory logics that structure how they enact their science. Specific laboratory logics depend on the social location of laboratories and field sites, and they change when cross-fertilizations with other sites develop. Writing a history of science that traces the intersections of conceptual logics is difficult. These intersections take the "natural course of an excited conversation among several persons all speaking simultaneously among themselves and each clamoring to make himself heard, yet which nevertheless permitted a consensus to crystallize" (Fleck 1979, 15). Such a conversation also permits consensus to refract. The coming chapters alternate between crystallization and refraction.

CHAPTER 1

Framing the "Opium Problem": Protoscientific Concepts of Addiction

What American publics and institutions define as worthy cures for drug addiction depends on who is perceived to be addicted, on what drugs addicts depend, on the meanings attributed to addiction, and on patterns of social status. The modal late nineteenth-century American addict was an upper- or middle-class white woman maintained on morphine by her physician. Respectable "medical addicts" gave way to an urban underclass that used narcotics for "nonmedical" purposes or "recreation." These new addicts were culturally distinct from their precursors: these poor, working-class, increasingly African American and white ethnic males were viewed as part of the "dangerous classes."[1] How addicts are treated very much depends on their membership in specific social groups; they cannot be lumped together as raceless, classless, or genderless. Historian David Courtwright has written, "What we think about addiction very much depends on who is addicted" (1982/2001, 4). The associations between illicit narcotics and "delinquent" subcultures worked against recognition that addiction might be a matter for scientific research or clinical investigation and that even "nonmedical" addicts might use narcotics to medicate themselves in absence of legitimate alternatives. Today, the distinction between "medical" and "nonmedical" has become blurred (DeGrandpre 2006). The long-standing division between "medical" and "nonmedical" obscures the historical dynamic of self-medication among "nonmedical" users.

The social transformation of the addicted population is sometimes attributed to the 1914 passage of the Harrison Act, which abruptly criminalized physicians' dispensing of narcotics. Narcotic use actually began to decline before that law was enacted (Courtwright 1982/2001). Social and professional learning about the negative organic, social, and economic effects of drug use was primarily responsible for the decrease (Musto 1973/1999). However, patterns of law enforcement and the demographics of criminalization affected how addiction was thought of as a medical and scientific subject. After the constitutionality of the Harrison Act was established in 1919, physicians became reluctant to maintain patients on opiates, for fear of prosecution. Shying from legal entanglements, physicians received little education about how to treat addiction. The medical profession entered a state of sanctioned ignorance during which only a handful of physician-researchers and scientists pursued systematic knowledge about addiction. This book is about those who dedicated scientific careers to studying the neurophysiological processes—but not the social dynamics—of opiate addiction. This chapter characterizes the state of addiction knowledge prior to the mid-1920s, when addiction research was first organized as a cooperative scientific enterprise.

CLINICAL ENTREPRENEURIALISM: THE EARLY STAGES OF A PROTOSCIENCE

Early on, competing theories took root about the underlying neurological and physiological processes of addiction and the disturbing propensity to relapse. The disease concept of addiction goes back to a cultural emphasis on abstinence and temperance that emerged as early as the 1780s. The concept did not really come into clinical and scientific vogue until the late nineteenth century, when animal tests and autopsy studies were first conducted to establish the effects of opiates on tissue. Early clinical studies on intact organisms yielded little scientific consensus. Nineteenth-century and early twentieth-century treatment took the form of clinical techniques for withdrawing individuals, taking up practical questions of whether patients required confinement—or even quarantine—due to the socially contagious nature of their disease. Physicians concerned themselves with the nature of the addicted person's diet; use of proprietary remedies, ranging from hypnotics (e.g., chloral hydrate) to purgatives (e.g., strychnine) to dilute opiates (e.g., laudanum or paregoric); and participation in practical therapies that supplied "an occupation of an absorbing kind" (Terry and Pellens 1928/1970, 546).

Addiction treatment reflected medical sectarianism in microcosm (Starr 1982). Clinical sectarianism was fought out at the level of practical decisions about whether or not to employ opiates and other "heroics," how best to regulate dosage, and what the etiology and progression of the disease was supposed to look like. Public debate over the social implications of maintaining addicts on "another poison" arose in the wake of the Harrison Act. Drug maintenance has been the most contested treatment modality, continually constructed not as treatment but as tantamount to condoning drug use or being "soft on addicts." In the late teens and early 1920s, clinics were briefly established to "maintain" opiate addicts. However, *Webb et al. v. U.S.* (1919) barred physicians from maintaining patients, forcing medical practice to change even faster than it otherwise would have (Courtwright 1982/2001). Changes in clinical practice came out of physicians' experience with iatrogenic addiction and a culture that did not construct narcotics use as a "public problem" except when it occurred among the so-called dangerous classes. When opiates were one of the few effective weapons in the medical armamentarium, physicians were represented as progenitors of addiction, nefarious purveyors of dope who preyed on innocent, largely female patients. Due to relatively unfettered access to narcotics, medical professionals themselves were subject to addiction at high rates. Developing reliable therapeutic expertise for withdrawing people safely and insisting on abstinence comprised one defense against the charge of iatrogenic addiction leveled at their profession.

Studies in which researchers administered drugs to themselves, family members, or close associates were the primary form of research that supplemented learning from clinical experience during this stage of "clinical entrepreneurialism."[2] Clinicians developed a bewildering variety of therapeutic innovations in relatively private settings. Because clinicians themselves were the first "addiction researchers," many did not take kindly to the emergence of an organized, public research apparatus. One of the first U.S. Public Health Service investigators, Clifton K. Himmelsbach, explained:

> Many individual, excellent physicians attempted to do something about [drug addiction], and their approaches had to do with devising new ways of treating withdrawal. They felt that if they could treat withdrawal effectively, that would cure drug addiction. So that was the era of many, many new and weird kinds of treatments of withdrawal, including causing an individual's skin to blister and withdrawing the blister fluid and injecting that into them. All sorts of weird things were done—purgation, the use of atrophy and alkaloids, etcetera, just some perfectly astounding things, most of which did more positive harm than good so far as the suffering of the individual is concerned during withdrawal.[3]

Nineteenth-century treatment modalities, nostrums, and techniques were purveyed through private practitioners; franchises, such as the Keeley Institutes; or congregate institutions, such as the New York State Inebriate Asylum in Binghamton, New York (White 1998). These were founded on the notion that alcoholism and opiate addiction were curable, despite there being no systematic technique by which physicians could assess the extent of addiction or predict its degree of curability.

Should modern readers doubt that a vast amount of empirical research was conducted on drug addiction in nineteenth-century and early twentieth-century clinical settings, even brief perusal of *The Opium Problem* (Terry and Pellens 1928/1970) should set such doubts to rest. This controversial compendium, produced in 1928 by the Bureau of Social Hygiene in New York City, summarized over four thousand treatises in more than a thousand pages. Aptly characterized as "diffuse" (Acker 2002, 59), *The Opium Problem* attests to the sheer multiplicity of uncoordinated and individualistic efforts to cast drug addiction as a matter for systematic clinical and scientific investigation. After the bureau had supported addiction research for three years, the Rockefeller Foundation took responsibility for the systematic study of drug addiction, before courting the National Research Council (NRC). The NRC, an organ of the National Academy of Sciences, was initiated to coordinate war-related research during World War I. In 1929, the NRC merged its Committee on Pharmacological Research with the New York bureau's Committee on Drug Addictions (Acker 2002, 77).

The resulting NRC Committee on Drug Addiction was constituted to take an "increasingly extended intellectual approach and a corresponding decrease in emotional, commercial, and other interests," in order to provide a sound and well-founded basis for national and international drug control. The authors of *The Opium Problem* concluded that until policy was placed on scientific footing, "we should look with disfavor upon dogmatic statements and arbitrary and unscientific rulings relating to either groups or individuals, while seeking in the experiences of all earnest and intelligent workers such elements of fact as may be uncovered and utilizing them in the gradually evolving plans for prevention and control that unquestionably will develop with an increased knowledge and eventually supersede the chaos of contradictory opinion that marks present-day activities" (Terry and Pellens 1928/1970, 928). The newly incarnated NRC committee adopted a singularly pharmacological research agenda: developing a nonaddicting analgesic as a "technological fix," as Caroline Acker aptly termed it, for the opium problem. However, to achieve that narrow yet still elusive goal of medicinal chemistry, useful knowledge of how addiction worked had to be produced.

Like other Progressive disease typologies,[4] early twentieth-century scientific investigations were directed at determining whether or not there were physiological or psychological markers useful for distinguishing addicts from nonaddicts (Acker 2002, 42, 50). By 1925, there was a consensus that there were no distinguishing physiological attributes that provided clinicians a reliable guide to identifying addicts (Acker 2002, 50). Lawrence Kolb advanced convincing explanations based on underlying psychopathology, which were implemented in the 1930s in the treatment regimen of the Public Health Service narcotics farms. Disease models of addiction came into clear relief against competing constructions of addiction as a moral problem (i.e., a vice, sin, or crime)—notions that Kolb undertook to dispel. In 1925, he published three papers based on work at the federal government's Hygienic Laboratory in Washington, D.C., in which he set out diagnostic criteria—called the K-classification scheme—to assess the degree of psychopathology exhibited by drug addicts (Kolb 1925a, 1925b, 1925c).[5] Used to categorize addicts for decades, the Kolb classification system was based on state-of-the-art psychiatric diagnostic categories that were modified with the passage of time (Kolb 1925c).

Kolb's goal was to dispel popular associations between drugs and crime. He argued that opiates inhibited aggression and demonstrated that changes in law enforcement—not an increase in violent crime—had increased the number of addicts behind bars. He divided addicts into two primary categories: (1) those accidentally addicted via medical treatment but otherwise normal and (2) those predisposed by psychopathology to the "vicious" pleasures and consequent "deteriorations" of narcotic drugs. Assuming that the Harrison Act was making occupants of the first category an endangered species, Kolb argued that occupants of the second category, suffering from mental disease, be treated humanely. He adopted a language of psychopathology to protest punitive criminalization. His theory that psychoneurotic deficits predisposed individuals to addiction aligned with those of his contemporaries who attributed addiction to "constitutional psychic defects" (Acker, 2002, 152). Kolb's construction of drug addiction as stemming from psychiatric problems was a strategic construction absent compelling physiological data. Production of that data and techniques and metrics for producing it would become the mainstay of the Addiction Research Center, which was housed at a thousand-acre congressionally mandated narcotics farm (nicknamed "Narco") in Lexington, Kentucky, where Kolb served as medical officer in charge from its opening in 1935 until the beginning of World War II.

Settlement of the physiological question by 1925 did not propel greater knowledge of addiction. Indeed, Caroline Acker shows that it acted as a limit against which proponents of criminalization asserted themselves. Treatment institutions founded on the notion that addiction was a treatable medical condition declined, leading to a decline in private addiction research (Acker 2002, 62–63). In her account researchers found themselves stymied, and addiction research stalled to become the backwater science that it would remain through much of the twentieth century. Acker claims that "no front in physiological research seemed to offer promising leads for understanding addiction" (2002, 63). Not until the opiate receptor research of the 1970s and even later use of medical imaging technologies for studying the effects of opiates on the brain, she argues, was there a promising physiological front. My story differs in that I argue that the early neurophysiological research established the knowledge base necessary for neuroscientific approaches ascendant today.

Addiction research had to become a highly interdisciplinary knowledge formation to get around technical obstacles, the obduracy of addiction as a social problem, and the politicization of that problem. Ongoing attempts to integrate physiological with psychological conceptualizations of addiction might be seen as "failures" but also stand as an early example of problem-oriented research and the attempt to base treatment and the politics of drug control on science. Scientific knowledge production about addiction took multiple forms during this period of seeming neglect. Enthusiasm for the multiple modes of clinical entrepreneurialism documented in *The Opium Problem* was dampened by the emergence of the national coordinating committee headed by the NRC. *The Opium Problem* concluded by raising the epistemological problem of policy making on the basis of uncertain and contradictory data. None of the fundamentals of the opium problem were sufficiently well established in 1928 as to be beyond doubt, according to the NRC committee. After reviewing a vast amount of data, the committee stated that the apparent honesty and intelligence of those who advocated contradictory positions convinced it to accept some "partial truth" from each of the statements, studies, opinions, and unproved theories that formed the data set (Terry and Pellens 1928/1970, 926).

Setting out this pluralist and constructivist account of the scientific knowledge of "chronic opium intoxication," the committee advocated the "most elastic administrative measures possible" given the "default of exact knowledge" (Terry and Pellens 1928/1970, 926). The authors of *The Opium Problem*, physician Charles Terry and his wife, Mildred Pellens, were sympathetic toward opiate addicts and had a sense of urgency about the declining availability of treatment in the wake of the Harrison Act. They believed that an opportunity for a more systematic knowledge of addiction was disappearing. Noting that maintenance clinics offered opportunities for further scientific study of the kind that might place policy on a more rational footing, Terry and Pellens recommended the development of a research program by qualified individuals to apply existing knowledge in the clinic (1928/1970, 927).

Physiological models of addiction were multiple, converging only on the hope of a cure. For example, autoimmune theories based on the idea that drugs are "toxins" were advanced independently in the 1910s by George E. Pettey (Terry and Pellens 1928/1970, 548–52) and Ernest S. Bishop (Acker 2002, 39–40). These theories owed much to bacteriological models underlying the germ theory of disease.[6] Proponents of autoimmune theory considered addiction the direct correspondent of infectious disease. One of them wrote in 1910 that "morphinism is a disease as really [*sic*] as is typhoid fever or pneumonia" (quoted in Terry and Pellens 1928/1970, 145). Proprietary "antitoxic" treatments arose, including Narcosan, a mixture of lipoids, nonspecific proteins, and vitamins that was responsible for a number of deaths. Based on the theory that narcotics call forth protective or neutralizing substances when introduced into the body, Narcosan was thought to protect against these unidentified substances in the blood and reduce the discomfort of withdrawal. One critic of Narcosan, George S. Johnson, found that the mixture added no value to the withdrawal process. Another criticism of Narcosan was based on the theory that addiction was an endocrine disturbance or hormonal imbalance. Proponents of this theory advised injections of testicular and ovarian "proteals," which were inexpensive and easily manufactured since they were not patented.[7] The Narcosan debate illustrates how unregulated competition sometimes caused grave public health problems during the era of clinical entrepreneurialism.

Hoping to identify the underlying structural pathology of addiction, clinicians unsuccessfully tried to locate an essential "toxemia" or even brain lesions, which many claimed existed but none could prove. Agonistic contestation over the merits of various therapeutic approaches and etiological theories led Terry and Pellens to complain: "The most apparent conclusion to be reached from the material reviewed is that, for the most part, treatment of this condition has not emerged from the stage of empiricism" (Terry and Pellens 1928/1970, 428).

After a thorough review of the extant literature, they found that few proponents of treatment procedures offered rationales for measures they urged others to adopt. Like most Progressives, Terry and Pellens evidenced more faith in the research enterprise than its findings warranted, and they failed to locate sufficient proof to warrant the unqualified acceptance of any theory. Thus they urged more research, including laboratory experiments designed to yield generalizable conclusions.

Scientific rationalists saw themselves as particularly opposed to moralists, for whom addiction was simply a bad habit or a vice. Judgments about whose views were most scientific mapped onto positions regarding which treatments worked best. Pettey wrote scathingly that those who held addiction to be a "perversion of the will" advocated coercive, abrupt withdrawal "notwithstanding the fact that others who have tried it have wound up with a maniac or a corpse to testify to the success of their efforts" (quoted in Terry and Pellens 1928/1970, 146). Those who constructed themselves as scientists scolded their unscientific brethren for holding the position that addiction resulted from emotional or psychological defects: "When will it be realized that all the derivatives of opium, whatever they are, have the same objections, the same dangers, and lead to the same addiction, and that the only way of curing an addict is not to give him another poison, but to remove the one he is taking?"[8] Most, if not all, early studies recognized both "psychic" and physiological components at work in the production of addiction.

A bewildering welter of theories, definitions, and models of addiction arose. Attempts to define the pathology, symptomatology, and prognosis of the disease were so heterodox that they were easily displaced by the set of newly dominant ideas that became the "official model" of the 1930s (Acker 2002, 32, 38). The official model was a mosaic crafted from an array of conceptual approaches and clinical phenomena, consisting of both physiological pieces (e.g., the phenomena of tolerance and withdrawal) and psychological pieces (e.g., explanations based on psychopathy or personality deficit). The dynamic proliferation of theories about addiction as a disease process meant that researchers could pursue their own ideas without having to integrate or account for those of others (Caroline Acker, personal communication with the author, August 18, 2006). However, the physiological model put forward by the particular thought collective described in chapter 3 was able to define the parameters within which more research would take place (Fleck 1979).

The search for a technological fix proceeded in an opportunistic, uncoordinated, and heterodox fashion prior to the advance of the "official model" of the

1930s. Just as Terry and Pellens feared, an opportunity for systematic clinical study was lost with the abrupt closure of the maintenance clinics in the early 1920s. The decay and dismantling of the treatment infrastructure and the deskilling of physicians meant that clinicians emerged from the era of clinical entrepreneurialism less knowledgeable about addiction, treatment, and pain management than they had been before the Harrison Act.

PSYCHOANALYSIS, "NARCOTIC BONDAGE," AND REPETITION COMPULSION

Coexisting alongside clinical entrepreneurialism was a second important inquiry into addiction, that of psychoanalysis. No longer considered scientific (and disdained by many scientists), psychoanalysis has just about disappeared from drug historians' gaze and might be considered unworthy of attention in a book like this. In its day, however, psychoanalytic interpretations garnered more attention than did prescientific, empirical studies of addiction. Psychoanalysis could be considered to have been the primary professional domain for the study of drug addiction in the first several decades of the twentieth century.[9] The legacy of psychoanalysis lingers, which is not to say that the lineage is straightforward or simple. Today, the powerful drive to repeat seemingly irrational acts is couched in the unassailably naturalized neurobiological and behavioral vocabularies of putative "pleasure genes"—not in terms of Freud's pleasure principle. Drug users now enjoy endorphin rushes, which require no recourse to the concept of libido. Operant conditioning explains repetition but not, perhaps, compulsion. There are nevertheless common structures of belief between now-discredited pseudoscience and neurobehavioral and genetic accounts: (1) addicts are inexorably driven to repeat unintelligible acts by internal and external forces beyond their control; (2) these acts have undeniably negative consequences; (3) the underlying internal mechanisms take psychopathological form; and (4) addicts are not masters of themselves but are instead in thrall to the external forces of suggestion, substance, and impulse. These beliefs persist even in scientific accounts cleansed of the language of psychoanalysis. Despite the declining cultural salience of psychoanalysis, it has provided a wellspring of beliefs about addiction as an artificial or unnatural state of dominance by the id and dissolution of the ego.

Through psychodynamics, an American branch of psychoanalysis with medical ambitions and scientific pretenses, some of these beliefs still have traction today. The persistent vestiges of psychoanalysis can best be explained by recourse to Ludwik Fleck's idea of thought collectives, each of which form thought styles, defined as a "readiness for directed perception, with corresponding mental and objective assimilation of what has been so perceived." These thought styles undergo social reinforcement, a feature of all social structures, which then constrain the individual by "determining 'what can be thought in no other way'" (Fleck 1979, 99). According to Fleck, whole eras are ruled by particular thought constraints, which later leave "remnants" in the form of multiple ties or historical connections to thought styles that dominated previous eras (1979, 100). The history of addiction science can thus be narrated as a succession of thought styles that displace one another yet conserve some aspects of the previous structure of social and cultural constraints on cognition.

As early as 1897, Freud regarded drug addiction as a substitute for masturbation, the "primary addiction" (Rosenfeld 1965). Believing there was a chemical basis for psychosexual behavior, Freud posited that endogenous or "toxic" mood alterations freed individuals from the "compulsion of logic" and made them enter "suggestible" states over which the pleasure principle no longer presided. He argued that repetition compulsion, now independent of the pleasure principle, gave the appearance of a "hint of possession by some 'daemonic' power" (Freud 1961, 26–30). In *Three Essays on the Theory of Sexuality* (originally published in 1905), Freud sketched clinical similarity between neurotic disorders of sexual life and the "phenomena of intoxication and abstinence that arise from the habitual use of toxic, pleasure-producing substances" (Freud 1975, 82). Freud's followers categorized addiction as a disorder of desire; a psychosis or neurosis; a borderline state; a perversion or fetish; an impulse neurosis; a form of narcissism, mania, or melancholia; or an outcome of castration fears, "dismemberment motives," paranoia, schizophrenia, sadism, and masochism. One of the most coherent psychoanalytic explorations of addiction can be found in the corpus of Sandor Rado, an orthodox Freudian who advanced an influential account of the "pharmacogenic orgasm" prior to emigrating to the United States from Germany (Rado 1926, 1933). After a decade at the New York Psychoanalytic Institute, Rado's ambivalence toward Freud led him to found the Columbia Psychoanalytic Clinic for Education and Research, the first U.S. graduate psychoanalysis center that was under medical auspices. His writings illustrate the discursive shift between the psychoanalytic vocabulary of desire and a psychodynamic vocabulary more resonant with biomedicine.

Finding an inexact science in the pharmacology of the 1920s, Rado advanced a "metaerotic" theory to penetrate the "obscure region" of morbid cravings (1926, 396). He suggested that the artificial technology of the hypodermic syringe displaced "natural" libidinal discharge by short-circuiting addicts' biological sexual apparatus. The "potent poisons" they ingested forced the natural genital organization to surrender to an unnatural form of erotic gratification, the "pharmacotoxic" or "pharmacogenic" orgasm, equivalent to the diffuse, pregenital alimentary orgasm of the baby at the breast.[10] A siege metaphor pervades Rado's writings on the subject, in which the id conquers the ego and erects an "absolute monarchy" (1926, 405). Drug addiction was framed as the outcome of a battle between a weak ego and an imperialist id that deranged the dependable regulation of pleasure and pain.

In his classic 1933 paper, Rado argued that drugs subsumed addicts' reality and allowed an artificial "pharmacothymic regime" to triumph, causing altered libido, mental atrophy, and sexual impotence (68–70). He retained Freud's insight that addiction substituted for masturbation, claiming that the pharmacothymic regime "initiates an artificial sexual organization which is autoerotic and modeled on infantile masturbation" (71). Those who used drugs in an auxiliary or "prosthetic" manner were excused from full-blown pathology: for instance, normal coffee drinkers and smokers exhibited "abortive forms of this illness" (79). Among the first to propose that drug addiction was a functional (if maladaptive) attempt to self-regulate "tense depression," Rado viewed drug use as the libido's attempt to take what it could get in the absence of actual gratification. He maintained that the problem with the "spurious pleasures" of drugs and alcohol was their false inflation of the action self, which managed self-awareness and hedonic control in contrast to the "dark unexplored continent" of the physiological processes of bodily pleasure (Rado 1969, 24). A theory of "narcotic bondage" provided Rado a touchstone throughout his lengthy career. His dedication stood in marked contrast to his contemporaries, most of whom considered the subject uninteresting.

Addiction interested Rado because he was part of a movement to place psychoanalysis on an experimental, hypothesis-driven—or "basic" science—footing (Rado and Daniels 1956). A leading proponent of the movement called "adaptational psychodynamics,"[11] Rado emphasized that the self-awareness and organismal integrity of the "action self" was propped up by physiological mechanisms or "neural activating systems" (1969, 52). "According to my hypothesis," he wrote, "the action self is the organism's systemic picture of itself, derived from the information it receives about its own activities by means of its sensory equipment" (1969, 49). He argued that the action self was directly affected by the pleasures of consumption: "If a man cannot derive a kick out of what he does, if he cannot feel happy and satisfied through his successful actions, he has nothing to feed his action self with because the action self is nourished upon the pleasures experiences derived from successful activity. Factors that go into developing this certainly include genetics and past experience" (1969, 50).

Adaptational psychodynamics attempted not only to cleanse psychoanalysis of its dependence on Freud but to incorporate biochemical and behavioral elements of systems theory. Elucidating basic laws of behavior in biobehavioral systems, Rado went so far as to construct a taxonomic table of behavioral disorders along the lines of organic chemistry (1969, 173–75). His general theory of "narcotic bondage" was a search for the essential pathology underlying all "drug dependence," a term he and others substituted for "addiction" in the 1950s. Rado maintained that self-medication was "a malignant form of miscarried repair artificially induced by the patient himself" (1957, 165). Self-government, he proposed, was an evolutionary framework that culminated in mature human adults fit for the levels of cultural cooperation exacted by democratic systems (1957, 167). In adaptational psychodynamics, "the organism [was viewed] as a biological system operating under hedonic control" (Rado 1957, 167). Similar to his contemporary Roy S. Grinker, who espoused a theory of functional anxiety, Rado thought that pain, stress, and deprivation were necessary to stimulate growth. He considered addiction almost a "natural experiment," because it interfered with hedonic regulation, a cumulative process modified by culturally specific patterns of reward and punishment: for example, sophisticated individuals could accept "delayed reward in lieu of immediate reward," but the less sophisticated could not (Rado 1957, 167). Both pleasure and pain took more culturally specific form in adaptational psychodynamics than in the experimental approaches of behavioral analysis (see chap. 7). Reward, however, indicated successful performance in both lexicons.

Rado explained that narcotic bondage resulted from the failure of gratification to travel the normalized pathways of reward in systems where "effort and performance are spurred by the pains of deprivation and are directed, facilitated, and rewarded by a variety of pleasures" (1957, 167). He maintained that conduct within regimes of hedonic control required the predication of education on "reward and punishment, that is, offering pleasure and inflicting pain" (1963, 164) and that reward varied between individual and species: at the physiological level, the "alimentary orgasm" signaled nutritional satisfaction; at the reproductive level, the sexual orgasm signaled insemination (1957, 167; 1963, 164). Rado argued that narcotic bondage threatened the species because it represented a failure of the entire regime of hedonic control. He observed that absent "standard (hetero)sexual union," masculine failures, including impotence and homosexuality, appeared in addicts (1963, 163). Rado explained that in the "adaptive struggle for existence" waged between a primordial desiring-self and a reality-tested self, the reality-tested self normally triumphed (1957, 166); and he noted that the "superpleasure" of narcotic bondage deposed the reality-tested self and enthroned the grandiose desiring self, a process that reduced highly evolved individuals to infantile states. In Rado's view, social and legal regulation could not control this failure; indeed, law enforcement, policing of affect, or imposition of punitive policies produced bitterness, defiance, and rage in addicts. Rado maintained that prohibition produced and incited the very behaviors it sought to repress.

Relating narcotic bondage to new research on the physiology of pleasure emerging from behavioral and experimental psychiatry, Rado claimed that psychodynamics foreshadowed the search for physiological mechanisms, pathways, and "pleasure centers" in the brain. He corroborated his theory with the work of James Olds, who made the well-publicized discovery that rats would electrically stimulate the "pleasure centers" in their brains up to two thousand times per hour and were highly motivated to work for such "brain-stimulation rewards."[12] Optimistic that a biochemical immunization would be developed to guard against the dangers of superpleasure (Rado 1957, 169), Rado believed that only psychodynamics reached the underlying disorders that made subjects susceptible to narcotic bondage. Rado observed that these currently remained inaccessible to biochemistry, which lacked a method for the "human biological study of mental life" (1963, 160). Rado's writing took on an increasingly strident tone as he witnessed the exclusion of psychodynamics from the "medical core" of addiction studies in the 1960s. Lamenting Freud's mystical romanticism as a dangerous "revival of ancient animistic speculations" (Rado 1963, 161), Rado undertook a lifelong effort to make an honest biomedical science of psychoanalysis.

Marginalized and delegitimated by the mid-twentieth century, psychoanalytic constructions of addiction are puzzling in their ubiquity and tenacity. Psychoanalysts constructed addiction as a libidinal relation—a craving or overpowering desire—between persons and substances. Even where there was only a skeptical embrace of psychoanalytic concepts, craving, euphoria, and repetition compulsion were still called on to explain anomalous, intangible, obscure, or problematic relations between persons and their objects of desire. In the United States in the mid-twentieth century, psychoanalysis was also called on in courts of law, the popular press, and policy hearings, to explain otherwise unintelligible acts. When psychoanalysts incorporated into their thought a vocabulary of stress informed by cybernetic systems theory and advances in endocrinology, they essentially smuggled psychoanalytic discourse into behaviorist, biological, and sociological explanations for the behavior of drug addicts—explanations that became dominant even as the cultural authority and persuasive power of psychoanalysis waned.

Constructions of addiction as a disorder of desire—resulting from disinhibition, regression, and the substitution of artificial pleasures for real ones—inhered not only in therapeutic discourse and cultural parlance but in global and domestic policy instruments. Official antipathy toward psychological constructions of addiction was well established. Yet the nation's first "drug czar," Harry J. Anslinger, chief of the Federal Bureau of Narcotics from 1930 to 1963, sounded like Freud when he wrote: "[Addicts'] intense overexcitement of the nerves and emotions leads to incontrollable irritability and irresponsible acts due to irresistible impulses of suggestive origin. . . . In the earliest stages of intoxication the willpower is destroyed and inhibitions and restraints are released; the moral barricades are broken down and often debauchery and sexuality results" (Anslinger and Tompkins 1953, 21). Even outspoken critics of psychoanalysis adopted the assumption that addictions are rooted in early childhood experiences that predispose some individuals to lives of violent crime, constitutional mental instability, or misdirected aggression.

Psychoanalysis could account for the force of repetition compulsion and explain why addictions were so notoriously difficult to overcome depending on personality type: "An egotist will enjoy delusions of grandeur, the timid individual will suffer anxiety, and the aggressive one will resort to acts of violence and crime. Dormant tendencies are released and while the subject may know what is happening, he has become powerless to prevent it. . . . The drug has a corroding effect on the body and on the mind, weakening the entire physical system and often leading to insanity after prolonged use" (Anslinger and Tompkins 1953, 22–23). Trying to contain a "potent weapon of aggression" wielded by amoral nations seeking to spread addiction to the "free people of the world," narcotics law enforcers placed themselves in the heroic position of defending democracy (Anslinger and Tompkins 1953, 10–11, 25). By contrast, those who could not deny themselves drugs were considered weak links in the modern project of globalizing democratic freedom through the cultivation of individual self-mastery.

Moral deterioration was the major threat that drug addiction was said to hold for democracy. Its sources were those of which Rado—and Freud before him—spoke: habitual substitution of chemical satisfactions for real ones. Psychoanalysis was losing its grip over the ownership of the problem; it was cast as "crude" in contrast to the new conceptual framework of experimental psychology (Lindemann and Clarke 1952). For American ego psychologists, "satisfaction of basic drives or tension states" underlay the motivation for using addictive drugs (Lindemann and Clarke 1952). They maintained that addicts simply did not have the proper tools for integrating perceptions, memories, and expectations; that the more realistic and mature an organism was, the more functional it would be, and the less likely it would use drugs to "depart from the plane of reality" or regress to "primitive forms" (Lindemann and Clarke 1952). According to the psychologists, how well individuals defended against emotional pressure depended on whether the ego had access to an arsenal of social skills: if pressures exceeded individual capacities, the result might be imbalance, regression, or drug use; addiction had become the failure to solve problems with proper tools or social skills. Recurring portrayals of drugs as technologies mediating between artificial and natural states, normal and abnormal desires, and self and other represent the continued presence of a psychoanalytic past that was deeply interred in addiction science.

In the psychoanalytic literature, dependency was figured as a survival technique—dating from infant experiences—in which adults magically responded to the infant's simultaneous states of helplessness and omnipotence. The magical state of dependence was preempted by self-sufficiency, organization, and independence in most, but not all, adults. Maladaptive dependencies signaled the unconscious retention of infantile states. Dependent adults were considered problematic in a competitive society that equated masculinity with strength, dominance, and superiority, while equating femininity with weakness, submission, passivity, and inferiority.[13] These pathological dependency formations were not just gendered but racialized by such psychiatrists as Joel P. Fort (1954), who described addiction as a perverse link between dependency and masculinity that formed in the "matriarchal circumstances" of most male African American heroin users. He concluded that pathological mother-son relations and father absence produced addiction, especially in urban African Americans. In the mid-1950s Fort was a psychiatry resident at the U.S. Public Health Service narcotics hospital in Lexington, Kentucky (1997). There he encountered a growing population of black and Puerto Rican patients and founded a chapter of the American Civil Liberties Union in Lexington.

The figure of a domineering mother was thought to cause heroin addiction by weakening masculine identification and creating within the child a dependency that was later transferred to drugs. In his therapeutic encounters with heroin-addicted men and boys, Fort saw a strong "desire to revolt against a feminine identification," which he sought to release in the therapeutic encounter. This often opened tirades of invective against domineering mothers: "The resulting engram of masculinity in their minds was usually one of hostile, evil identification. The mothers often fostered a considerable sort of dependency which later on increased the young man's guilt over being a man. As these patients grew up, they tended to have to cover up their basic lack of masculine identification and dependency with violent aggression" (Fort 1954, 255). Fort maintained that heroin took the edge off fear, guilt, and doubt by providing a "phantasmagoria of psychic effects" that allowed subjects to achieve their desired goal, orgiastic pleasure; he argued that gang activities offered them a compensatory but "false" masculinity that supported individual gang members' "doubtful decision to be a man" (1954, 257). Fort saw the pharmacological orgasm as an erotic discharge of guilt, aggression, and "frankly incestuous interests": "The drug becomes an object in itself, and ultimately the only desired object" (1954, 253). Surprisingly, the idea that addictive substances subsume all other forms of gratification became a means through which psychoanalytic interpretations were extended into explanations of addiction that centered the role of social stratification in producing and sustaining patterns of drug use.

Multiple social worlds contended for problem ownership of drug addiction. The core group of addiction researchers repudiated psychoanalysis, as illustrated by a 1958 symposium of the National Institutes of Mental Health, where prominent researchers from the Addiction Research Center in Lexington, Kentucky, vented their frustration with psychoanalysis. They favored neurophysiological explanations that centered on the brain, disdaining "toxic theories," clinical confusion, and public hysteria.

> [T]he brain is the instrument governing social as well as individual physiological integration. We need to know particularly about the limits and opportunities of an addicted person's behavior, his internal value system of appetites, rewards and punishments relating to narcotic drug abuse, the predisposing factors, the relationship of addiction to his past experiences and future prospects, the internal and external lures and deterrents as seen from his point of view. (Livingston 1958, 185)

Psychoanalysis was chief among the "toxic theories" to which they referred. Yet when addiction was cast as a neurological matter rendered through the behavioral language of reward and punishment, there remained a residual psychoanalytic emphasis on appetites, childhood experiences, and predisposition. Objectively measurable degrees of drug dependence gradually displaced the earlier lexicon of psychopathology denoted by subjective states of consciousness—craving or pica, narcotic bondage or habituation. Yet the historian of science Ludwik Fleck reminds us:

> [W]e can never sever our links with the past, complete with its errors. It survives in accepted concepts, in the presentation of problems, in the syllabus of formal education, in everyday life, as well as in language and institutions. Concepts are not spontaneously created but are determined by their "ancestors." That which has occurred in the past is a greater cause of insecurity—rather, it only *becomes* a cause of insecurity—when our ties with it remain unconscious and unknown. (1979, 20)

The repression of psychoanalysis was the necessary backdrop against which addiction research constituted itself as "scientific." To those who had dedicated their careers to the study of addiction, basic brain research appeared to offer a clear pathway out of a muddled arena.

Narcotic addiction researchers emphasized the scientific nature of their inquiries because they were operating from marginal social locations. Except for a toehold in applied departments of pharmacology, such as the Department of Materia Medica at the University of Michigan (which became the Department of Pharmacology discussed in the next chapter), they were unrepresented in any medical school curriculum or department of psychology. Addiction research was not an academic enterprise but a governmental one, borne out of the official response to the "opium problem." The NRC Committee on Drug Addiction induced alkaloid chemists and pharmacologists to look closely at the chemical structure of morphine, separate what produced addiction from what relieved pain, and develop compounds that promised reduced abuse liability and could be tested in animals and humans. Psychoanalysis was the backdrop against which addiction research moved onto the experimental stage and into the social worlds of laboratory science. Although neurophysiology and pharmacology dominated twentieth-century addiction research, vestiges of psychoanalysis stuck in scientific as well as popular constructions of the concept of addiction or drug dependence. Even as addiction research became the experimental science described in the chapters to come, psychoanalytic and psychodynamic explanations arose to account for why only some individuals who are exposed to drugs become addicted to them. Such accounts shaded into older moralistic constructs of alcoholism and addiction as "diseases of the will" (Sedgwick 1993; Valverde 1998). Addiction researchers set out to refute previous explanations of addiction they considered "unscientific," which included both moral and psychopathological accounts of individual variation.

CHAPTER 2

Creatures of Habit: Feeding the "Junkie Monkeys" of Michigan

Sociologist Howard S. Becker observed: "Science works when you make the world into the kind of place where that kind of science will work. That's the purpose of creating laboratories" (2005).[1] Scientific communities become committed to particular laboratory logics that form the practical basis of how they go about their work. Concepts alone do not guide scientific commitments, for the research materials, technologies, and methodologies available exceed the conceptual boundaries of theoretical approaches. A broad shift to experimental physiological research was under way during the 1920s and 1930s, when the addiction research enterprise came into being (Clarke 2005, 286). Monkey colonies were first organized as part of developing the infrastructural capacity to maintain reliable access to experimental subjects for a variety of scientific projects. The monkey colony can be seen as a project to create a research site where a particular kind of science could work—an experimental science designed to elucidate the neurophysiology of tolerance, dependence, and withdrawal.

Faced with psychological, or "subjective," desire for drugs, pharmacologists had either to incorporate desire into their experimental models or find some method to disqualify it. They turned to animal models both to bracket desire and to place their research on the more objective ground sought by the NRC Committee on Drug Addiction. Seeking to place drug policy on solid footing, the committee turned to the basic sciences, a move that effectively cut out social scientists and clinicians from the addiction research enterprise in its formative moments. Animals presented an expedient route to determine toxicity, of course, but some researchers set about using monkeys to learn more about desire. Questions immediately arose as to whether animals and humans responded similarly to drugs.

Animal models relied on a set of laboratory logics that enabled researchers to attribute meaning to their observation of the visual manifestations of animal behavior and to their measurements of physiological responses. Animals were interpreted as "addicted" once they reached a steady state of maintenance on morphine—for example, when administration of morphine produced no change in heart rate or respiration. They were then abruptly withdrawn from morphine, and another test compound, or "challenge" drug, was administered. Depending on the profile of effects observed during this substitution, the animals would either proceed through withdrawal or have withdrawal arrested by the test compound. Data produced on the basis of this logic of substitution revealed which drugs produced tolerance and withdrawal, and these drugs were considered "addictive."

Working collaboratively and conflictually with the pharmaceutical industry, the NRC committee systematically set out to review all compounds that promised to achieve analgesic effects without producing physiological symptoms of tolerance and withdrawal. When companies wanted to market drugs as painkillers, the committee would subject the drugs to human and animal testing to determine whether releasing them onto the market would pose a threat to public health. The idea that opiate addicts could be shielded from the consequences of their own physiological needs and psychic desires was central to the committee's efforts to contain the "opium problem" by identifying a nonaddicting painkiller and getting people to substitute it for morphine-based compounds. While industry supplied interesting compounds, the committee was never in thrall to the pharmaceutical industry, acting instead as an independent, nonregulatory source of oversight. Shuttling between basic medicinal chemistry, animal pharmacology, and clinical research, the committee was placed in the role of synthesizing competing findings between research sites. One of the research sites most integral to the committee's efforts was the monkey colony built by pharmacologist Maurice (Mo) H. Seevers at the University of Michigan to document primates' affinities for addictive substances.

Remarkably for his era, Seevers became a "harm reductionist" across a half century of laboratory life and long before the term was fashionable. He wrote, "The only realistic and achievable objective is to confine excessive drug use to a minimum and find better ways for society to live with it." He encouraged his colleagues that they should not become "puppets in international drug control" and simultaneously that they should combat the "plethora of pseudoscientists, false prophets, quasi-intellectuals, instant experts, self-seeking politicians, beaurocratic [*sic*] ignoramuses, soft-headed educators, and others of similar ilk" spreading a "hedonic plague" of drug abuse. Against this plague, he thought that scientists of his ilk should "educate individuals to have long range concern for health in the face of strong hedonistic desires" (Seevers 1972, 12). As a public spokesperson for pharmacology, Seevers was unusual in several respects. Most pharmacologists neglected the study of drug addiction, due to the stigma attached. Seevers's interest in all things drug-related spanned his career from the 1920s to the 1970s, during which the fates of pharmacology and addiction research fluctuated. The remainder of this chapter explores the changing situation of pharmacological research as enacted in the laboratory life of Seevers and in the monkey colony he brought to life.

Based on the laboratory logic of substitution, Seevers refined a technique whereby compounds were administered blind to a colony of morphine-dependent monkeys to determine whether human beings were likely to use or abuse them. The roots of the logic of substitution are located within the pharmacological enterprise and attempts to establish animal models for addiction (DuMez 1919; DuMez and Kolb 1925, 1931; Eddy 1973). Those studying the "junkie monkeys" of Michigan were obviously using animals in instrumental ways. Seevers is credited with the idea of establishing and maintaining a colony of morphine-dependent monkeys used as research tools.[2] In *Creating the American Junkie,* Caroline Acker argues that the "search for a nonaddicting analgesic emerged as a project typical of the 'classical pharmacology' of the 1930s, in which bioassay of compounds revealed therapeutic or toxic effects and their related dose ranges" (2002, 94). However, there was more to it. Whereas Acker argues that addiction research conducted in the laboratory reinforced the supply-side emphasis of drug policy of the classic era, Seevers himself was interested in the structure of desire, the demand side of the drug problem. Lacking a common language for thinking about desire for drugs, pharmacologists designed laboratory logics that enabled them to study desire without turning to the contested vocabulary of psychoanalysis. This chapter describes these logics as a prelude to reconstructing the use of human subjects in addiction research.

EMBODYING PHARMACOLOGY: THE TURN TO ANIMAL MODELS IN ADDICTION RESEARCH

Interdisciplinary since its inception, pharmacology has been "a multifaceted discipline that has gained strength and vitality from its dependence on and relationship to other disciplines as they have grown and developed" (Bass 1969, 157). Well into the mid-twentieth century, pharmacologists found it difficult to "circumscribe a specific body of scientific knowledge and say, this is the substance of, and therefore belongs exclusively to, the science of pharmacology" (Seevers 1969b, 208). Rooted in botany, experimental biology, chemistry, and medicinal chemistry, pharmacology bore some relation to clinical medicine yet enjoyed far less prestige. As late as the 1960s, according to Seevers, "a majority of the leaders in the biomedical sciences viewed pharmacology as an applied branch of physiology or biochemistry, not worthy of recognition as an independent discipline" (1969b, 208). Several factors converged to expand opportunities for U.S. pharmacologists prior to World War II, including movements toward drug standardization and the wholesale reform of medical education in the United States. Today, pharmacology plays the role of a respectable basic science; others determine its therapeutic applications, clinical relevance, and policy implications.

On January 28, 1939, the Rockefeller Foundation, which had assumed funding of the addiction research project from the New York Bureau of Social Hygiene in 1932, transferred responsibility for the "opium problem" to the federal government (May and Jacobson 1989, 186). The newly constituted NRC committee operated under the name Committee on Drug Addiction and began to expand and consolidate the pharmacological research infrastructure in the United States.[3] The committee chose the University of Michigan Department of Materia Medica, under the direction of Charles W. Edmunds, as one of the premier laboratories for its purposes. According to Reid Hunt, a Harvard pharmacologist instrumental in getting the NRC involved, Edmunds now had "the most active department in this country, and, I presume, in the world."[4] In 1930, Edmunds hired Nathan B. Eddy to oversee the pharmacological testing of compounds provided by Lyndon F. Small's chemical laboratory at the University of Virginia. Eddy took on the role of liaison between members of the coordinating body, a part he played for the remainder of his distinguished career as one of the world's leading pharmacologists of the opioid drugs. In 1939, Eddy moved from Michigan to the National Institutes of Health (NIH), from which he steered the research agenda of the NRC committee for the ensuing decades.

The laboratory life of Maurice H. Seevers began with some of the earliest systematic animal studies on the effects of morphine and cocaine. While awaiting admission to Rush Medical School in 1925, he studied with Arthur Lawrie Tatum, MD, of the Department of Pharmacology and Physiological Chemistry at the University of Chicago, for whom he injected morphine into rhesus monkeys (Deneau 1970). Tatum was a "virtual consulting machine" whose research was tightly tied to commercial interests (Swann 1988, 103, 116). He started working on antimalarials for Parke-Davis in 1937, five years before the start of government-coordinated collaboration on antimalarials (Swann 1988, 112–13). However, his interest in morphine, cocaine, and the use of barbiturates as an antidote to cocaine overdose predated any commercial sponsorship. In 1929, Tatum became chair of the pharmacology and toxicology department at the University of Wisconsin at Madison. Seevers followed him, and they continued studying chronic morphinism (addiction) and the actions of barbiturates and central nervous system depressants in monkeys. Predating Seevers's 1930 dissertation, their early publications concerned experimental cultivation of chronic morphinism in rhesus monkeys and cocaine addiction in dogs, monkeys, and rabbits (Tatum, Collins, and Seevers 1927, 1929; Tatum and Seevers 1929). They observed morphine's paradoxical "dual effect," consisting of "a strange mixture of simultaneous stimulation and depression on different parts of the central nervous system" (Tatum, Collins, and Seevers 1929, 459). They found two lethal doses of morphine in rhesus monkeys: a lesser dose that killed by respiratory depression and a greater dose that killed by convulsions. Although these early experiments resulted in the death of animal subjects, Seevers and Tatum later tried to keep research subjects alive in order to study the long-term effects of repeated cocaine use, seeking to determine whether cocaine built tolerance as did morphine.

Questioning whether taking larger and larger doses of cocaine was evidence of tolerance or simply individual variation in the amount necessary to cause intoxication, Tatum and Seevers embarked on longitudinal experiments but reported that they were unable to bring about the "psychologic effects which are so characteristic of chronic cocainism in man" or the "sexual irregularities" observed in humans (1929, 403, 405). Concerned with extending their animals' lives, they administered intravenous cocaine to four dogs (one female and three males) for more than two years. Mere sight of the syringe excited the dogs, in whom they observed priapism and "nymphomania," but there was no evidence of abstinence symptoms when the researchers withdrew the drug (1929, 405). They reported that monkeys, in comparison, evinced neither desire for the drug nor abstinence symptoms but instead "presented a picture of extreme terror entirely resembling that immediately following the injection of the drug and during the course of its action" (1929, 407). Tatum and Seevers concluded that only dogs exhibited a "true cocaine psychosis with marked desire for the drug," while other species, including humans, were "sensitized rather than tolerant to cocaine when habitually administered" (1929, 409). They reported experiments similar to those of Claude Bernard,[5] who administered combinations of morphine and cocaine, codeine, thebaine, caffeine, strychnine, or barbital to dogs and other animals.

The goal of these animal studies was to create an experimental system useful for elucidating how morphine and cocaine affected humans—studies complicated by the human subject's state of mind. Preoccupied with separating psychological drug effects from physiological effects, the researchers raised no ethical questions. By controlling laboratory conditions, Tatum and Seevers believed they could carry out experiments with "no preconceived opinions but with the idea of gathering facts from close observations that might ultimately lead to a rational and consistent view of chronic morphinism" (1929, 447). Finding it puzzling that monkeys appeared to lack desire for the drug, they tried to turn to human subjects. To demonstrate cross-tolerance (i.e., when the "activity of one drug renders another drug, chemically unrelated but pharmacologically somewhat similar, less than normally effective"), they described a "chronic morphinist" who betrayed no change in blood pressure, respiration, or subjective symptoms when barbital sodium was administered (1929, 462–63). They interpreted this lack of change to mean that morphine made the subject "cross-tolerant" to the barbiturate. However, Tatum and Seevers rarely worked with human subjects. Their animal experiments were designed to control for confounding variables present in humans due to state of mind or desire.

The animal experiments conducted by Tatum and Seevers were meant to model human addiction, which they defined as a "condition of mind or body induced by drugging which requires a continuation of that drug, and without which a serious physical or mental derangement results." For them, "habituation" meant becoming accustomed to a drug but not being seriously dependent on it; "tolerance" meant that more and more of a drug was required to produce equivalent effects. They defined "true addiction" as a condition in which "the organism needs a repetition of the drug . . . in order to approximate normality more nearly and, in the case of man, also to satisfy conscious desires or to escape painful sensations or painful thoughts" (1929, 466). Seeking to reconcile the vast and disconnected facts produced by observers into a "harmonious schema," Tatum and Seevers presented a diagram depicting a well-integrated nervous system that balanced depression and stimulation (1929, 467, 472). Addiction, they postulated, was a vicious cycle in which increased dosages augmented nervous excitability to the point that sedation was required; it was the result of subjects' attempts to address states of physiological imbalance. Citing all previous European and American attempts to experimentally addict dogs, mice, and monkeys (DuMez 1919; DuMez and Kolb 1925), Tatum and Seevers advanced the "dual-action hypothesis" to make sense of the paradoxical coexistence of central nervous system depression and stimulation.[6] This hypothesis attempted to render the imbalance induced by morphine as physiological, not psychological.

Seevers's 1930 dissertation, "Acute and Chronic Narcotic Drug Poisoning," disproved an accepted belief that tolerance was the result of the organism building up a "general cellular immunity to the drug." Instead, Seevers postulated that some people needed increasing doses of morphine just to maintain normal equilibrium. He explained in his dissertation abstract, "Thus, by ever increasing doses a vicious cycle is established, and a state of exaggerated excitability of the central nervous system is reached with a raised threshold for depression whether it be by morphine or other depressants, allowing an individual to withstand doses of morphine that would cause fatal depression in the unaccustomed." Seevers's dissertation argued that abstinence symptoms were the body's signals that a depressant was needed in order for the subject to maintain physiological equilibrium between stimulation and depression; thus the severity of abstinence symptoms would be in direct proportion to the overall increase in the organism's nervous irritability. This work described the physiological need states apparent in morphine abstinence phenomena, but not the nonphysiological needs displayed by those deprived of cocaine. Lacking a scientific vocabulary for need states that were not physiological, Seevers's dissertation attributed them to "deranged mental conditions" and intense states of "subjective desire" experienced by regular users of cocaine.

Concluding that morphine addicts were simply seeking to maintain equilibrium led Seevers to think there might be something functional about the use of central nervous system depressants. Users of such other drugs as cocaine and cannabis, however, desired a dysfunctional disequilibrium. Venturing into the ongoing controversy about the nature of addiction as a scientific problem, Seevers and his contemporaries placed the study of addiction on a scientific footing to counter negative images of it in the medical profession and popular media. He explained, "To the average medical layman lacking firsthand experience with addiction, the term 'drug addict' may conjure a mental image of a sallow-skinned, hollow-eyed Oriental, who in his utter depravity is clutching with bony, long-nailed fingers at the throat of a young girl or suckling babe. Such a picture of addiction is commonly portrayed in the Sunday supplements or in the literature of the professional reformers" (Seevers 1939, 91).[7] Scientists identified with addiction research countered these representations by invoking hardheaded physiology and disavowing any connection with psychoanalysis or psychology.

Differentiating between states of physiological need induced by morphine and states of desire for cannabis or cocaine, Seevers spoke with the confidence of science.

> Addicts to cannabis and cocaine are of a different stripe. Addiction, in [the case of stimulants], is usually a manifestation of a psychopathic desire to escape from reality—a sequel to vicious associations—or the need for an inflation of the personality. . . . Peculiarly enough, no definite and characteristic physical signs or symptoms follow withdrawal from these compounds, as is the case with the opiates. The cocaine addict is subjectively depressed and desires his drug intensely; he may even commit murder to obtain it; yet the physical manifestations of withdrawal are not characteristic. The same may be said of the addiction to the resin of the hemp plant, Cannabis. (1939, 95)

Seevers divided drugs into three categories: those that produced habituation (caffeine); depressants that produced a "definite train of physical, as well as psychic, disturbances" if withheld (morphine); and those, such as cocaine, that produced excitatory or stimulant effects but only "psychic addiction," which, Seevers noted, was no less severe or difficult to cure than physical addiction (1939, 95). Psychic addiction was, however, more difficult to model in the laboratory.

The scientific interests of Seevers's laboratory clearly lay with depressants that produced addiction and characteristic symptoms of abstinence in monkeys. In 1936, he published two classic papers titled "Opiate Addiction in the Monkey" in the *Journal of Pharmacology and Experimental Therapeutics.* Far from declaring cocaine, cannabis, or caffeine nonaddictive, he simply designated them as beyond his scientific purview. He told a 1938 lecture audience:

> Few of us would like to admit that we are caffeine addicts; yet, I will venture to say that there are many in this room who will develop a headache before noon if they are deprived of their habitual cup of breakfast coffee, or its equivalent in caffeine from tea or coca cola. Do we have, then, in caffeine, a drug which possesses in a small measure the requisites of a drug of addiction? Do the blood vessels of the brain become dependent on caffeine so that its presence is necessary to relax them and permit an adequate blood flow to this organ? These are questions which I will not assay to answer. (95)

Such remarks indicate the everyday routine of drug addiction, as well as Seevers's belief that misrepresentations could be countered by public presentation of factual knowledge.

Ironically, Seevers had begun to notice that his chosen profession was dwindling, and he nearly defected to do clinical research on anesthesiology. He later derogated pharmacology as the "weakling of the medical sciences" (1969b, 130). Describing American pharmacology as having been "in the doldrums" during the 1930s, he explained: "The older generation was discouraged; the field was unattractive to young men and few were trained; those who were contemplated moving to more promising fields; industrial pharmacologists were excluded from Society membership; important chairs were being filled by people from other disciplines" (1969b, 129). Seevers joked that in the 1930s, the main research question in pharmacology was, "What is the matter with pharmacology?" (1969b, 209). He was attuned to the low social status that dogged the field of pharmacology through much of the twentieth century (discussed in the next section of the present chapter).

Gaining experience with monkeys in Madison,[8] Seevers began to make what he called "monkey movies."[9] He shared their scripts with psychologist Harry Harlow, whose experiments on deprivation of maternal love are among the most notorious examples of primate research.[10] Based on the laboratory logic that "such slight differences exist between the signs of abstinence in this animal and those of the human addict that the monkey surpasses any other animal as a test object for the study of experimental addiction," these movies explored the puzzling problem—as Seevers wrote in the margins of one of the scripts—that "monkeys fail (usually?) to show signs of desiring injections of narcotic drugs."[11] Despite showing physiological symptoms of abstinence and possessing "sufficient cortical development to associate the administration of the drug during abstinence with relief of its distressing symptoms," these monkeys, "addicted" to codeine, morphine, heroin, and Dilaudid for periods ranging from nine to twenty-one months, did not appear to "desire" injection. The animals displayed grossly visible signs—sunken eyes, prostration, or muscle twitching—but they also showed social responses that researchers had to interpret, such as opposition to capture, desire for handling, discomfort, irritability, and quarrelsomeness.

The monkey movies joined other attempts to document visible markers of desire or develop methods to measure "desire or striving" (Spragg 1940). What Seevers called "positive desire-responses" were based on a conditioned, positive association between the needle and relief of symptoms. Because monkeys generally associated the needle with negative events, such as "disturbance at being caught" or the pain of injection, the total experimental situation worked against monkeys making overt, positive expressions of desire for the drug.[12] To get around the problem of negative associations, another primate researcher, S. D. S. Spragg, working under Robert M. Yerkes at the Yale Laboratories of Primate Biology in Orange Park, Florida, developed a "choice procedure." He trained chimps to cooperate with morphine injections by first adapting them to saline injections and rewarding them with fruit, praise, and patting (Spragg 1940). The chimps were then trained to "readily cooperate" for injection, with "only verbal approbation as reward," before they began receiving injections of morphine (which were not followed by reward). This "preliminary adaptation" was, in Spragg's view, responsible for his successful demonstration that chimpanzees would "work" for a dose of morphine (Laties 1986). Sheer force would not have worked, because the chimpanzees were heavy and active, but "preliminary adaptation" enabled twice-daily injections to become routine in Spragg's pathbreaking studies.

Once Spragg's experimental subjects were habituated to morphine injections, situations could be set up in which they could follow the dictates of desire, by choosing a color-coded key to unlock either a white box containing a syringe filled with morphine or a black box containing a banana. Their choices depended on whether they had most recently been deprived of food or morphine. When morphine-deprived, not only would the chimp unlock the box containing the syringe, but the animal would hand it to Spragg in urgent anticipation of injection. Another demonstration of the strength of animal desire was a movie made by Spragg showing a chimp forcefully pulling on a rope to drag the white-coated scientist into the injection room.[13] Similarly, Seevers's monkey movies tried to capture identifiable expressions of desire, which were seen as central for drawing connections between human and nonhuman primates. This strategy was part of Seevers's overall effort to keep pharmacological work in the animal laboratory relevant to the all-too-human problem of desire for drugs. Seevers wanted to augment pharmacology's public relevance by expanding beyond animal studies. His selection of research questions reflected these desires, but his laboratory logics were trained on animal models.

While still at the University of Wisconsin, Seevers continued to build toward establishing the biochemical basis for the action of morphine and its derivatives by seeking support from the NRC Committee on Drug Addiction.[14] Rather than request financial subsidies, he sought the "large quantities of confiscated opiates that are destroyed by the Narcotic Division," for use in studies of "chronic morphine poisoning" in monkeys.[15] Researchers on the committee program enjoyed courtesy appointments with the U.S. Public Health Service that enabled them to obtain "quantities of condemned material from the Bureau of Prohibition of the Treasury Department" and "to receive alkaloids in interstate commerce" from chemist Lyndon F. Small (Acker 2002, 75–76). Seevers's request was relayed to Lawrence Kolb, who had done some of the earliest experiments on monkeys and who was then chief of the Division of Mental Hygiene of the Public Health Service. Kolb granted Seevers a portion of the purified morphine and appointed him a consultant to the Public Health Service. In return for the morphine, William Charles White, then chair of the NRC committee, requested that Seevers share his results with the committee. He placed no other conditions on Seevers "except a footnote in the publication recognizing this correlation [with the committee] without mention of the specific grant of the morphine."[16] White praised Seevers and closed his letter with the hope that great care would be exercised as to the security of the material.

The quest to organize a reliable supply of research material yielded Seevers far more than a source of purified morphine. The monkey colony would place him squarely within the social network of addiction researchers. From his vantage point within the scientific and policy-coordinating bodies, Clifton Himmelsbach saw Seevers as helping "break down barriers between individuals and individual institutions so that a correlated attack may be made on the problem as a whole."[17] As Seevers replied in a 1941 letter to Himmelsbach, "I have spaded up a lot of oysters in the past three years and it begins to appear as if a 'pearl' or two might be forthcoming when they are opened. If so, it must be applied to the human, [and] the only logical way to do it, I believe, is at your institution [Lexington] through some sort of cooperative venture." He saw this cooperative approach as "clear[ing] the way for pharmacology."

Advent of war officially suspended the NRC committee's work on June 19, 1941. That year, Charles W. Edmunds died suddenly, and Seevers was recruited from Wisconsin to assume the reins of the University of Michigan department. Several principal members of the addiction research network were asked to participate in the government-coordinated development of antimalarial drugs. Drug toxicity and efficacy was assessed in rhesus monkeys by various government contractors, including Seevers from 1944 to 1945. The antimalarial program absorbed the efforts of those few scientists who had pursued the subject of drug addiction prior to the war. Although personnel were temporarily diverted from the nascent addiction research enterprise, the war ultimately enhanced the feasibility of federally coordinated scientific assaults on such problems as venereal disease (Brandt 1985), the anemias (Wailoo 1997), and addiction, all once considered outcomes of sin and vice.[18] Ultimately, the renamed NRC Committee on Drug Addiction and Narcotics (CDAN) resumed meeting in 1947. By then, Seevers and Samuel Irwin had set up shop to use monkeys as preclinical bioassays to test the abuse liability of compounds, based on the logic of substitution established by Himmelsbach and Eddy prior to the war. However, they also continued to pursue the basic mechanisms, including "desire," that brought about addiction.

In its attack on the "opium problem," the postwar CDAN aimed, first, to reduce the socially legitimate use of habit-forming drugs, by convincing physicians not to prescribe them and by convincing the public to steer clear of proprietary remedies containing such drugs. Second, the committee wanted to replace "each use of habit-forming drugs with a substance not habit-forming but capable of producing the medicinal action required of the habit-forming product." The committee maintained that through substitution, industrial production of alkaloids could be "reduced to a minimum," thus lessening the "police authority necessary to control the situation."[19] The logic of substitution transcended the laboratory. As illustrated by the committee's sense of its goals, substitution was a public health measure designed to reduce reliance on law enforcement. The problem, as the committee saw it, was the lack of viable substitute drugs that it could recommend to physicians or the public. Failing to grasp the social meaning of "habit-forming drugs" and cultural aspects of their use, the committee set to work in the fields of pharmacology.

AT WORK IN THE NEW FIELDS OF PHARMACOLOGY: DISEASE AND DISEQUILIBRIUM

Prior to World War II, U.S. pharmacologists weathered a formative "identity crisis" during which they feared "engulfment" and the "unethical" taint of commercial enterprise (Seevers 1969b, 210). The founding fathers of U.S. pharmacology recognized the lack of research infrastructure and set out to build one. In 1924, John J. Abel wrote to Abraham Flexner that pharmacology should not be subordinated to physiology. He defined "drugs" as the proper object for the field, writing: "I am fully aware that they also constitute the field of study for the physiologist, the pathologist, and other medical scientists. The scope of this domain is so large that there is ample opportunity for all the above-named individuals to work without ousting the pharmacologist or subordinating him to some other field." Abel described pharmacology as a vibrant enterprise that was "almost daily making new additions to our armamentarium of drugs, which cannot be subordinated to physiology which has its own problems which may or may not interlock with pharmacology" (Seevers 1969b, 209).

Famously, Abel advocated pluralism. He called for the scientific community to "let one pharmacologist be more of a chemist, another more of a physiologist, another more of a clinician," in a unified, cumulative, and—most important—independent enterprise within the broad field of experimental medicine and biology. His vision went unrealized for several decades. The differentiation of pharmacology from physiology occurred earlier in Europe. By the 1930s, European pharmacologists had a coherent sense of identity and a degree of organizational autonomy. Cognizant of their relatively underdeveloped state, their American counterparts set out to raise the field's reputation through ambitious research programs. This effort propelled pharmacology and medicinal chemistry into becoming the "most frequent foci" of research collaborations by the onset of World War II (Swann 1988, 3). Pharmacology expanded its emphasis on experimental therapeutics, although the leadership resisted moving toward practical, therapeutic application. "For us to go clinical is, to my mind, as disastrous as to remain what we are," wrote the editor of the *Journal of Pharmacology and Experimental Therapeutics* (quoted in Chen 1969, 131). The main engine for growth proved to be the general expansion of biomedical research during and after the war.

Postwar pharmacology was characterized as immature but growing rapidly. One thing that was emphatically not a part of its growth was overlap with addiction studies—when perusing the membership of the American Society for Pharmacology and Experimental Therapeutics (ASPET) in its first sixty years (1908–69), it was rare to find anyone but Seevers who worked primarily on opiate addiction. The differentiation between toxicology and pharmacology came about in the early 1960s, when the first society devoted to toxicology was established. Finally, the evolution of tools in biophysics and molecular biology allowed pharmacologists to explore drug action at the subcellular and molecular levels. The 1950s and 1960s witnessed a proliferation of new forms of neuropharmacology, psychopharmacology, and neuropsychopharmacology that incorporated experimental psychology and biological psychiatry. There was, however, a postwar workforce crisis in the field.

Expansion of pharmacology departments and a higher profile of pharmacology in the medical school curriculum had been among Abel's goals during the formative stages of ASPET. As the main professional society in the field, ASPET lobbied for federal investment to strengthen graduate education and increase the number of pharmacologists produced through NIH training grants (Bass 1969, 167). Public visibility grew due to the popular press's portrayal of Frances O. Kelsey, the FDA pharmacologist who prevented thalidomide from becoming a public health disaster in the United States.[20] Organized pharmacology had a contradictory relationship with the FDA. Although increased drug regulation meant more work for pharmacologists, many believed that the FDA hampered innovation, so ASPET's Public Affairs Committee sought to influence health legislation and broaden the FDA's interpretations of regulation. ASPET strengthened professional networks not only among academic pharmacologists but among their industry counterparts. The private sector absorbed most of the pharmacologists produced by federal workforce investment. Although ASPET initially barred industrial pharmacologists from membership, they were admitted starting in 1941, and by 1969, the organization boasted there was "no difference between academic and industrial pharmacologists" (Chen 1969, 151). Academic pharmacologists increasingly worked as industry consultants. No longer Seevers's "weakling of the medical sciences," pharmacology is synergistic with the pharmaceutical industry and with other fields concerned with drugs and drug-cell interactions. The level of analysis in which pharmacology should be engaged has long been contentious, with scientists questioning how knowledge of the molecular-level activities of a drug could be best situated within the "whole organism," much less how whole organisms could be best situated within the complex social contexts in which humans ingested drugs or became addicted to them.

Pharmacologists sought to insert their expertise into the periodic social controversies in which drugs were increasingly embroiled. In the wake of the war, Seevers helped the Japanese government control a popular epidemic of amphetamine use. He participated in the Second U.S. Medical Mission to Japan, in May 1951, and initiated an ongoing capacity-building educational exchange with Japanese pharmacologists that persists to this day (Domino 2004, 149). Seevers played a similar role in the postwar heroin crisis in the United States and later claimed to have been privileged to examine the problems endemic to the "drug scene in most of the principal countries of the world" (1972, 5). He was often the only pharmacologist at gatherings convened to respond to drug addiction as a social problem or cultural crisis. "Drug use is a symptom or sign, not the primary disease," Seevers intoned at the New York Academy of Medicine conferences titled "Drug Addiction among Adolescents" held in the fall of 1951 and the spring of 1952. "The adjustment of these individuals to society," he added, "is in inverse relation to the stress to which they are subjected." Rather than define adolescent addiction as "crime" or "disease," Seevers interpreted it as an abnormal psychological response to modern stresses—such as "fear of the future, fear of impending war, fear of atomic bombs, and fear of military service"—that exceeded the individual coping skills of adolescents. Finding rising heroin use unsurprising, Seevers confidently stated that adolescents were unusually susceptible to outside influences and "dominated by herd instincts" (Committee on Public Health Relations 1952, 109). He concluded that stress took its greatest toll among the most maladjusted—and hence least immune—individuals.

During this period, disease was coming to be redefined in pharmacological terms as disequilibrium within a homeostatic system, borrowing language from cybernetics. Drug use was an attempt to restore homeostasis or an equilibrium of the kind that Seevers posited in his dissertation. His earlier definition of addiction as a "condition of desire" had shifted to an explanatory model in which stress and anxiety played a leading role. By the mid-twentieth century, there were other sources of the idea of homeostasis, such as neuroendocrine research and systems theory. Addiction researchers drew on these despite drug addiction being thought of as a social problem that manifested in clinical abnormality. Some characterized pharmacology as a clinical science from its inception, and pharmacology departments were generally housed in medical schools. For Seevers, clinical medicine played an interpretive role for pharmacology: "it is important to pharmacology as a discipline that it be interpreted to the clinician by one who knows from experience how the problems of the clinic differ from those of the laboratory" (1969b, 215). The problem was sorting out the division of labor between the clinic and the laboratory.

Seevers maintained that pharmacologists played an interpretive role for the effects of drugs and chemicals. "True" pharmacologists "spoke for" drugs and might come from several disciplines.

> The biochemical pharmacologist fragments the organism in order to study its component parts; the organ-oriented subdivisions of pharmacology are engrossed with specific technics and interests; the clinical pharmacologist, while dealing with drug effects on man, is also a specialist; toxicology is too often identified only with small animal pharmacology. In order to bring perspective to medical and health problems concerning drugs, information from all sources, subcellular to the whole organism, must be evaluated with a minimum of bias. Often the pertinent information is found only in indigenous

> medicine. Often the picture must be constructed primarily from witnesses from the past. Competence for such reconstruction requires a broad background in the laboratory with more than a passing knowledge of the clinic, a "composite" pharmacologist, if you please. *This* is pharmacology. (Seevers 1969b, 216)

Differentiating between "true pharmacology" and "pseudopharmacology," Seevers disdained extrapolations based on "inconsequential" or "inadequate" data obtained through "unrealistic doses in small animals" (1969b, 212). He did not respect hasty moves from drug-cell interactions to human therapeutics by persons with "little, if any, knowledge of the principles that govern such interactions or the complexity of the biological systems with which [they are] dealing" (1969b, 211). The knowledge production problems to which Seevers pointed sharpened with the separation of preclinical from clinical research. The conflict between researchers who used intact organisms and those who worked at cellular or subcellular levels went beyond training or laboratory technique—the conflict was about the public value of pharmacological knowledge claims and the social status of those who made them.

Seevers argued that individual pharmacologists could only be expected to make significant contributions in very limited areas, in which they should persist until they became "masters" (1969b, 213). Thus the broader pharmacological research enterprise was one in which the components of "clinical-pharmacological knowledge" were coordinated (as illustrated in the quote that follows). Having survived the doldrums of earlier generations, Seevers saw pharmacology as an autonomous discipline that should define itself so as to remain publicly visible without being subsumed by clinical medicine.

> If pharmacology is submerged it will be in institutions where the pharmacologist, even though medically trained, identifies pharmacology only in laboratory terms. It is not likely to happen where pharmacology occupies an important position in the basic and clinical teaching of medical students throughout their educational program; where clinical pharmacology conducts training programs at the postdoctoral level and is recognized as a bridge between general pharmacology and clinical medicine; where the clinical pharmacologist is trained in both; where he/she is formally and physically associated with both; where he/she interprets laboratory findings in clinical terms and serves as a coordinator in all things of a clinical-pharmacological nature. In the long run, it may be that this type of cooperative activity will be a principal reason why general pharmacology as an independent discipline will survive in medical schools. (1969b, 21–22)

By the end of his career, however, Seevers felt pharmacology "received little but scorn in the scientific and medical communities" (1972, 3). Because he positioned himself as the embodiment of his science, an affront to pharmacology was a personal affront to him. Pharmacology remained a subordinate research enterprise. Within pharmacology, addiction research was even more easily tarred with the brush of an illegitimate science (Clarke 1998).

ANIMATING A RESEARCH ENTERPRISE: THE LABORATORY LOGICS OF ANIMAL DESIRE

Sorting out animal models to clarify relationships between physiological need and psychological desire occupied Seevers and his colleagues for decades. Along with Lauren Woods and James Wyngaarden, Seevers used six monkeys in a 1947 comparative study of methadone and morphine. The process made him eager to continue work on abuse liability of the opiates with monkeys, which required overcoming the technical difficulties of organizing and maintaining monkey colonies (Swain 1991, 21). Such colonies were part of the developing international primate research infrastructure integral to experimental physiology (Clarke 2006, 286). The morphine-dependent monkeys of Michigan literally embodied this emerging institutional form but took specific shape for the purposes of addiction research. Ensuring the monkeys were tuberculosis-free plagued Seevers, as monkeys are so susceptible to the disease that entire colonies can be quickly wiped out. Then as now, moreover, primate research facilities were expensive to operate because they involved ongoing costs that were hard to justify to external sponsors and university administrators. The university initially invested three thousand dollars in the laboratory, and Seevers turned to CDAN (at the committee's sixth meeting after war's end) for another twelve hundred dollars. On March 10, 1950, CDAN agreed to fund both Henry K. Beecher's research at Massachusetts General Hospital, discussed in chapter 4 of the present book, and Seevers's project, titled "Studies in the Monkey Designed to Determine the Value of this Animal for Predicting Addiction Liability to the Newer Synthetic Analgesics" (Committee on Drug Addiction and Narcotics 1950, 112).

Perennially underfunded due to industry reluctance to pay for testing, CDAN was looking not to fund research infrastructure but to obtain short-term results. But Seevers wanted continuous funding, because he planned to "carry out in the monkey all of the procedures at present employed at Lexington for the study of addiction liability" (Committee on Drug Addiction and Narcotics 1950, 112). He intended to build up a colony of between sixty and seventy animals.[21] The real reason that CDAN could not guarantee Seevers continued funding was that some of its members were unconvinced that animal results corresponded to human addiction in any meaningful way. Taking every opportunity to reassure the committee that the similarities between animal models and humans were significant enough to warrant further work on animals, Eddy and Seevers patiently explained what results in the monkey meant for humans. For instance, when Isaac Starr, chair of the committee, asked what morphine-addicted monkeys looked like during withdrawal, Seevers replied: "They are very like man in withdrawal. It shows nausea, vomiting, rise of temp, etc. It is the only time an otherwise wild monkey seems to become tame, amenable to handling. The animal wants relief of his discomfort and seems to associate that in some way with the handling" (Committee on Drug Addiction and Narcotics 1950, 114). Still, the committee had to be repeatedly convinced that Seevers's results were relevant to problems within CDAN's purview.

Interpretive work was necessary to render animal behavior meaningful, and thus Seevers had to translate what he was observing into a comparative catalog of drug effects that drew parallels between animals and humans. Desire for the drug was evidenced by an animal that would "come and hang on to the attendant's clothing as if seeking something" (Committee on Drug Addiction and Narcotics 1950, 114). Perhaps in response to the question of animal desire, Seevers began to make data films in the early 1950s like those he made previously in Wisconsin. The films depict monkeys in various stages of withdrawal and show vomiting, convulsions, seizures, hallucinations, tongue biting, and abdominal cramping (monkeys holding their abdomens tightly). Even hard-to-observe peripheral neuropathy, which occurs in extreme cases of alcohol dependency, could be glimpsed. One film made in the early 1950s showed "sick" (withdrawing) monkeys housed individually and in groups. When housed together, monkeys that feel healthy "pick on" those who are "sick" (going through withdrawal). According to James Woods, who later inherited the colony, group-housed monkeys can be aggressive toward each other. Noting inequality in nutritional intake and other problems relating to social behavior, he said, "We don't group house at all now; if we ever do again it will be in a very limited way" (2005).

Films from the early 1950s depict the first high-throughput system for testing addictive potential of new compounds. The films show a lab technician who administered shots four times a day to each monkey. Housed in groups of six, the monkeys were released in a fixed order. The animals entered a corridor, jumped through a trap door, and received their dose. Speedy administration meant that the technician handled each monkey only long enough to inject it before moving to the next animal. The University of Michigan laboratory maintained about twenty morphine-dependent monkeys in the 1950s, giving them the capacity to determine dependence liability for between fifty and sixty drugs each year. They used a scoring system to measure severity of withdrawal based on the morphine abstinence syndrome described in chapter 3 of this book. The work in the monkey colony was modeled on studies of human beings coordinated by CDAN and conducted by the Public Health Service.

Students and colleagues of Seevers continued his tradition of making monkey movies. One such film, *Studies on Drug Dependence in the Monkey,* was filmed in 1979 at the Central Institute for Experimental Animals of the Medical Research Laboratory in Nogawa, Kawasaki, Japan. Foregrounded inside a box-like apparatus, the monkeys in the film undergo effects of stimulants, hallucinogens, and depressants. The narrator intones that a monkey, seemingly engrossed in stereotypical and repeated activity, "never forgets to press the lever when the red light is on." The films depict monkeys self-administering cocaine to the point of convulsions, something no longer allowed. A narrator explains that one experimental subject died two hours after filming, from exposure to high doses of meperidine (Demerol). It is difficult to watch these films, with their lone subjects engaged in their own "experiment perilous" (Fox 1959/1998). As the voice-over occasionally points out, their expressions are pained, and some of their gestures are suggestive of human beings.

Respectful of their animal subjects and protective of their scientific practice, behavioral pharmacologists have something of a siege mentality, given some of the tactics that animal rights activists have adopted toward them. When I watched the monkey movies with researchers who work with monkeys today, the researchers engaged in interpretive work: they pointed out with irony when animals on-screen were said to "appear to be visually hallucinating," and they instructed viewers on the observable phenomena they use as the basis for interpretations. The researchers were and are careful not to attribute human-like traits to the monkeys. At one point, a film narrator carefully said: "The monkey is here presumed to be experiencing visual hallucinations. Observe here the eyeball movements." Subjects in the film were profoundly alcohol- and opiate-dependent monkeys who were used to demonstrate the comparative lack of objective signs of abstinence when withdrawing from drugs that do not produce physiological dependency (such as LSD). In the making of these movies, observables had to be interpreted for audiences to make sense of what they are viewing. For example, the Japanese film narrated what was thought to be going on in the brain when central nervous system depressants were administered. The film's narrator explains: "[The brain] requires the presence of the drug to retain normal cellular activity. . . . Thus the nerve cells are never drug free and the brain becomes resistant to drug action to the point that the drug becomes necessary for normal functioning." A tension between observation and interpretation, practice and theory, runs through these visual texts.

Few viewers of these movies would dispute the profoundly visual effects of withdrawal from high doses of intravenous ethanol on the monkeys. These were particularly obvious in a film titled *Behavioral Effects of Alcohol in the Rhesus Monkey,* made in the 1960s at the Southern Research Institute in Birmingham, Alabama, by Barbara McEwen and Gerry Deneau, who had recently departed Ann Arbor. During filming, the "drugged monkeys," normally curious when not drugged, were administered curiosity and dexterity tests that documented poor coordination and lack of interest in their surroundings. The film showed not only delirium tremens during withdrawal but also the peripheral neuropathies that accompany severe dependence on alcohol. As the monkey reached the twenty-ninth hour of alcohol withdrawal, severe tremors began. At forty-eight hours, the animal appeared to be picking cobwebs out of space and seemed to be undergoing visual hallucinations. Woods noted that monkeys "do this under the circumstances that you would think, the same circumstances that you would expect in people. Hallucinations in alcohol withdrawal are only observed in humans who are quite strongly dependent" (2005). The film ended with a happily anthropomorphic event, the animal's recovery and restoration to normalcy.

This sequence of films in the tradition of Seevers, to my knowledge the only monkey films that remain extant, depicted evolution in the technical apparatus used to study animal models of addiction. The technical problems initially posed in drug self-administration studies were considerable because the original metal harnesses were heavy and could chafe the monkeys, who were quite capable of reacting in ways that damaged harness or tether. Rubbing wounds made by the original metal harnesses were painted with medications. Today's polyester jackets, harnesses, and lightweight aluminum springs allow more freedom of motion than the formerly used tubular tethers, and the animals chew the jackets to "customize" their fit. Another condition that had to be in place for drug self-administration studies was an apparatus allowing animals to self-inject. In 1961, James Weeks, a cardiovascular pharmacologist working at Upjohn Pharmaceuticals in Kalamazoo, Michigan, invented an indwelling intravenous catheter system for rats (Weeks 1961, 1962). The apparatus was adapted to monkeys by Tomoji Yanagita in Seevers's lab. A late 1960s film made by Seevers and Yanagita on self-administration of pentobarbital showcased cages, harnesses, and tethers. The monkeys in the film clearly manifest symptoms of drug intoxication; pensive, yawning monkeys repeatedly press a lever until they nod off, their hands abruptly falling to the floor. Present-day viewers told me that one would very seldom see a monkey intoxicated so severely these days, because researchers work with smaller doses and get the same effects without having to worry about such gross effects.

Research methodologies have evolved with changes in the technical apparatus. Behavioral pharmacology laboratories are currently set up to examine the propositions of behavioral economics and choice models (Hursh 1991). Early studies simply allowed animals to self-administer extremely high doses in order to establish the pattern and schedule of ingestion and to determine the effects and consequences of that pattern. The seizures, convulsions, and self-injurious behaviors seen in the relatively crude studies are no longer produced. Although the FDA drug approval process required lethal dose (LD-50) studies in animal models, such studies were performed by toxicologists, not by substance abuse researchers. Those who study addiction have moved on to more nuanced approaches that allow them to get at the drug effects that result from chronic use, which are far more subtle than death. Such approaches rely on the reliable reproduction of drug dependence in animals, which is based on the laboratory logic of concordance.

Over the years since animal self-administration models became more precise, they have also become more predictive of "abuse potential" or "addiction liability" among human beings. Pharmacologists have discovered and documented animal preference for the same drugs that humans use in socially problematic ways. The establishment of correlations between human and animal drug consumption, "liking" or preference, and effects became more compelling. Once validated, that laboratory logic has given way to a preoccupation with the persistence of drug-seeking behavior in the face of negative consequences. These topics are taken up again in chapter 7 of this book, which situates behavioral pharmacology as the pivot point between older theories of conditioning and newer theories drawn from neuroscience and genetics. The research infrastructure developed by Seevers at the University of Michigan successfully marshaled enough resources and social status to continue (although its existence came under pressure in the 1960s and 1970s as animal research became more controversial).

Interestingly, Seevers was a proponent of gathering "minimal animal data" and guarding against overgeneralization from animal studies to human beings. He did not seek to expand the domain of animal research but instead argued against the waste of animals inherent in what he saw as "slavish adherence" to the large-scale studies that were becoming customary practice in the pharmaceutical industry by the early 1960s.[22] Limitations on animal research are closely linked to the expansion of clinical research on human subjects: Seevers's ethical stance toward the minimization of animal research was based on his belief that studies should be performed in humans as soon as feasible. He argued that drugs of low toxicity in humans produced undetectable effects in animals unless they were administered in amounts "far in excess of those ordinarily used in human therapy." Seevers claimed that "human disease counterparts are rarely available for study in animals," although it was his lifelong goal to provide one (1960, 6). Thus he advocated the earliest possible clinical trials once toxicity in animals was determined to be low. This ethic of the minimal use of animals lost out in the regulatory emphasis on large-scale studies set into FDA policy by the 1962 amendments. However, Seevers's performance of ethicality was partly due to his belief in the partiality of knowledge claims based on animal research: there were limits to what could be learned about addiction through animal models.

Compared to the broader shifts within experimental therapeutics, biology, and pharmacology, the addiction research arena was a tiny enclave. However, the animal models produced by addiction researchers have enjoyed remarkable tenacity. Believing monkey studies of morphine-like compounds predicted qualitative responses in humans, Seevers nevertheless recognized the technical and philosophical difficulties of translating research methods and findings across species. He noted that "direct extrapolation or interpolation of results from one species to another is not only impossible but entirely misleading" (Seevers 1960, 6). At times, he even identified differences in drug effects between species of monkeys (Committee on Drug Addiction and Narcotics 1953). The scientific limitations lay with the difficulty of correlating pharmacological and psychological variables to explain drug-induced behavior or drug seeking (Seevers 1960, 6). Hitting squarely up against desire, Seevers turned to experimental psychology and behavioral analysis, fields that were in the process of evolving "drug self-administration" techniques based on a different set of laboratory logics than those of classical pharmacology. The results of the testing program were "usually so unspectacular, so difficult of attainment, and so unrewarding in a scientific sense" that good scientists were uninterested in them (Seevers 1960, 9). For the monkey colony to yield on its scientific promise, a new set of laboratory logics would have to arise that used the "junkie monkeys" to mimic human self-medication and drug seeking. By the time that behavioral pharmacology arose to make use of the research platform constructed by Seevers, there were new cultural conversations and an emerging sense of the ethics of both animal and clinical research. These are related in the ensuing chapters; chapter 7 resumes the story of the "junkie monkeys."

Archives sometimes come to life in ways that serendipitously animate aspects of the historical moments they enshrine, as does a film made sometime in the early 1960s by the University of Michigan audiovisual department, *Morphine Physical Dependence in the Monkey.*[23] Rather than a data film geared toward the research community, this film was meant to convey seriousness of purpose to a wider—even public—audience. This film is an aesthetically pleasing documentary with high production values, set in a fashionable living room in which Seevers presides over a coffee table littered with artifacts, including opium pipes, books, and a small Japanese statue. Joining him are four men in suits: Nathan B. Eddy, who had been the linchpin of the NRC committee for thirty years and was perhaps the world's leading pharmacologist of the opioid drugs; University of Michigan pharmacologists Sam Irwin and Gerry Deneau; and Duncan McCarthy, a Parke-Davis executive closely associated with the University of Michigan Department of Pharmacology. When the conversation turns to individual susceptibility to drug dependence, Irwin explains that millions of people undergo anesthesia without developing "emotional ties" with the drugs administered. Eddy explains that physical dependence cannot be reduced to tolerance, in response to which Seevers jokes, "Have we spent all our lives just fooling around?" Irwin and Deneau proceed to explain the research question being studied in the monkey: How are psychogenic dependence, individual susceptibility, or "emotional ties" related to or different from physiological tolerance? They chart out the rationale for using monkeys, who behave in ways "much easier for us to interpret" and "more similar to man" than other animal models, such as the rat or dog.

The monkeys play a role in this film that resembles that of domestic pets rather than laboratory animals. They are encircled by flimsy, circular wire cages quite unlike the boxes in which they were actually housed. The animals stretch, doze, yawn, and cry, becoming more and more obviously exhausted and pathetic as withdrawal proceeds inexorably. Deneau narrates their progress, stating at the crucial moment that "one never fails to be impressed by the rapidity with which morphine reverses the course" of the withdrawal. Indeed, the sick animal responds almost immediately by returning to a state of comfort before the viewer's eyes. Eddy intones, "Since results in the monkey are very like man, producers and legal people accept them as unequivocal evidence of what would happen in man." Surprisingly, he states, "A nonaddicting analgesic would *not* solve our problem with drug abuse by any means"—an admission indicating that the NRC project had run up against a limit marked by the presence of human desire and social context. As Eddy elaborated later, physical dependence was inadequate to explain the drive that underlay drug-seeking behaviors in monkeys and men.

The protobehavioral primate laboratory described in this chapter was to later serve as an entrée for a full-blown behavioral logic of drug self-administration by animals, a logic that transformed the field in the 1960s. Nascent behaviorist principles underlay the laboratory logic of the physiological investigations by Seevers and his fellows. However, they did not possess a vocabulary for the scientific analysis of behavior other than the discredited lexicon of psychoanalysis. Preoccupied with studying physiological dependence, they built a pharmacological research infrastructure that became instrumental for behavioral pharmacologists to come (Balster and Bigelow 2003; Schuster 1976). Interestingly, Seevers recognized the potential of behavioral models of drug self-administration even as they proved threatening or unpersuasive to other pharmacologists. "Seevers was smart enough to know that psychology was going to have something to say about these things" (Woods 2005). When it came to drugs beyond his self-defined purview, Seevers recognized the limits of the laboratory logics of substitution but did not yet see how to move toward establishing concordance.

One of the limitations that Seevers hit up against was how to define "addiction" as a scientific object capable of holding together heterogeneous elements. "It has become impossible in practice, and is scientifically unsound, to maintain a single definition for all forms of drug addiction and/or habituation. A feature common to these conditions as well as to drug abuse in general is dependence, psychic or physical or both, of the individual on a chemical agent"—thus began a 1965 article by Eddy, Halbach, Isbell, and Seevers, "Drug Dependence: Its Significance and Characteristics," which was written by a powerful scientific coalition seeking to shift the older, protoscientific terminology toward a newer scientific terminology of "drug dependence of this or that type."[24] Applying the term *dependence* to habitual drug use represented a scientific consensus and a lasting conceptual shift in the field.[25] The Committee on Drug Addiction and Narcotics concurred with the semantic shift on July 1, 1965, by voting to change its name to the more scientifically credible Committee on Problems of Drug Dependence.

Despite the rising fortunes of pharmacology, Seevers remained concerned about his field's status. He wrote: "Today pharmacology no longer needs to be sharply circumscribed to find its place in the scheme of things. In this era of molecular biology defining pharmacology to encompass the action of all chemicals on all living matter is accepted with little debate" (1969b, 210). At the time, some pharmacologists felt that molecular biology might subsume their discipline and become "the only thing that really counts" (Seevers 1969b, 211). Seevers was critical of the gap between the promises of molecular pharmacology and "application of pharmacologic knowledge to human therapeutics or the public health" (1969b, 213). His concerns were twofold: that those who did not use biochemical approaches would be relegated to second-class citizenship and that knowledge of molecular approaches did not truly qualify one as a pharmacologist (1969b, 212–13). Indeed, he argued against exalting molecular pharmacology, because other pharmacological approaches were equally likely to contribute to public health. Bringing perspective to public health problems involving drugs or chemicals was, in Seevers's view, the unique domain of pharmacology, given the problems of alcoholism, drug dependence, air and stream pollution, and the ubiquitous presence of pesticides, food additives, and over-the-counter drugs (1969b, 216). Producing useful and usable knowledge for the sake of these public health problems was the overarching goal at the heart of this research enterprise.

The "junkie monkeys" of Michigan were maintained on morphine as a means by which to render them useful to the project of categorizing drug effects and classifying the elements of drug dependence. The monkey colony was brought into being for this purpose, and its existence allowed researchers to begin raising questions about the underlying structure of addiction. The "junkie monkeys" thereby invoke the ethical specters typically associated with utilitarianism and the instrumental use of animals as research subjects. These specters have increasingly come to haunt the pharmacological research enterprise, which relies on intact organisms even in the age of molecular pharmacology. They loom especially large when scientific work on intact animals must be coupled with research on human beings, as is necessary for research on drug dependence. The next few chapters look further into the thought collectives that became central to the social organization of the clinical research infrastructure, which relied on prisoner patients rather than "junkie monkeys" for "research material."

CHAPTER 3

"A New Deal for the Drug Addict": Addiction Research Moves to Lexington, Kentucky

Systematic research on the effects of narcotic addiction on human beings began at a federal penitentiary annex at Fort Leavenworth, Kansas, where several thousand drug addicts were housed in the U.S. Army Disciplinary Barracks. In 1930, the U.S. Public Health Service (PHS) was granted statutory authority to run medical services in U.S. prisons.[1] A medical detail was dispatched to Leavenworth the next year. There, a small biochemical laboratory was established to "determine the more exact nature of the chemico-physiological changes occurring in connection with drug tolerance and addiction" (NIMH 1971, 9). The ethical ambivalence lodged at the heart of this origin story was expressed in a caution by Assistant Surgeon General Walter L. Treadway.

> It is not assumed that Federal prisoners should be used as experimental animals for the furtherance of medical knowledge. However, a large prison may be regarded as analogous to a laboratory, subject to control, where observations and scientific studies should be made possible. (1930, 8)

The injunction against using federal prisoners as "experimental animals" simultaneously gestured toward a level of social control over research subjects that was possible only in structurally coercive settings, and the urge to put captive populations to use in the production of knowledge.

The laboratory at Leavenworth came into being under the direction of a young PHS clinical investigator, Clifton K. Himmelsbach, whose work was coordinated by the NRC Committee on Drug Addiction (CDA), described in chapter 2.

> [I]t immediately struck me that this was a very, very dependable kind of illness, that things happen almost by the clock. You could predict, you could just almost tell what was going to happen, when it was going to happen, and when it was going to fade. So I got the idea of reducing this to numbers of some sort and getting a picture of this illness. And I started with a 1, 2, 3, 4, plus, based on the appearance of signs that occurred, and this was the first feeble attempt to quantify the morphine abstinence syndrome. (Himmelsbach 1972, 8)

Himmelsbach developed a method to track withdrawal, which he called the "morphine abstinence syndrome" (1941). He found that all patent medicines marketed to "cure" addiction or relieve withdrawal symptoms were ineffective. His first scientific paper (1933) concerned high rates of malaria among addicts due to shared syringes. After Leavenworth, Himmelsbach conducted clinical trials of analgesics on cancer patients at Pondville Hospital in Massachusetts before moving to Lexington, Kentucky (Acker 2002, 86–89).

Laying the methodological foundation for the laboratory logic of substitution described in the previous chapter, Himmelsbach pioneered the prediction of a drug's "addictive potential" by systematizing the progress of abstinence symptoms. If a "less addictive" candidate drug was administered to a chronic morphine user, the experimental subject could be observed for whether that drug alleviated or promoted withdrawal symptoms. This logic of substitution was applied in the unique circumstances of a laboratory that opened in 1935 under Himmelsbach's direction in Lexington, Kentucky, on the rural, thousand-acre campus of a federal prison-hospital that served narcotic addicts who resided east of the Mississippi River.

"Narco" was one of two U.S. narcotics farms operated jointly by the PHS and the federal Bureau of Prisons (BOP), in Lexington, Kentucky, and Fort Worth, Texas. Congress changed the name from "U.S. Narcotic Farm" to "U.S. Public Health Service Hospital" soon after Lexington's opening on May 29, 1935. The new name became effective on July 1, 1936, but the nickname "Narco" stuck. Designed as treatment hospitals to quarantine addicts far from urban temptations (Musto 1973/1999, 204–6), these hybrid prison-hospitals were presented to the public as a "New Deal for the drug addict" (Conhurst 1935, 1). The Porter Bill (1929), their enabling legislation, contained a research mandate pursued at Lexington from its opening in 1935 until 1979.[2] Construction of the Lexington facility cost $3.6 million and was portrayed as an institutional solution to a social problem of national scope that crosscut racial, ethnic, and class divisions: "Dope plays no favorites and has no pet hunting grounds in this country, Government men say. Over 100,000 addicts are scattered up and down the whole scale of life in fairly regular ratios regardless of color or race or economic position. They constitute a very real and solution-demanding problem" (Conhurst 1935, 1). This chapter brings back to life the larger institution of Lexington and the laboratory that brought into being the drug addict as a scientific subject and an object of knowledge.

Once settled in Lexington, Himmelsbach hired what became the core group of scientists in the addiction research enterprise, although World War II would split the first generation into two groups. The initial group consisted of ranking PHS officers, most of whom had worked in penal institutions where there was a high incidence of narcotics addiction. The first collaborative research team consisted of biophysicist Howard L. Andrews, who made one of the first electroencephalographs and was invited to Lexington to "find out what's going in the brains of these addicts"; Ralph Brown; Robert H. Felix, who later became director of NIMH; Justin K. Fuller, previously chief medical officer at Leavenworth; Michael Pescor; biochemist Fred W. Oberst; surgeon William F. Ossenfort, who later became chief medical officer at the Atlanta Penitentiary; Victor H. Vogel, a clinical psychiatrist; and physiologist Edwin G. Williams.[3] World War II took so many of the first group to Washington that when the second group began to arrive in the early 1940s, only fifteen staff remained in the research unit (Martin and Isbell 1978, 27). The second group included Harris Isbell, who did an internship at Lexington in the early 1940s and succeeded Himmelsbach as director in 1945; Abraham Wikler, who came as a psychiatry resident in 1940; Anna J. Eisenman, a chemist hired during the war and one of few women researchers there; biophysicist Karl Frank; H. Franklin Fraser, a clinical researcher; Harris Hill, Conan Kornetsky, and Richard Belleville in psychology and psychometrics; and William R. Martin, who became director of research in 1963, when Isbell, Fraser, and Wikler retired. In 1948, the research unit became the first basic research laboratory of the newly formed National Institute of Mental Health (NIMH) and was named the Addiction Research Center (ARC).

The history of substance abuse research is inextricable from the story of Lexington. Despite their geographic isolation—or perhaps because of it—researchers at Narco had access to a large pool of drug-experienced subjects from which they could select subjects who fit eligibility criteria. Constituted as an elite corps, they made formative conceptual contributions. Even their technical and custodial staff was handpicked, because Himmelsbach believed they had to be "thoroughly sold" on the idea that their work contributed to scientific progress if he was to achieve the levels of control he believed necessary to the research process. Himmelsbach wanted "no one [to] ever come into the unit except [his] people": "[They were] my eyes and ears twenty-four hours a day, seven days a week, 365 days a year, as long as we stayed open, and I was in constant touch with them, and they with me, by telephone, so that this was a continuous kind of controlled situation in which they felt perfectly free and comfortable with me and I with them" (1972, 15–17). This dream of perfect control and a total situation of round-the-clock observation were integral to the research ward at Lexington, which was the only laboratory in the world entirely devoted to the study of drug addiction. Bringing back to life the material, discursive, and organizational arrangements of this institution demonstrates how the social organization of knowledge production enabled rapid moves from clinical observation to testable hypotheses, making basic and even molecular mechanisms of addiction discernible.[4]

The central question driving addiction research was why individuals varied in the propensity to addiction and relapse. Haunted by variation in the "subjective" effects of drugs, researchers turned to animal models to produce "objective" accounts of the physiological mechanisms involved, including tolerance, addiction or dependence, withdrawal, and relapse. Yet human questions remained the driving force as the field came into being: Why were some individuals more or less susceptible to addiction than others? What accounted for high rates of relapse, which have been documented since the earliest days of institutional response? Did some people experience the pleasures of drugs or the pains of withdrawal differently from others? Did some experience the anticipation or effects of pain differently than others? Did drugs work differently in some people? To answer such questions in what they considered "objective" terms, the ARC relied on a steady stream of "research material"—including human subjects and nonhuman entities, such as animals and chemical compounds—around which institutional routines, metrics, and protocols were developed. The human subjects were supplied by the surrounding institution, the compounds by pharmaceutical companies via Nathan B. Eddy, the biological coordinator of the NRC/NAS Committee on Drug Addiction and Narcotics (CDAN).

Although the ARC was the only place in the United States where drugs were tested in human subjects, its paramount scientific goal was to understand the underlying neurophysiology of drug addiction. However, in the course of pursuing basic questions, the ARC provided a much-needed drug-testing service to the U.S. government, the pharmaceutical industry, the World Health Organization, and the United Nations. Small-sample clinical drug trials used experienced drug addicts to compare the abuse potential of new compounds. The roster of companies whose drugs were tested on human and animal subjects at Lexington by the mid-1950s includes Abbott Labs; Burroughs-Wellcome; Ciba; Endo; Hoffman-LaRoche; Lederle; Eli Lilly; Merck; Parke-Davis; Schering; Smith, Kline and French; Squibb; Upjohn; Winthrop-Sterling; Wyeth; and others. The ARC's evaluative capacity was crucial to the pharmaceutical industry, which lacked the infrastructure, research capacity, and techniques to determine whether its products were addictive or not. Industry submitted compounds to the NRC coordinating committee for administration at Lexington—there was only indirect contact through CDAN between researchers and industry representatives. Compounds tested at Lexington included many in regular use today: alcohol; barbiturates; buprenorphine; clonidine; codeine; cyclazocine; Demerol; Dilaudid; heroin; LSD; mescaline; methadone; nalorphine, naloxone, naltrexone, and other narcotic antagonists used to reverse opiate overdose; major and minor tranquilizers, such as Miltown and Equanil; sedative-hypnotics, such as Seconal; marijuana and delta-9-THC; and cough syrups. Buprenorphine, a pharmacotherapy for opiate addiction not FDA-approved until 2003, was pioneered at the ARC by Donald Jasinski, who first glimpsed its potential in the 1970s.

Postaddicts were the ARC's primary "research material," a role not unusual for U.S. prisoners even after the 1949 adoption of the Nuremberg Code (Rothman 1994, 62–63). Postaddicts were experienced drug users who detoxed on entry to the institution and whose sentences exceeded six months (no subject could be administered a drug within six months of release). Lexington housed several kinds of patients, among them a couple hundred neuropsychiatric patients who were not drug addicts, several hundred convicted felons with a history of drug taking, and "volunteers," addicts whose peers or relatives urged them into treatment but who were not serving sentences.[5] People who voluntarily sought treatment at the Lexington Hospital never participated in research. They could not be held against their will, and nearly 70 percent signed out against medical advice (Rasor and Maddux 1966). By the late 1950s, administrators perceived voluntary patients as thorns in their sides, regarding women housed in the "Jenny Barn" as especially troublesome (Campbell 2000, 120–25).[6] Women were not used in research, for they were considered "unreliable" subjects or worse, as the term *jenny* is a pejorative signifying a female donkey. Nor were young people, the mildly addicted, or the mentally ill considered to provide valid testimony necessary for research. Neither their words nor, apparently, their bodies could be trusted, and thus they were saved from the exploitation to which seasoned male narcotic addicts were invited.

Implementation of a federal civil commitment program for narcotic addicts in 1967 relaxed security at Lexington, a topic explored further in chapters 5 and 6 of this book. After 1968, convicted felons who volunteered to participate in research were transferred to the ARC from federal penitentiaries elsewhere, and the research ward expanded its operation and heightened its security. Reluctant jailers, the ARC researchers were far more interested in science than security, yet they were caught holding the keys to the miniprison that was their laboratory in the scandal-saturated atmosphere of the 1970s. Born in the crucible of New York State's murderous assault on Attica prisoners in 1971, the Stanford Prison Experiment of 1971, the coverage of the Tuskegee Study of Untreated Syphilis in the Negro Male in the summer of 1972, and Jessica Mitford's 1973 book *Kind and Usual Punishment: The Prison Business,* the debate over prison research undid the ARC. Federal prison research ended in 1976, after the PHS had turned Lexington over entirely to the BOP, which cut off access to human subjects.[7] The social context did not lend itself to careful understanding of what was actually happening in the laboratory life of Lexington, nor did it address who should organize, monitor, or pay for clinical trials of abuse liability once they became impossible to conduct at Lexington. Forced out of bluegrass country, the ARC was absorbed into the National Institute on Drug Abuse in 1974 and was renamed the Intramural Research Program in the 1990s.

INSTITUTING ADDICTION RESEARCH AT THE NARCOTICS FARM

The Lexington narcotics farm came out of the modern project to infuse penalty with a moral or rehabilitative mission. This new form of restraint—or "discipline," as Foucault famously dubbed it—brought in a "whole army of technicians": "warders, doctors, chaplains, psychiatrists, psychologists, educationalists." Foucault wrote, "[B]y their very presence near the prisoner, they sing the praises that the law needs: they reassure it that the body and pain are not the ultimate objects of its punitive action" (1979, 11). Psychiatry occupied a central position within the proliferation of this swarm of subsidiary authorities through which the state extended its power. As the quote from Walter L. Treadway at the beginning of this chapter indicates, the institutionalizing urge out of which Lexington came was propelled as much by the will to knowledge as by the attempt to reform prisons as sites for rehabilitation and vocational training.

The narcotics farms were the brainchild of two reformists—Treadway and James V. Bennett, an up-and-coming assistant director of the BOP who later directed the agency for a quarter century (J. Roberts 1996). Appointed to the Committee on Drug Addiction in 1929, Treadway shortly became head of the newly created Division of Mental Hygiene. From this position, he oversaw site selection, construction, and the opening of the narcotics farms. The sites were selected to support agricultural activities with "some degree of satisfaction or profit" (NIMH 1971, 3). The first director of the BOP, Sanford Bates, who held that position from 1930 to 1937, credited Treadway with educating the government about the "wisdom and importance of professionalizing the type of public service" involved in treatment of the "dependent and delinquent classes."[8] Bates emphasized that Lexington was established and run as a hospital, institutionalizing a new therapeutic approach to the management of drug addiction: "No matter who succeeds to its administration, it cannot ever become an old-time prison."[9]

The administrative staff at Lexington referred to "patients," rather than "inmates" or "prisoners." They carried out rehabilitation and vocational therapy through such agricultural industries as farming and dairying and such prison industries as the "needle works" (for sewing prison uniforms and "going-home clothes"), a woodworking shop that manufactured chairs and office furniture for federal institutions, a laundry, a "microphotography" unit, and a print shop and book bindery. This hybrid prison-hospital delivered congregate care at an immense scale through the routines of a hospital with tight security. Although its rehabilitative mission was at odds with the broader criminalizing trajectory of U.S. drug policy, part of the project was to position the "dangerous classes" to receive "moral therapy" (Tomes 1994). Not everyone greeted the institutionalizing urge with enthusiasm, despite the political consensus out of which the narcotics farms were built. Until shortly before he assumed the helm at Lexington, Kolb had not supported specialized facilities for addicts (Acker 2002, 155, 163), despite advocating a strong federal role in mental health and hygiene. Lexington was the bricks-and-mortar incarnation of the idea that treatment, research, and rehabilitation should be linked.

By all accounts, Kolb assembled an enviable staff to run the institution, "raiding" both of the bureaucracies that oversaw Lexington's construction. In congratulating Kolb on the "fine character of [his] staff," Bates noted he was "somewhat aghast at the number of fine subordinates that you have selected from our institution."[10] The laboratory occupied a unique niche in the institutional ecology of the Lexington Hospital, which provided it with space and with laundry and dining services and "allowed us to borrow some of their patients" (Martin and Isbell 1978, 29). After attending a CDA symposium at Lexington on October 14, 1936, Bennett, by then commissioner of prison industries, complimented Kolb: "It seemed to me that you have a well-rounded, feet-on-the-ground research program which cannot but add much to our knowledge of drug addiction. For the first time in the history of the problem we are in a fair way to finding out at least what not to do and what remedies to abandon."[11]

Although prison officials apparently believed that the ARC was engaged in treatment research, it was not a clinical unit, nor did it conduct clinical research. It was a small, semiautonomous research unit that was unique in conducting basic and behavioral research on humans and animals in the midst of a large clinical and custodial facility. The unit also assessed the abuse potential of new drugs from the pharmaceutical industry, supplied by CDAN. The ARC never conducted research directly for the pharmaceutical industry, nor were there any contracts or financial arrangements with industry. The ARC had very different goals from the Lexington Hospital, which sought addicts who were good candidates for rehabilitation.

Despite U.S. drug policy resting largely on criminalization, the Lexington Hospital was set up to detoxify on entry, treat underlying illnesses, and attend to routine medical conditions (including dental problems typically encountered by addicts, among whom the dentistry practiced at Lexington had a fine reputation). After these basic issues were addressed, patient-inmates could engage in therapeutic vocational and recreational activities, including such skilled activities as haircutting, dairying, sewing, woodworking, or photography. Such activities were not typically encountered in prisons except through prison industries, so difficult interactions with the criminal justice system plagued the hospital from the outset. Determining which convicted felons would be assigned to Lexington was contentious because the institution had a reputation as a "country club." Federal marshals and judges were confused about how to define addiction, which drugs were addictive, and what kinds of addicts made good candidates for rehabilitation. At first, Kolb sought candidates among prisoners serving lengthy sentences, but sentence length turned out to be a poor guide for deciding who was to go to Lexington. The founding medical officer in charge did not interface well with law enforcement; he deplored criminalization as a "bad solution [to] a problem that has in a sense been created by governments."[12]

Later, as assistant surgeon general, Kolb testified before Congress that criminalization produced addicts as criminals. Echoing him, Conan Kornetsky, who started working at Lexington as a University of Kentucky graduate student in 1948, said in a 2003 interview with the author: "The government screwed up completely. If anything these long sentences made criminals out of noncriminals. They defined them as criminals because they're using drugs. Even in Kolb's definition, they were defined as criminals. . . . they were defined as psychopaths. . . . If you read [the Kolb classification scheme] carefully, they really weren't psychopaths, they were psychopathic-like. Only 5–10 percent were classic psychopath, and the others were various other types of personality disorders. Their psychopathy was that they didn't have the same sort of ethical ideas that the rest of us had. Basically, they used drugs. It was sort of a self-fulfilling prophecy. [They were] psychopaths because they [were] in jail for using drugs." Lexington produced a particular kind of addict identity and the behaviors, interpretations, and social definitions to go with it. The institution circulated a vernacular argot through which addicts and their parents, partners, and physicians understood addiction (Maurer and Vogel 1967).

Administrators and researchers at Lexington opposed the punitive direction of national drug policy engineered by the Federal Bureau of Narcotics (FBN) in the 1950s (McWilliams 1990). ARC personnel tried to direct federal policy toward a public health approach. In a 1959 speech before an audience of doctors and lawyers, Isbell argued, "A tug-of-war between one group advocating 'extremely severe repressive measures' and another group favoring liberality in dealing with addicts has been a block to progress on the problem." From a medical and scientific perspective, he stated, penalties for drug addiction were "far too severe, far too repressive" in the United States. Even as the principle investigators at the ARC argued against criminalization, lengthy sentences and more accurate screening enlarged the pool of eligible subjects, and the unit's scientific productivity rested on a regular supply of knowledgeable test subjects. The glory days of ARC research coincided with the mandatory minimum sentences imposed by the Boggs Act (1951) and the stiffened penalties that came out of the Daniel hearings of 1955–56.[13] A structural contradiction derived from the conflict between Lexington's rehabilitative mission and the ARC's distinctly unrehabilitative practice of experimentally readdicting people known to have been recently addicted to illicit drugs.

From the outset, Lexington administrators tried to influence law enforcement to populate the institution with only "suitable" convicts—those deemed capable of rehabilitation and reliable enough to serve as research subjects. World War II changed the addicted population with which Lexington dealt. Prewar morphine addicts and opium smokers differed from postwar addicts, who were mainly heroin users, younger, poorer, increasingly African American, and more commonly involved in minor, nonviolent criminal offenses. The war also took much of Lexington's administrative and research staff to Washington, due to Kolb's aspirations to build a federal infrastructure to conduct basic neuropsychiatric research. His efforts and those of his protégé Robert H. Felix, whose career began at Lexington, were central to the establishment of NIMH (Felix 1939, 1944; Felix 1979, 17; Grob 1991, 68; Harden 1986; Kleinman 1995). The laboratory at Lexington became the only active NIMH unit doing basic research in 1948, an affiliation that bought it more autonomy from the prison-hospital, and gained it a powerful ally that was more oriented toward basic biomedical research than toward custodial care. The research mandate was shaped by the imperatives of CDAN to find "a chemical substitute for opium which will give substantially the same amount of relief and not be habit-forming."[14] The laboratory at Lexington was the site for the coordinating committee's human studies, gaining a unique hold on scientific credibility, material support, and a steady supply of subjects in the wake of the war.

Rapid innovation coupled with lack of industrial capacity to test pharmaceutical products in human beings "forced" the ARC into the area of abuse liability assessment (Martin and Isbell 1978, 32). Such government entities as the Office of Naval Research and the U.S. Army also contracted with the ARC to evaluate drug potency (Wikler 1960, 17). Compounds tested at Lexington were first evaluated elsewhere, then brought to Lexington by Nathan B. Eddy of the NRC committee, the main external influence on the ARC testing program (May and Jacobson 1989). Testing served the purpose of decision making for domestic and international drug control, to which the ARC played an advisory and even regulatory role. ARC data and recommendations were tightly coupled to those of the Expert Committee on Drugs Liable to Produce Addiction of the World Health Organization (WHO; see World Health Organization 1950).[15] The WHO began contributing to CDAN's annual budget in 1961, turning to CDAN for advice on psychotropic drugs from the mid-1950s through the 1960s. During this time, the ARC was the main testing body for the WHO, the FDA, the FBN, and the United Nations, a role that ended with passage of the Controlled Substances Act (1970). Prior to that, the ARC enjoyed continuous access to a wide variety of compounds until industry began to develop its own evaluation capacity.[16] One observer noted: "Nathan Eddy used to come with his bag of medicines to try on the addicts, and they used to rate them. In fact the technique of drug discrimination in animals is really a technique of what they were doing in humans. They would rate them compared to morphine" (Kornetsky 2003b).

The testing load was overwhelming and time-intensive. Martin and Isbell wrote, "Our capacity to test these drugs was strained to the limit and only the development of screening methods in monkeys at the University of Michigan prevented us from being completely overwhelmed" (1978, 32). Not until the 1960s did animal models become all that useful for drug screening. Until then, human beings were the most valuable source of information about drug effects. Despite the testing program, however, researchers were never in thrall to the pharmaceutical industry; they were buffered from fund-raising and administration and granted latitude to do basic research by virtue of their PHS positions. They defined addiction in physiological terms, as the predictable outcome of social and psychological conditioning, and sought to unmask neurophysiological effects in isolation from "psychopathological" effects. That science was not done anywhere else, so it is worth a close look at how people found themselves part of the institution that surrounded the laboratory at Lexington.

PATHWAYS TO LIVING AND WORKING AT THE "FANTASTIC LODGE"

Lexington was regarded as an almost mythical destination. It was well off the beaten path. Patients were mandated there by courts east of the Mississippi, bused in from Chicago and New York City. Both naive researchers and addict "volunteers" described winding up at Lexington as if magically drawn to the spot. Federal prisoners sought to transfer there due to its reputation. Different hierarchies of credibility, social status, and evolving values developed between the research side of the institution and the custodial and clinical aspects of Lexington. Early in the institution's life, administrators sought to educate state and federal governments on the "wisdom and importance of professionalizing this type of public service" in order to keep Lexington from ever becoming an "old-time prison."[17] In this context, "professionalization" referred not only to the application of psychiatry to the "dependent and delinquent class" treated at the institution but also to the research effort.[18] Initially, it was hoped that professionalization would bring about moral as well as physical rehabilitation, through systematically implemented moral treatment regimens to "readjust" addicts (Acker 2002, 166–67). Over time, enthusiasm for modern moral therapy gave way to bureaucratized routines, more coercive procedures, and a "hardening" of the clinical staff's attitudes toward addicts and their beliefs about addiction (Acker 2002, 167). Despite Kolb's commitments to humane treatment, Lexington soon displayed a typical disjuncture that historians have identified in other large-scale institutions founded on humane visions: founding ideals give way to practices of social and behavioral control designed to manage large numbers of unruly subjects (Acker 2002, 162–63; Braslow 1997; Lunbeck 1994; Pressman 1998; Scull 1989, 22; Tomes 1994).

Ambivalent representations populate the historiography of "Lexington and its discontents" (Courtwright, Joseph, and Des Jarlais 1989, 296–318). Bipolar characterizations of the prevailing custodial and clinical environment at Lexington abound from both sides of the wall. The popular press promoted Lexington to country-club status: "Ringed by the fabulous Kentucky racing stables, the USPHS hospital (nicknamed Narco) stretches over a green hill like a country club. The inmates are called 'patients'; the guards, 'security aids'; and the disciplinary board is gently titled 'the adverse-behavior clinic.' The iron gates and window bars are painted soft colors of turquoise and rose" (Salisbury 1951, 60). Such depictions did not curry favor with the public, due to popular disregard for addicts. As radio personality Walter Winchell remarked in the 1950s, Lexington was regarded as a "multi-million-dollar flophouse for junkies."[19] The cultural milieus in which opiate addiction took root in the United States made the therapeutic culture at Lexington a celebrity culture. Musical instruments were purchased by the institution, and well-known jazz musicians played in a large auditorium dedicated to talent shows and concerts (Davis 2003). There was a branch of a medical society for physicians who succumbed to their occupation's typically high rates of addiction. Residents worked at a variety of jobs: families of the scientists and clinicians who lived on the grounds had access to Chinese cooks and African American domestics drawn from the inmate population (Senechal 2003).

During most of the institution's life, there was substantial differentiation between researchers and clinicians in terms of constraints, routines, and expectations.[20] The clinical environment was more bureaucratized. A heroin addict from Southside Chicago, Marilyn Bishop, whose audiotaped memoirs were published under the pseudonym "Janet Clark," described her arrival at Lexington: "It was a long, tiresome procedure. . . . They make you fill out all kinds of forms, form after form after form. Have you ever been in the institution before? Have you ever attempted cures before? What's your habit? How much were you using? That was the first time I ever had any contact with the Lexington attitude about junk [heroin]; you know, just very matter-of-fact, as though he would ask someone how many cigarettes they smoked in a day" (Hughes 1961, 210).[21] Indeed, the folders of forms in the federal archives in Morrow, Georgia, reveal that Lexington's highly bureaucratized day-to-day operation tracked everything from milk production to the whereabouts of every syringe. Application forms summarized which drugs qualified one for admission to Lexington ("opium, morphine, heroin, Demerol, methadone, dolophine, codeine, coca leaves, cocaine, Novocain, isonipecaine, and Indian hemp") and which did not ("sodium phenobarbital, amytal, nembutal, Seconal, luminal, chloral hydrate, bromides, paraldehyde, Benzedrine, elixir terpin hydrate, any other barbiturate, and ALCOHOL"). There was a two-page application to be filled out by the applicant, a two-page Medical Certificate of Drug Addiction to be filled out by the applicant's physician, and an additional form to be filled out by women applicants. The latter indicated the paternalism and institutional sexism of Lexington: a sample version was filled out by "Mrs. Violet Rose Buttercup" and granted the surgeon general, the medical officer in charge, or their designated representatives the authority to communicate with the applicant's next of kin.[22] Treatment was regimented; prisoners and volunteers were perceived as difficult if they did not comply with institutional routines (Hughes 1961, 216). The degree of social control reached coercive levels despite therapeutic intent. Clinical and support staff were hardly immune from the generalized social stigma pertaining to addicts; if anything, conflicts between staff and patients confirmed addicts as undesirable, unruly, or otherwise abnormal.

Over time, addicts who habitually made the trip to Lexington noticed both demographic shifts among the general population and attitudinal shifts among staff. "Brenda" noticed more African Americans from Washington, D.C., by the mid- to late 1950s. She recounted a drastic change in a young, white psychiatric aide who had been "very nice and sociable" during a previous hospitalization. By 1956, she was so changed that "Brenda" stated: "I couldn't believe it was the same person. She had toughened, and hardened, and wouldn't smile" (Courtwright, Joseph, and Des Jarlais 1989, 307). Despite this, Lexington occupied an almost mythic status for patients, who sometimes begged for admission. In a letter to "Dr. Cobb" (*sic*) addressed to the attorney general in Washington, D.C., an addict from Terre Haute, Indiana, wrote on behalf of himself and his wife: "This will be the last request I'll ask. The last time I was there complications arose, which forced me to leave before I was cured. . . . [This time] I feel sure we will manage to stay until we are completely cured."[23] The view of a well-run, genuinely therapeutic Lexington contrasted to portrayals in which addicts chafed against the strictures of institutional routine or invented ingenious ways to get around the rules—such as "kiting," the practice of sending notes between inmates (Maclin 2004).

The patient-inmate population became more diverse over the life of the institution. The diversity among residents outstripped the diversity among staff. Harris Isbell started the Social Science Section in 1962 to study demographic shifts in admissions to Lexington. That unit did a study in 1966 of all admissions to Lexington and Fort Worth from their respective openings in 1935 and 1938 through 1964, showing a marked drop in the age of male admissions (only 16 percent were under age thirty in the 1930s, compared with 50 percent in the 1960s). Southern admissions had fallen off, while those from northern cities (notably New York and Chicago) had climbed. The percentage of nonwhite inmates (which included Chinese) was less than 20 percent in the 1930s but more than 40 percent by the 1950s. By the 1960s, there were many more admissions among people with prior criminal records who were regularly engaged in illegal activities requiring more cash than most postwar addicts could muster. Postwar addicts were younger, less skilled, and less educated—they faced such structural constraints as the disappearance of viable employment. By 1960, the racial-ethnic transition was clear: out of roughly one thousand Lexington patients, eight hundred were male; 50 percent were white, and 48 percent were African American. Over 70 percent were addicted to heroin, less than 10 percent to morphine, and more than 13 percent to synthetic opiates (Rasor and Maddux 1966).

Negative impressions of Lexington often center on initial impressions of the institution. Heroin addict Marilyn Bishop said: "You never get over that first shock. After a while, they start looking like people to you, and everything, and you get used to it. You get used to looking at the sores, at women that are so thin that it just shouldn't be. I mean, they look like those pictures from Dachau and the concentration camps, of people who have been starving for hundreds and hundreds of years or so, and all hunched over and huddled-up and sick-looking" (Hughes 1961, 213). Despite this description, Bishop praised the food as "above jail par"—eggs, fresh fruit, dessert, and salad (Hughes 1961, 221). She noticed what Becker came to call "labeling," by which residents came to identify themselves as "junkies" and assume an identity they had not previously called themselves prior to Lexington: "After the first six, eight months that I was making it, I never said, 'Well, I'm a junkie,' as an excuse or as anything. But now I say it constantly. I always refer to myself as a junkie, even when I'm not hooked on anything. And when you're introduced to somebody for the first time, the first thing you find out is whether he's a junkie or not. It's like belonging to some fantastic lodge, you know, but the initiation ceremony is a lot rougher" (Hughes 1961, 214–15). Lexington produced "junkies" who were initiated into a "fantastic lodge," sharing a common language and a set of social norms that marked them as a separate class.

Classification by drug of choice and diagnosis was a major part of the Lexington routine, not only among medical personnel but also among residents. Old-style "medical junkies," whom Bishop described as Southern hypochondriacs, were distinguished from the new class of "illicit junkies" who considered themselves "members of the underworld" (Hughes 1961, 219). The two intermingled at Lexington, although they shared neither social experiences nor language to interpret them. Gradually, the number of "accidental" or "medical addicts" declined. To make the boredom of the institutional routines bearable, illicit junkies shared information about policing, drug markets, and technique; smoked cigarettes (which were ubiquitous among residents, staff, and researchers, all of whom received standard-issue heavy glass ashtrays on their desks on arrival); talked about shared interests in dope and jazz; did work assignments; or sought dental or medical care. "It's not exactly what you'd call an exciting routine," admitted Bishop, "but it's pure luxury, compared to most prisons" (Hughes 1961, 225). The construction of Lexington as "luxurious" was common among locals, U.S. marshals, convicted criminals, and potential patient-inmates (Senechal 2003, 184).

Routine was socially supportive for those who lived at Lexington. Postaddicts recounted feeling at sea upon leaving the institution, returning to the familiar life after taking "the cure." As noted earlier, Lexington was to junkies an initiation rite through which they became members of a "fantastic lodge." Lexington provided a sense of belonging that ironically transformed people into "incurable junkies" for the first time in their lives. Addicts were produced according to persistent and widely held beliefs in the underlying psychological—and psychopathological—basis of addiction. The "psychogenic" basis of drug addiction, established by Kolb, was in the process of being investigated and undermined by the basic scientists in the neurophysiological laboratory next door. Relationships replayed the typically hierarchical division between educated, largely white, middle-class male scientists in white coats and subjects from the ranks of the poor and working classes. With the exception of physician addicts, well represented at Lexington and somewhat favored at the ARC because they could assist in data processing in the age before computation, subjects came from very different social circumstances than did those who studied them. However, subjects possessed a broad range of experiences with the social circumstances surrounding drugs and drug markets, on which researchers depended for the production of valid results.

Becoming a subject in a research study marked a Lexington resident with distinction as a "real" addict whose condition was important enough to merit scientific inquiry. Subjects were housed on a separate ward when part of a study and not released into the general population. Separate housing was one of the chief incentives for participation in studies—even a small private room varied the tempo of institutional life. Financial incentives were minimal—the ARC never paid any more than other prison industries. Access to drugs clearly attracted some subjects, although they could not know if they would receive an active compound or a placebo.[24] Nor could they predict what drug would be administered.[25] Researchers reiterated beliefs that participants volunteered out of an altruistic desire to give something worthwhile back to society. A researcher who began in 1963 put it: "Obviously, they were gaining benefits from us. It wasn't treatment benefits. We never stated this in any way as being a therapeutic benefit. But these people were serving long sentences, they liked to have the variety, and some of them were altruistic. I believe that some of them really felt for the first time in their lives, where they had never done much good, that they could actually do something that was a benefit" (Gorodetzky 2003). The belief in the altruistic motivations of prisoner patients was central to researchers' construction and maintenance of their self-identity as ethical subjects.

Such safeguards as informed consent, eligibility criteria, protocols, and the Organizational Review Board were central to researchers' performance of ethical science. To participate in ARC studies, prisoner patients had to meet eligibility criteria: they had to be healthy; they could not be "naive" to the drug being tested (which meant they had to have formerly consumed drugs of its class); they could not be administered experimental drugs within six months of release; and they had to "volunteer" for studies about which they could know little beyond the fact that drugs would be administered, that they would be monitored physiologically, and that they would be asked to answer extensive sets of questions or to engage in various exercises. Undergoing pencil-and-paper tests was called "being on the sawmill," and these tests included a variety of psychometrics (Johnson 2005). Such instruments and protocols enabled the ARC to amass an unrivaled data set on the effects of drugs on humans. Thus Lexington has taken on an almost mythical status among researchers.

AN INTELLECTUAL MONASTERY: THE MEANING OF LEXINGTON TO ADDICTION RESEARCHERS

Members of the founding generation of addiction researchers were naive to the social contexts in which drug use took place. While later generations of addiction researchers entered the field knowing a bit about the social context of drug use or even being acquainted with peers who used narcotics or marijuana, none of the founding generation had social or familial connections to the "drug scene." They were completely reliant on their informants' veracity for narrative accounts of subjective effects and life histories, having no choice but to observe closely and listen attentively if they wanted to learn anything about addiction. They soon became involved in the process of building objective scales to measure the intensity and specificity of addiction, scales that became the ARC's hallmark.[26] The research ward was the researchers' primary conduit to their experimental subjects, on whom they relied to an unusual degree (Himmelsbach 1972, 1994). Those whose scientific careers began at Lexington recount flashes of insight garnered from casual conversation with participants in the dayroom of the research ward.

The topic of ethical limitations on work with human beings arose immediately due to the nature of clinical research on opiate drugs, such as morphine, Dilaudid (dihydromorphinone), codeine, hypnotics, and barbiturates, all of which Himmelsbach studied in the formative years of his career. His precocious awareness concerning informed consent was revealed in interviews separated by two decades, in which Himmelsbach maintained that gaining informed consent was a normalized practice in the research programs he built at Leavenworth and Lexington. The first interview was conducted in the late spring of 1972 (before the sensational story of the PHS role in sustaining the Tuskegee syphilis experiment broke).

> Early in research at Leavenworth, it became clear to me that the individuals participating in the research as subjects deserve some credit and deserve some consideration as well. I think this had been unheard of by any of my predecessors, but it seemed to me that they ought to do this willingly, not because they had to, not because they had lost their citizenship and were prisoners. So I got informed consent. I would tell them what we had in mind, the good, the bad, and the indifferent of it to the extent that I was able, and get their informed signatory consent before I would accept them as steady subjects. I don't know that that was the first time people got informed consent from study subjects, but it was right early in the course of research on man. I kept that up there and at Lexington as long as I had anything to do with clinical investigation, and I still do. (Himmelsbach 1972, 17)

Questioned shortly before his death (which occurred on March 20, 1995) about why he was thinking about informed consent in the mid-1930s,[27] Himmelsbach revealed that a lawyer with whom he had been friendly, James Kelly, had suggested that informed consent procedures could be easily built into the research process at Leavenworth. His 1972 interview detailed the paternalistic nature of what informed consent meant to Himmelsbach: subjects knew they could withdraw from studies if they so chose; subjects knew that he, the investigator, would not let anything "adverse" happen to them; and subjects trusted that he "would not let them suffer unnecessarily or to suffer any permanent damage" (1972, 18). Remorsefully, Himmelsbach recounted an "individual who died in my arms at Lexington from causes that I could never understand," eight to ten hours after withdrawal, despite administration of morphine. "Other than that instance," he claimed, "I don't know of a single individual that ever was harmed or was permitted to harm himself" (1972, 18).

Echoed through the years by researchers, such statements about the lack of mortality have been part of the ongoing construction of the research at Lexington as an ethical enterprise. Although there were occasional suicides at Lexington, and there was a morgue there, no deaths were directly linked to the administration of a drug under study. As recounted in chapter 5 of the present book, there were some close calls, but the ARC researchers pioneered the use of nalorphine and other narcotic antagonists to counter opiate overdose, the most common source of danger. The occasional suicides occurred among the general population, not among the small cadre of research subjects. The construction of ethical identity derived from status hierarchies in the PHS, of which most researchers were commissioned officers, and also from the researchers' position as physicians who espoused the injunction to "first do no harm." The informed consent process was applied not only to postaddicts but to the so-called normal individuals who served as controls to establish baselines. According to Himmelsbach, controls received no more than a single, ten-milligram dose of morphine, yet they, too, were asked for consent (1972, 18).

Postaddicts were not considered "normal" individuals within the ethical economy of Lexington or Leavenworth, because they had once been addicted to narcotics.[28] Instead, they were considered always already ill. Himmelsbach reported: "[T]hey all came in heavily addicted, and they were sick when they came in or about to get sick. . . . They were not normal, certainly, they were volunteers, they participated in what we wanted to do, willingly. As a matter of fact, they knew more about it than I did, much more. I learned from them. They gladly told me what they do. They gladly participated in these studies. As a matter of fact, they were enthusiastic about it" (1994, 11). Learning from those who knew the most about narcotics addiction—addicts themselves—was a basic tenet held by researchers who spent their early years at Lexington. Himmelsbach referred to this as "dealing the patient in," a locution clearly based on the card games that were a ubiquitous activity at all levels of the institution.

Years after departing Lexington, Himmelsbach participated in an elite gathering of clinical researchers convened in Atlantic City by the Law-Medicine Research Institute (LMRI) of Boston University to discuss the "concept of consent in clinical research."[29] He there argued: "[W]e must deal the patient in . . . so that he can participate in the judgment. There are some derivative values to him as a human being, and to the extent he can understand these, I think he should understand them. His consent should be in this frame of reference" (LMRI 1963, 36). Contrasting the broad responsibility of informing patients to the narrow act of gaining informed consent, Himmelsbach attested to "values that derive for the benefit of the individual that participates in research, the satisfaction that he gets from it when he has some comprehension of what he's done." Himmelsbach claimed: "I've seen this thousands of times. I've seen it in prisoners, and I've seen it in other people." A forceful proponent of this view, Himmelsbach stood in marked contrast to his fellows, who framed the benefits that accrued to research participants solely as "plain ordinary money" (LMRI 1963, 17). Insisting that the value of research to the participant-subject transcended money was prevalent at the ARC. It was one of the chief ways in which the white, male, middle-class physicians and scientists who worked there safeguarded their reputations and secured their social relations as ethical subjects.

The ARC attracted a succession of researchers of considerable scientific acumen. Jasinski remembered: "You're talking about an era when the Public Health Service could be extremely selective. The people who got into the Public Health Service in the 1930s and the 1940s—before the Second World War and through the Depression—were the best of the best. The smartest group of people I ever met in my life was at Lexington. Wikler was a genius, and Martin was probably among the most creative scientists I ever met. Probably the best of them all intellectually was Isbell. Abe used to describe [the ARC] as like an intellectual monastery because it was a wonderful place to do science. We were isolated from everything. You had a conglomeration of very bright, creative people, and you had a coalescence of forces happening at the same time, which led to a golden era" (2003). Those who contributed to the team enjoyed a sense of prestige. Himmelsbach recounted: "I think we learned some things together that we probably wouldn't have learned individually. Certainly the sum was greater than the total of the parts. This was one of the early multidisciplinary approaches in human research" (1972, 18).

Well into the 1960s, almost all significant drug addiction researchers spent time at the ARC at the inception of their careers. Budding researchers enjoyed an atmosphere of intellectual curiosity about how addiction worked, unremitting attention to research design, and the "low walls" touted for collaborative, interdisciplinary research environments today. Many recall Lexington as formative to their subsequent intellectual and professional development (Gorodetzky 2003; Jasinski 2003; Kleber 2004; Kornetsky 2003a, 2003b; Jaffe 2002, 2007). At the ARC's fortieth anniversary, Felix said: "As one stands here in 1975 and looks back at the beginning of this great research program as described in the words of the investigators, one can appreciate how frontiersmen in any field of endeavor must feel. Leaving familiar paths of endeavor which are accepted and 'respectable' the adventurers launched forth into an uncharted wilderness, hardly knowing which way was north and sure only that they were alone and they were expected to think better of their rashness after a while and return to 'civilization.' Certainly many of us had moments when we felt somewhat that way at Lexington" (Martin and Isbell 1978, 6). The symbolic status of Lexington as an origin story for the field should not be underestimated, despite its status as a total institution (Goffman 1981).

Lexington placed novice researchers in close contact with subjects and senior scientists. The latter were a close-knit group, whose familial bonds continue to this day and who remember the research culture in highly favorable terms. Their working environment was physically and conceptually separate from the rest of the institution; the ARC was described as a completely different universe. Although most researchers were PHS officers, social hierarchies at the ARC were flatter than those in the rest of the institution. Inexperienced researchers might suddenly find themselves in relationships of apprenticeship and mentorship to more experienced scientists. While they sometimes experienced their superiors as authoritarian or paternalistic, they retained reverence toward them.

Hired in 1948 as a psychology graduate student to administer clinical tests at the Lexington Hospital, Conan Kornetsky soon became involved in doing similar tests for the ARC and was able to wander freely about the research ward (unlike his imprisoned counterparts).

> I spent the evenings hanging around with them on the wards, just chatting with them. And they got to sort of accept me, I became sort of one of them. . . . I was called the "young doc" even though I was not a doctor. They would chat and tell me their experience. At first I thought I'd figure out how I was going to cure them, and really quickly decided I wasn't going to cure them. They'd tell me

> about their life's experience and where they grew up. At first, most of them were white, but then there was a big influx of black urban youth. A lot of the white patients were not from urban centers. Their life experience was they were drifters. . . . I got to be friendly with a lot of them. After a while they accepted me. First they would always try to tell me stories and exaggerate like mad, and after a couple of months the stories got less wild and more reality-focused. (Kornetsky 2003b)

Although such casual interchanges were permitted, formal research design was tightly controlled by senior scientists. Young researchers were granted latitude to toss ideas around informally during morning coffee sessions in the lab or the legendary Saturday seminars.

Researchers found their way to Lexington through either an informal social network or the accident of PHS assignment. It offered one of the first psychiatric residencies in the country. A rotating position as medical officer attracted "two-year wonders" just out of medical school who rarely knew what they were getting into. One of them, Charles Gorodetzky, reports:

> I got a phone call from Harris Isbell, must've been around October, November of 1962. I was an intern at Boston City Hospital, having graduated from Boston University medical school. He told me, "We've got a two-year position down here for medical officer, would you like to come down to Lexington?" Because I had asked for a research position, I was a candidate. . . . I said, "Where is Lexington, Kentucky? What is the Addiction Research Center?" (2003)

Gorodetzky's anecdote captures the happenstance with which many found their way to Lexington. First-contact stories are common in the interviews. Gorodetzky recalled arriving during a periodic renovation: "Everybody was moved out of their offices. They were all put up on the third floor where we had the volunteer research ward. All the desks were crowded side to side in the day room and they gave me a desk next to Abe Wikler, which is one of my dominant memories—to put me next to this giant in the field, me, this kid out of nowhere" (2003). The arrangement was temporary, as the retirement of Wikler, Isbell, and Fraser loomed. However, Gorodetzky's acquaintance with Wikler grew into a close personal and professional relationship, as they belonged to the same synagogue and spent two overlapping decades living in Lexington. When Isbell retired in 1963, neuropharmacologist William R. Martin took the reins, which he held until the "great hue and cry" of the 1970s (see chap. 6).

A DISEASE SUI GENERIS: THE CONCEPTUAL CONTRIBUTIONS OF ABRAHAM WIKLER

The founding generation at the ARC made addiction more tractable to the biologically oriented, experimental methods embraced by the postwar group that became the core of the addiction research enterprise. The career of Abraham Wikler, associate director of the ARC and chief of the section on experimental neuropsychiatry, exemplified the "basic" orientation of the postwar core. Raised in a close-knit, working-class Jewish family in New York City, Wikler was an intellectual whose writings reflect an awareness of his position between different generations. He credited his forebears with establishing addiction as a real physical and psychiatric disorder while deflating myths about "sex-crazed dope fiends" (Wikler 1944, 4). He valued the animal studies that Kolb had done at the Hygienic Laboratory in collaboration with A. G. DuMez to refute the theory that autoimmune disorder resulted in addiction (DuMez 1919; DuMez and Kolb 1925, 1931). This work had laid the "ground work for Himmelsbach's investigations at the Leavenworth Penitentiary and subsequently those of the Research Division at the Lexington hospital" (Wikler 1960, 2).

Knowing neither addiction nor research prior to doing his psychiatry residency at Lexington, Wikler listened closely to addicts' stories about relapse when they returned to old neighborhood haunts after leaving Lexington "cured." Based on cues and conditioning, Wikler's model of addiction remains an important touchstone. Although his ideas often emerged in conversations with prisoner patients, his passion for Pavlovian conditioning theory structured his experimental design.

> Abe, in talking to a number of patients, recognized the phenomenon for the first time that people could be detoxified for a long period of time, then in certain circumstances could experience what appeared to be withdrawal, triggered by a number of external stimuli. . . . Wikler viewed drug seeking and withdrawal [as something that] could be learned. He first saw this in 1948 and did both animal experiments and some human stuff on the idea that craving and withdrawal could be conditioned, à la Pavlov. . . . Abe would arrive at the same conclusion you would, but by a different logic, a circuitous logic that was always amazing. (Jasinski 2003)

Integrating insights drawn from conversation and observation was typical of the Lexington group. This capacity was central to Wikler's integrated model of the interplay between physiological and "psychogenic" factors, external "cues" and internal sensations.

Laboratory logics of substitution and mimicry were based on access to seasoned drug users, who were used as bioassays to gather data on drug effects. Rating scales and experimental techniques were designed at the ARC to translate "subjective" effects into quantitative, "objective" scales. These ultimately became the Addiction Research Center Inventory (ARCI), a scale still used in modified form today for assessing drug abuse liability (see chap. 7). Describing the ARC program to Congress, Wikler wrote that the research relied on prisoner patients "with histories of repeated relapses to narcotic drug use and very poor prognoses for cure who volunteer for such research" (1960, 10). Compounds were administered so that if tolerance were going to develop, it would do so within a month, a tedious and time-consuming method that required "a supply of eligible patients that is not always readily available" (Wikler 1960, 11). The ARC developed an efficient "substitution technique," also called the "Lexington test," but "direct addiction" was also used (Wikler 1960, 9–10). Experimental readdiction worked according to a laboratory logic that mimicked the process leading up to addiction, instead of the process of withdrawal that was central to the laboratory logic of substitution.

That Lexington researchers were in the business of readdicting prisoner patients for the sake of science was as clear to Congress as to the researchers and their subjects. Experimental readdiction was openly used to assess how "addictive" a given compound might be. This determination provided information used by pharmaceutical companies seeking to bring drugs to market. However, as indicated earlier, that was not the main reason for experimental readdiction. Answering the basic questions to which Wikler devoted his scientific career—defining the neurophysiological mechanisms of drug addiction based on a model of classical conditioning underpinned by "cues" central to social learning—required a laboratory logic in which the physiological process of experimental readdiction mimicked the process of addiction within its social and cultural context. He saw physiology and psychology as inextricably linked in the process of addiction, and he sought a method to disentangle their separate contributions.

Early in his career, Wikler became skeptical of purely psychogenic approaches to mental disorders. During the first year of his psychiatry residency at Lexington, Wikler diagnosed a basal ganglion disorder in a professional billiard player by using an unconventional diagnostic technology—a movie camera. The patient, a fifty-four-year-old white male, had repeatedly relapsed and been admitted several times in 1940 and 1941. Doctor and patient attributed each return to morphine's calming effect on a tremor that affected the patient's exercise of his profession. He first noticed the tremor after the death of his wife, to whom he was "greatly attached" despite her disdain for the "unfortunate associations" necessitated by his chosen profession (Wikler 1942, 399). Preoccupied with resolving whether the tremors and tics were of an organic or psychogenic nature, Wikler administered standard bioassays, such as the Wasserman test for syphilis, as well as various drug preparations, including morphine itself. He took moving pictures of the patient, which were shot at regular speeds and in slow motion, before, during, and after the administration of morphine. "The slow motion pictures revealed fine coordination and rhythmicity of the tremor characteristic of an organic disorder. After injection of morphine the patient was able to write, bring a glass of water to his lips without spilling and to perform test acts fairly well, but the tremor remained unchanged objectively" (Wikler 1942, 400). Wikler concluded that the patient's apparent grief masked the basic organic picture.

Undiagnosed brain lesions, Wikler became convinced, were often responsible for "mental disorders" but were masked by "psychogenically determined emotional factors" (1942, 400).[30] Accurate diagnosis depended on eliminating confounding emotional tensions that complicated patients' lives and finding the true disease, whether it be malaria, a brain tumor, or the surprising instances of cerebral *Candida* infection found among drug addicts (Wikler, Williams, and Weisel 1943). Thus fortified, Wikler embraced experimental approaches and set out to revise the basic concepts and terminology of Freudian psychoanalysis, to "bring closer together the now widely separated so-called 'organic' and 'psychogenic' schools of psychiatry" (1942, 402). His goal was conceptual integration—not elevation of one school of thought over another. He was steering clear of errors of diagnostic classification. For instance, he noted a characteristic loss of emotional inhibition among the addicts with whom he spent his working life. Sounding strangely prescient in his very first published talk, Wikler listed conditions that could account for lessened inhibition, many of which looked "psychogenic" but were not: trauma, epilepsy, disturbances of brain metabolism, hormonal changes, toxic psychoses from other drugs (e.g., bromides or barbiturates), multiple sclerosis, and neurological disorders. He argued, "[W]e still do not know how many 'constitutional psychopaths' or 'feeble-minded' cases may be attributed to birth injury, unrecognized intracerebral hemorrhages at birth or cerebral complications of childhood virus diseases." Citing promising results from electroencephalography, the imaging technology of the day,[31] he noted that such factors might account for a large proportion of "problem children" (Wikler 1942, 404). Rather than turn to an elaborate analysis of psychogenic motivation, Wikler urged more thorough neurophysiological assessment as a way to account for patients' turn to narcotics.

Himmelsbach sent Wikler on a yearlong training sabbatical before putting him in charge of the neuropsychiatric laboratory at Lexington.[32] During this time, Wikler gravitated toward experimental attempts to produce states resembling human neuroses through autonomic, somatic, and behavioral disturbances in animals (1942, 400).[33] Despite believing animal models to be limited in explanatory utility, Wikler developed practical techniques to get them to work (1948b). He focused on designing experimental situations to test his hypothesis that emotional disturbances could change "body chemistry" (1942, 401). Drawing on behavioral work, including conditioning theory, scheduling, and experimental extinction of conditioned responses (Anderson and Parmenter 1941; Pavlov 1927, 1941), he also read and cited the psychiatric literature on "war neuroses" and experimental production of anxiety.[34] He came to divide the world of psychological research into work based on "unassailable" psychoanalytic theories and work based on conditioned reflexes (1957). Both explanatory frameworks—psychoanalysis and conditioned reflex theory—relied on social learning and environmental adaptation but adopted distinct narrative practices, laboratory logics, and techniques. Wikler maintained that both the neural theories of Pavlov and the mental theories of Freud had led to misunderstandings and "dissipated the energies of investigators in endless polemics about the 'mind-body' pseudoproblem" (1957, 209). He came to see physiological mechanisms as embedded in complex patterns of change that depended on the meanings attributed to them, as well as individual biography, social environment, and observational goals.

Something about addiction evoked such hybrid approaches, which also appealed to Wikler's synthetic mind. The multidisciplinary thought collective that formed at the ARC perceived it to be impossible to get anywhere on the "opium problem" by taking any one route. There was not a deep conceptual split between concepts of physiological and psychological dependence: the goal was to integrate physiology and the "psyche," a division Wikler questioned so thoroughly that skeptical quotation marks littered his writings. For him, "psyche," or "personality organization," shaped addiction and the abstinence syndrome, the intensity and duration of which varied in relation to the personality of the addict (Wikler 1948a). Indeed, he argued that addiction only became

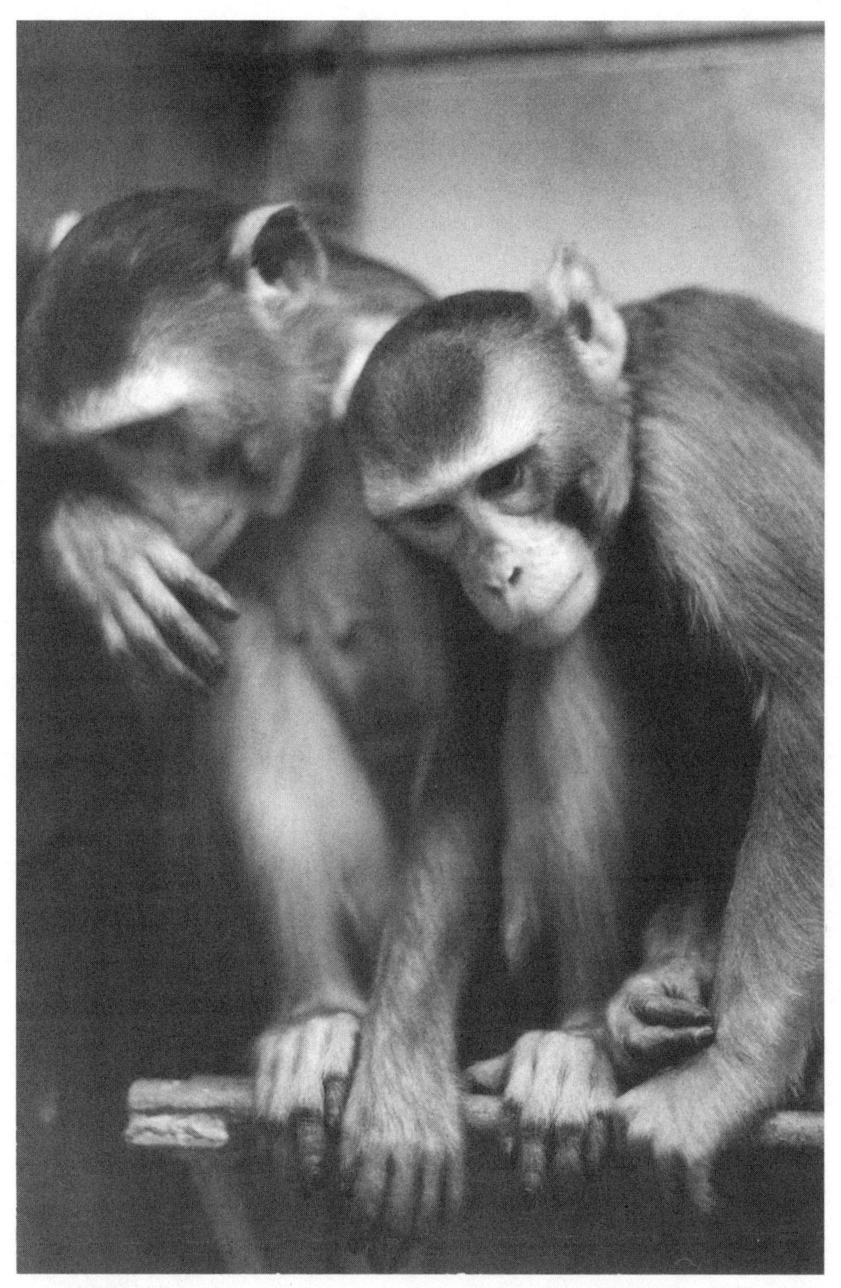

The monkey on the left received his first injection of morphine one hour before this photograph was taken. His expression and posture indicate moderate depression, which corresponds to what human beings call "being on the nod." The monkey on the right had received no drug (1964). (Photograph by Bill Eppridge/LIFE/©Time Inc.)

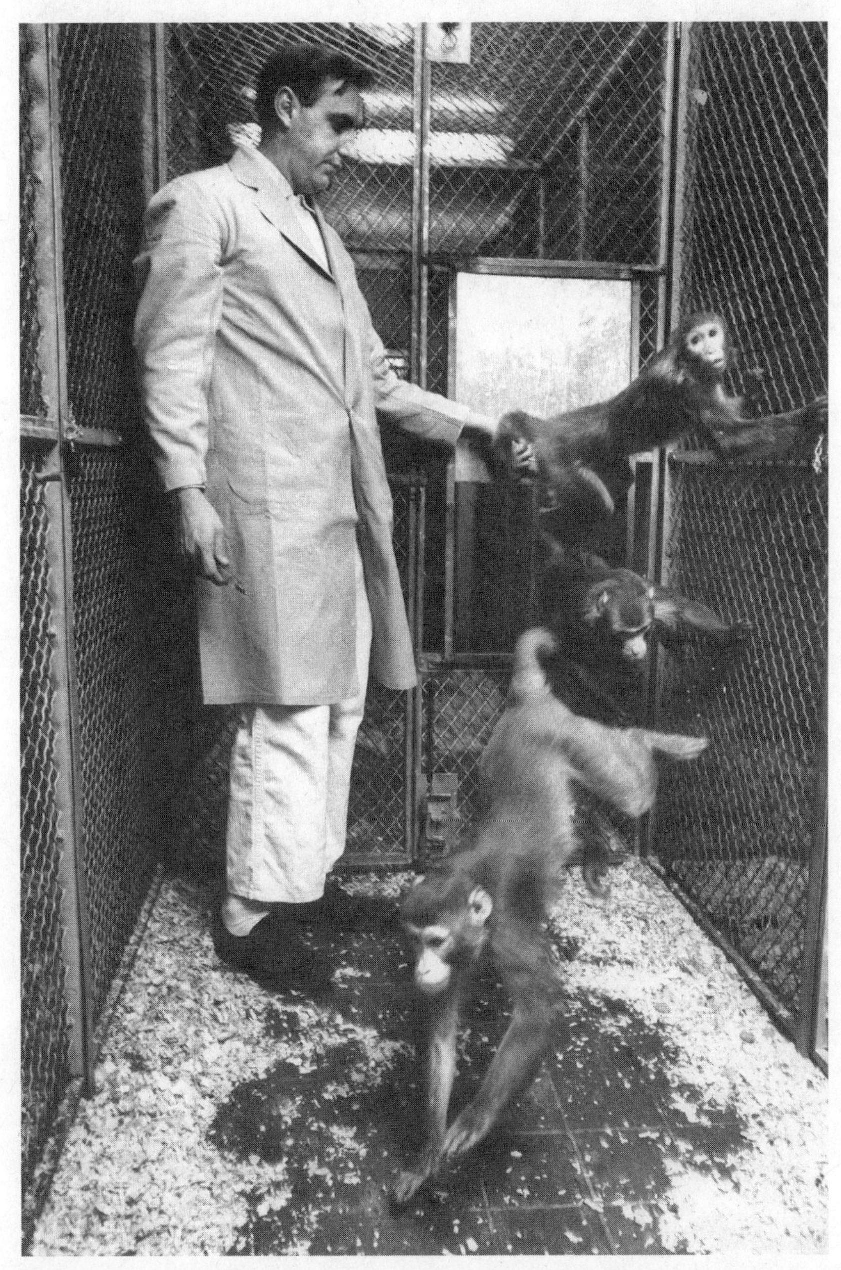

The University of Michigan "junkie monkeys" jumping into place to receive morphine injections from a lab technician holding a hypodermic syringe (1964). (Photograph by Bill Eppridge/LIFE/©Time Inc.)

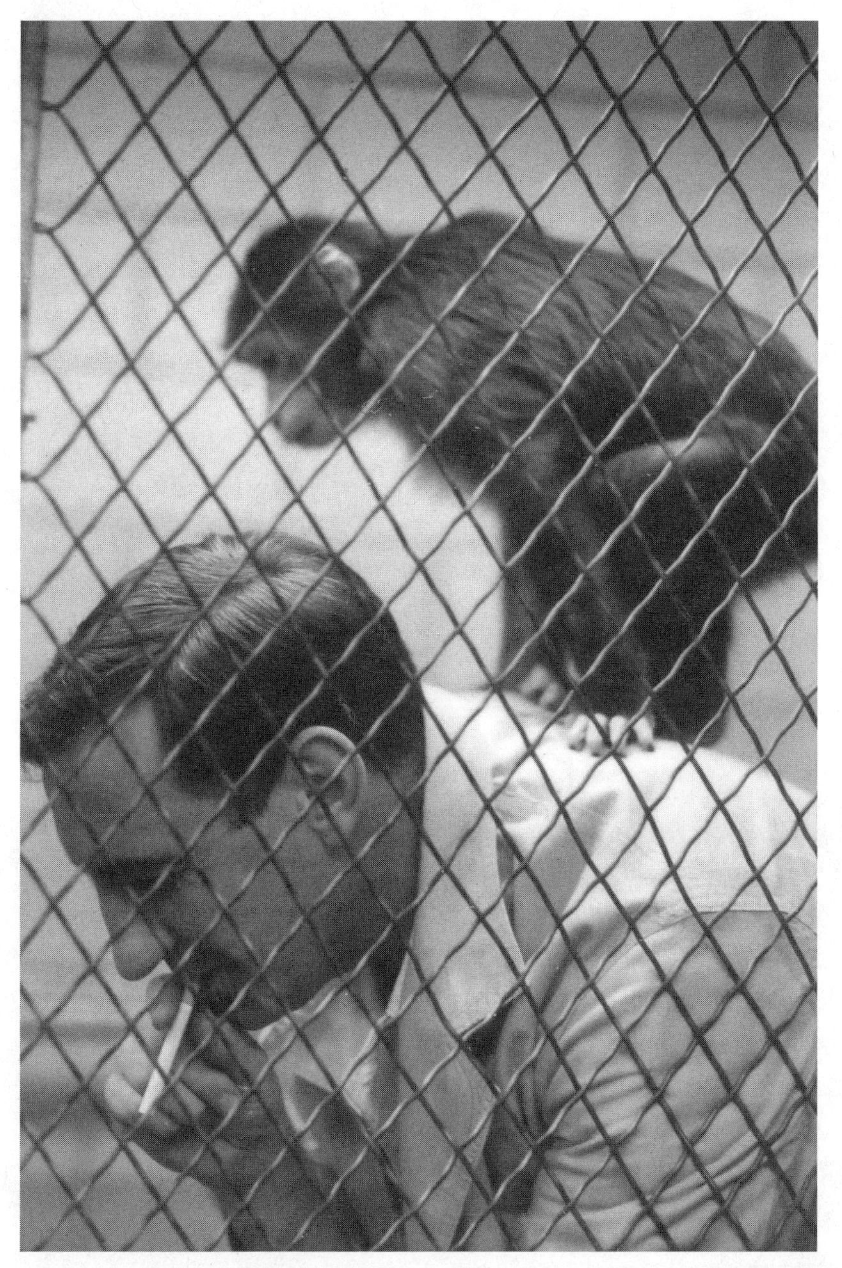

One of the monkeys of Michigan on the back of the lab technician responsible for administering regular morphine injections to the animals (1964). (Photograph by Bill Eppridge/LIFE/©Time Inc.)

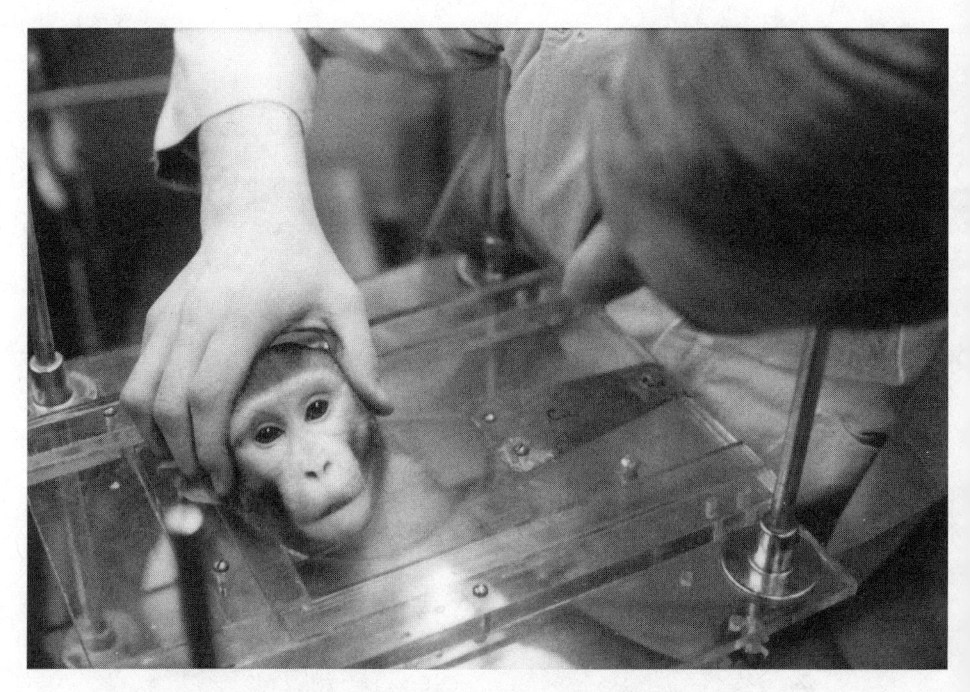

A researcher of the University of Michigan Department of Pharmacology positioning an experimental subject in a restraining chair (1964). (Photograph by Bill Eppridge/ LIFE/©Time Inc.)

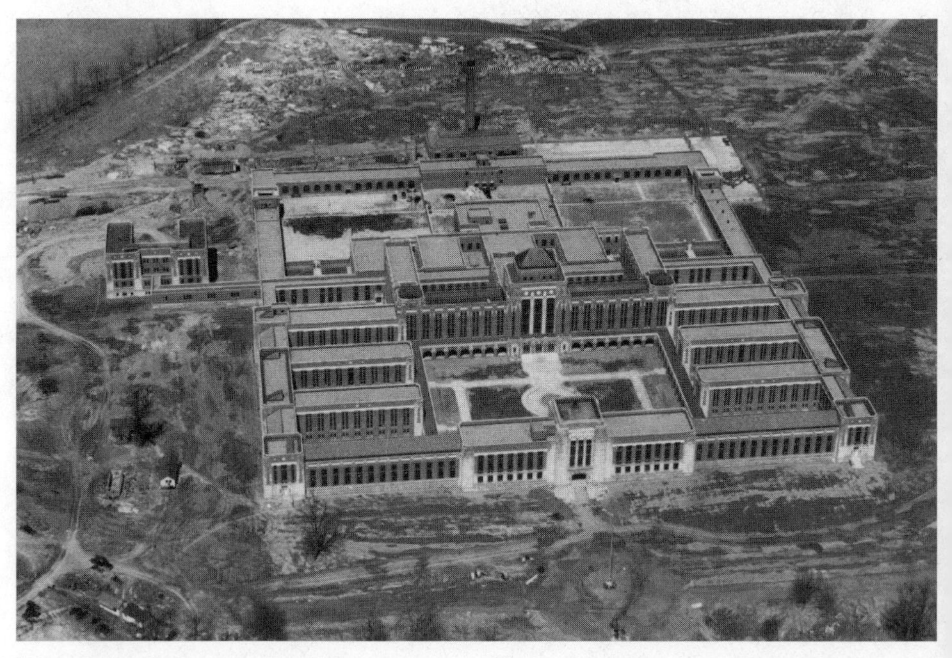

Aerial view of the institution at Lexington (1935). (Courtesy of the National Archives.)

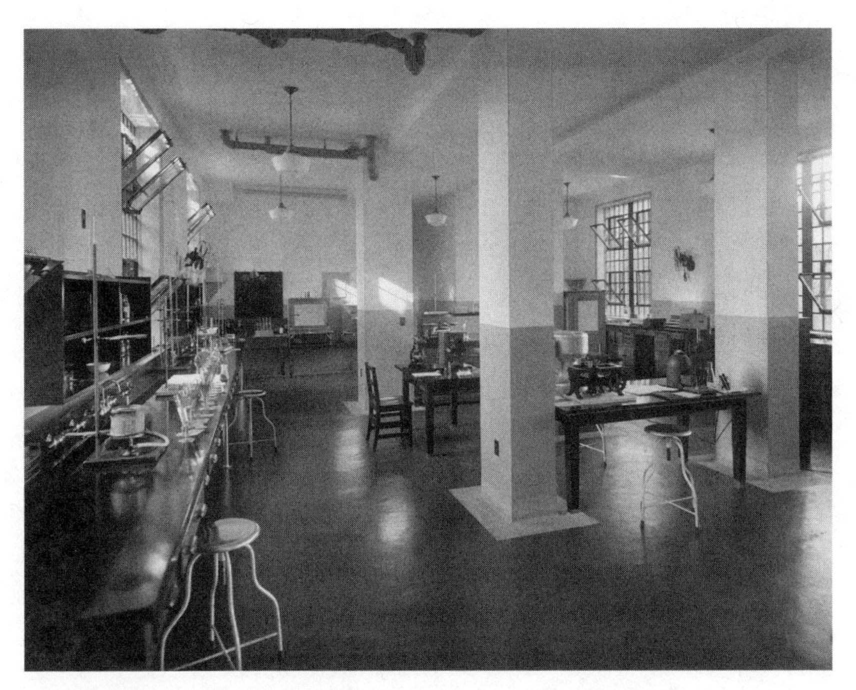

The laboratory at the U.S. narcotics farm in Lexington, Kentucky, upon its opening in 1935. (Courtesy of the National Archives.)

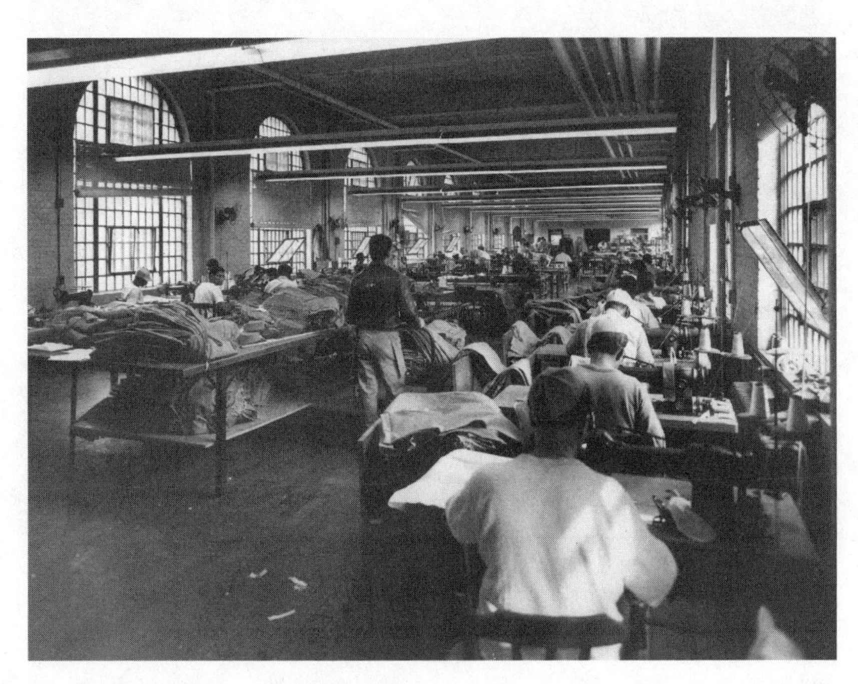

The "needle works" at Lexington (ca. 1956–58). (Photograph by R. C. Fuller. Courtesy of the National Archives, Southeast.)

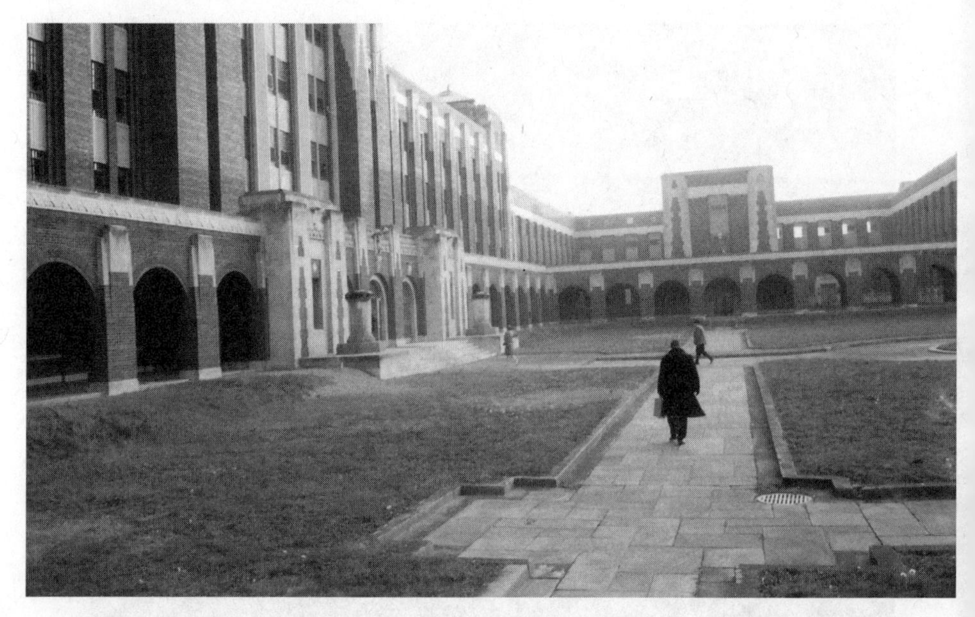

Walkway leading to the main entrance at the Lexington Hospital (1964). (Photograph by Bill Eppridge/LIFE/©Time Inc.)

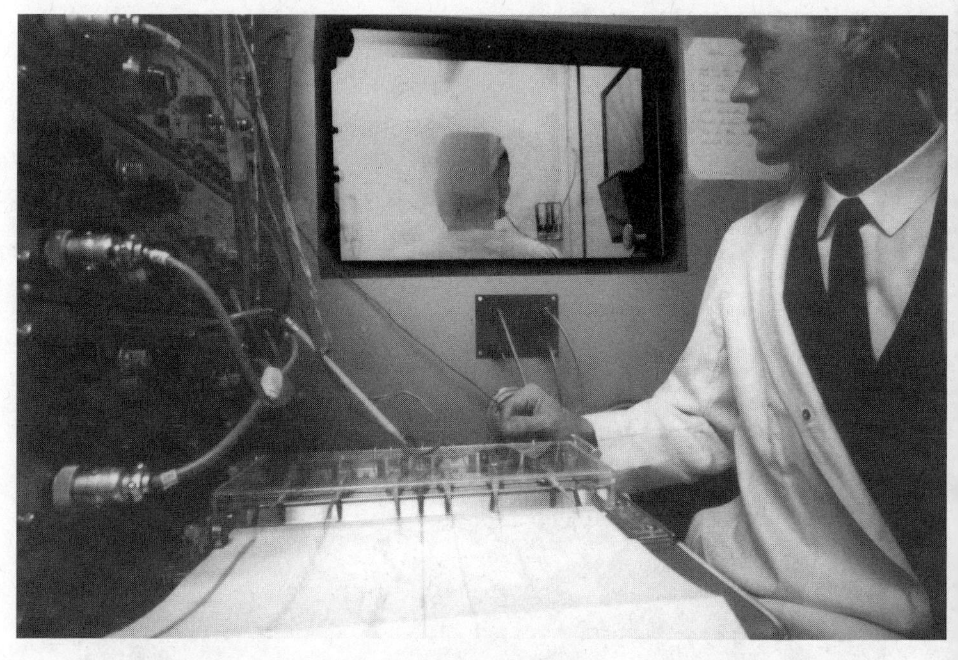

The government surplus ink-writing electroencephalograph machine depicted here was obtained by the Addiction Research Center for sleep studies and pain studies and for recording the effects of drugs on anxiety (1964). (Photograph by Bill Eppridge/LIFE/©Time Inc.)

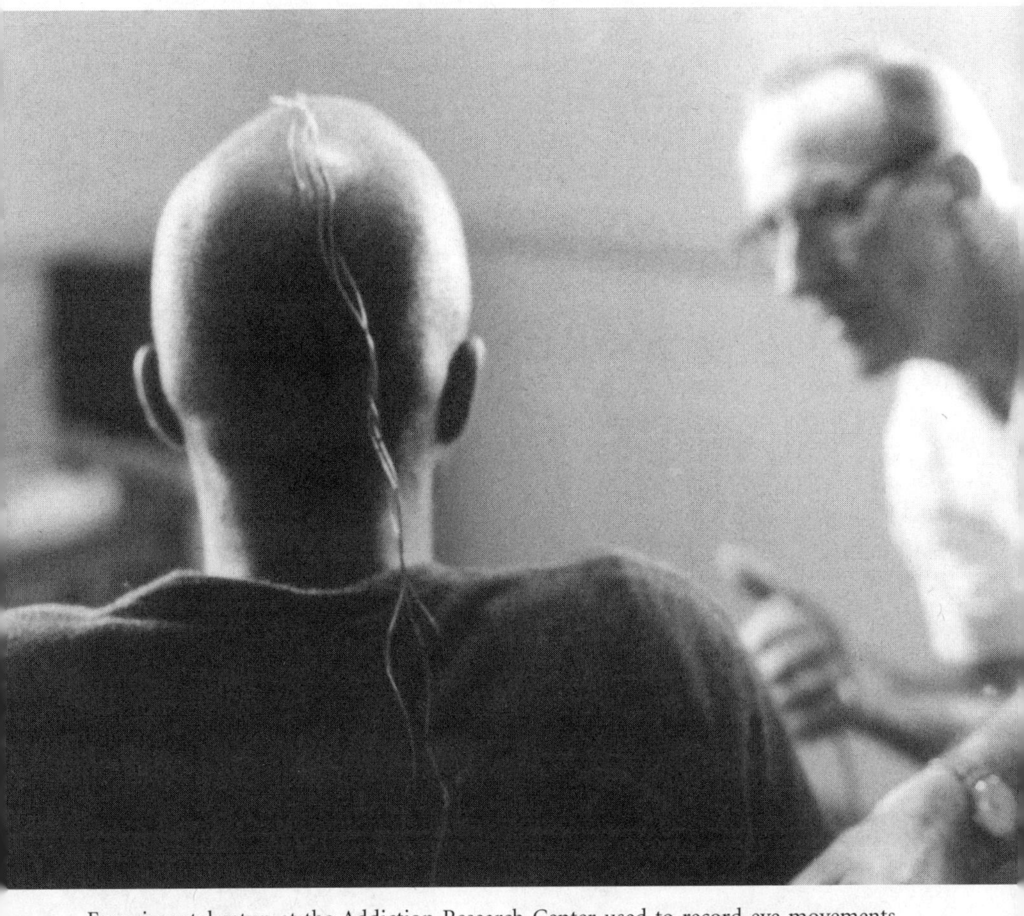

Experimental setup at the Addiction Research Center used to record eye movements while subject is spinning, an objective test for barbiturate effects (1964). (Photograph by Bill Eppridge/LIFE/©Time Inc.)

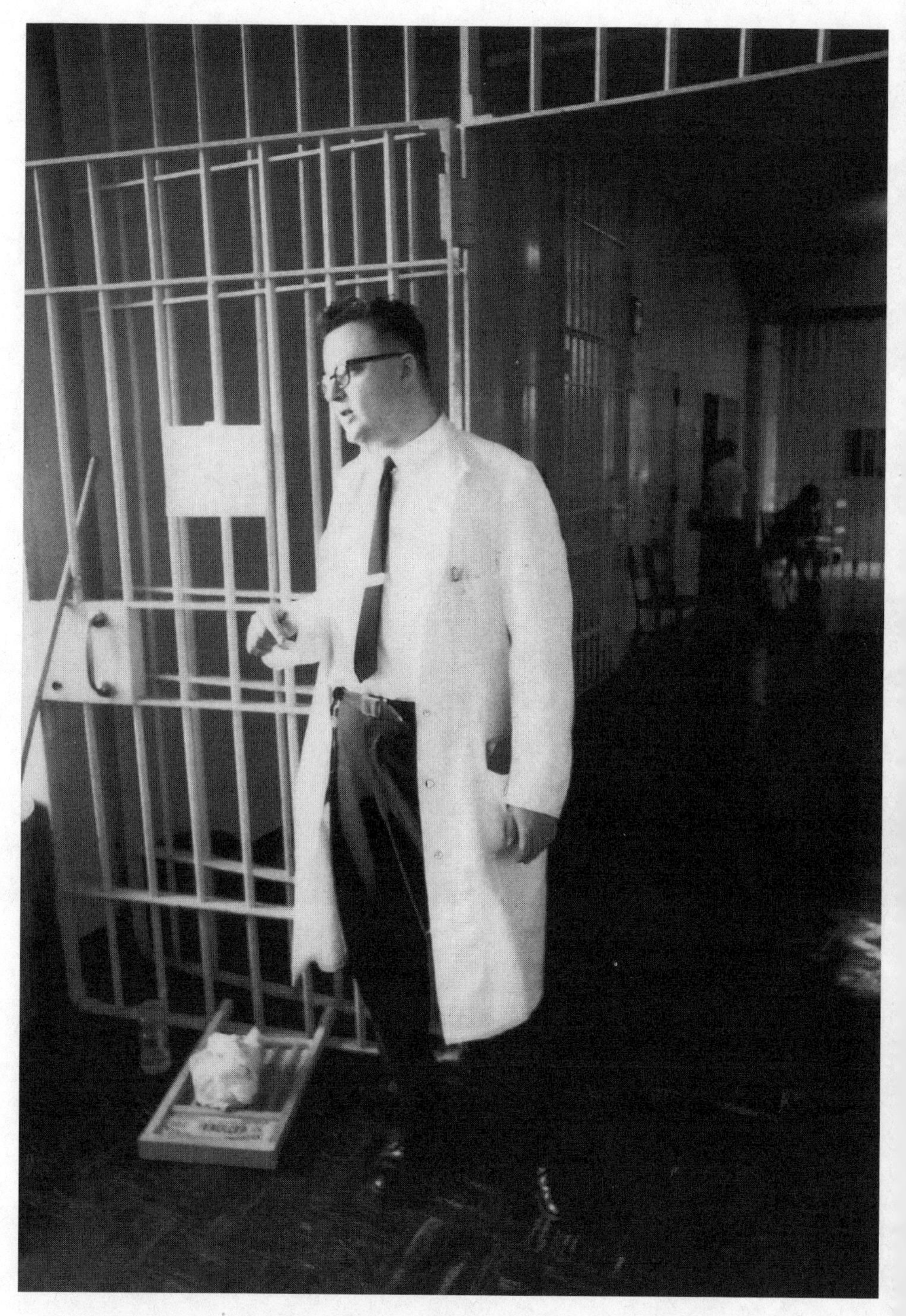

Clinician Frederick B. Glaser, MD, in a corridor inside the Lexington facility (1964). (Photograph by Bill Eppridge/LIFE/©Time Inc.)

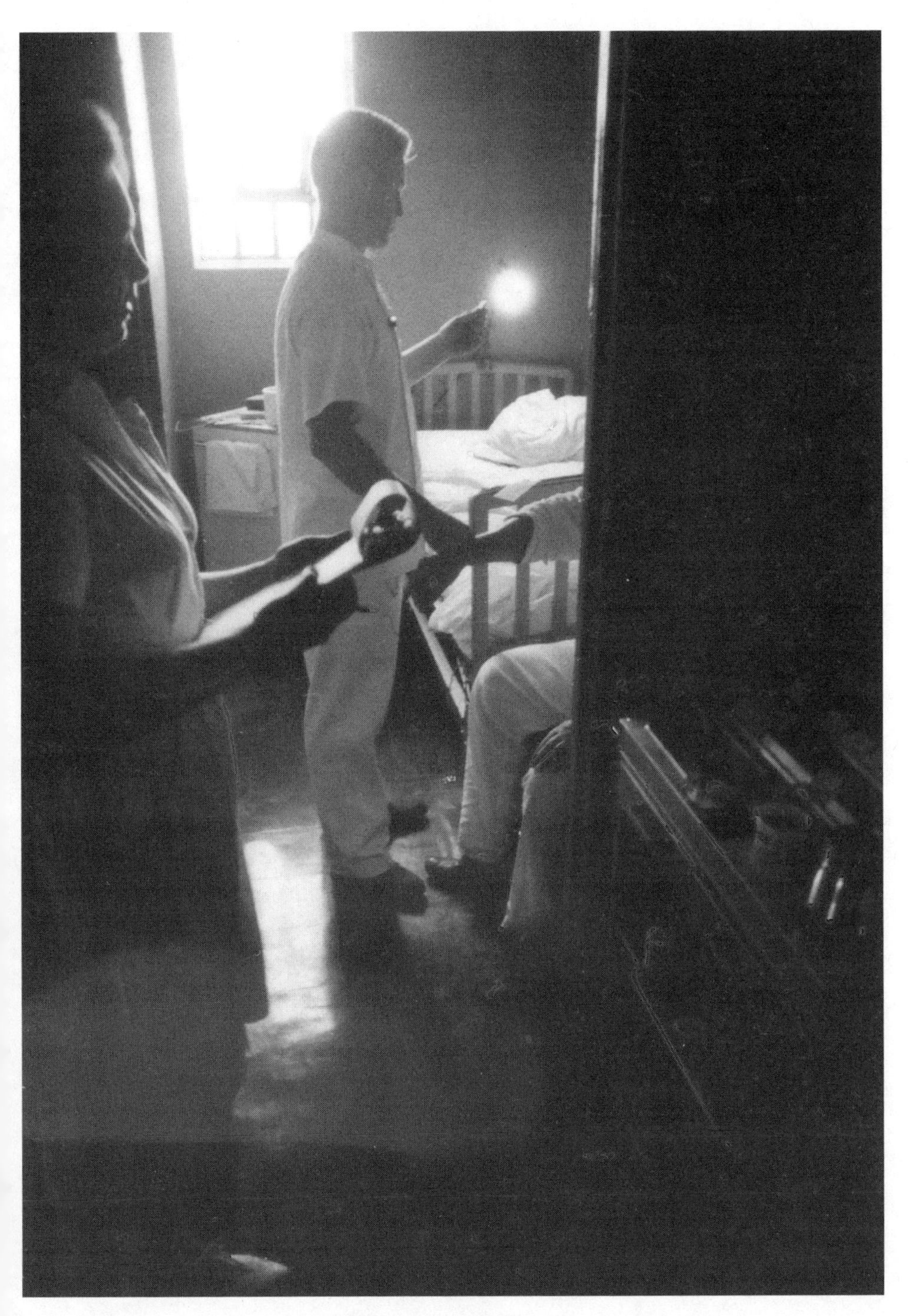

The room of a patient-inmate, whose blood pressure is being read by staff members at the Lexington Hospital (1964). (Photograph by Bill Eppridge/LIFE/©Time Inc.)

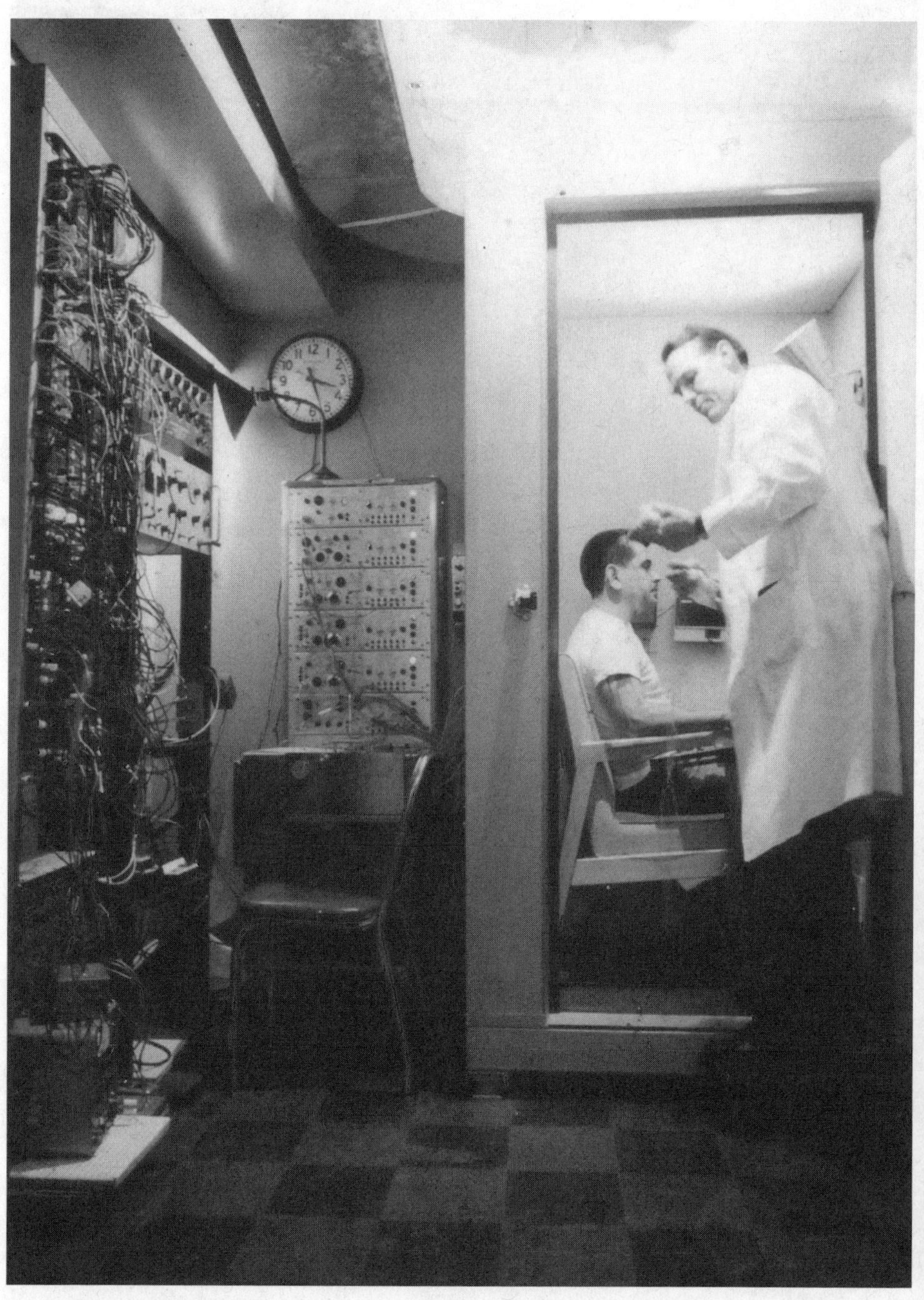

An experimental situation at the Addiction Research Center, showing subject in profile (1964). (Photograph by Bill Eppridge/LIFE/©Time Inc.)

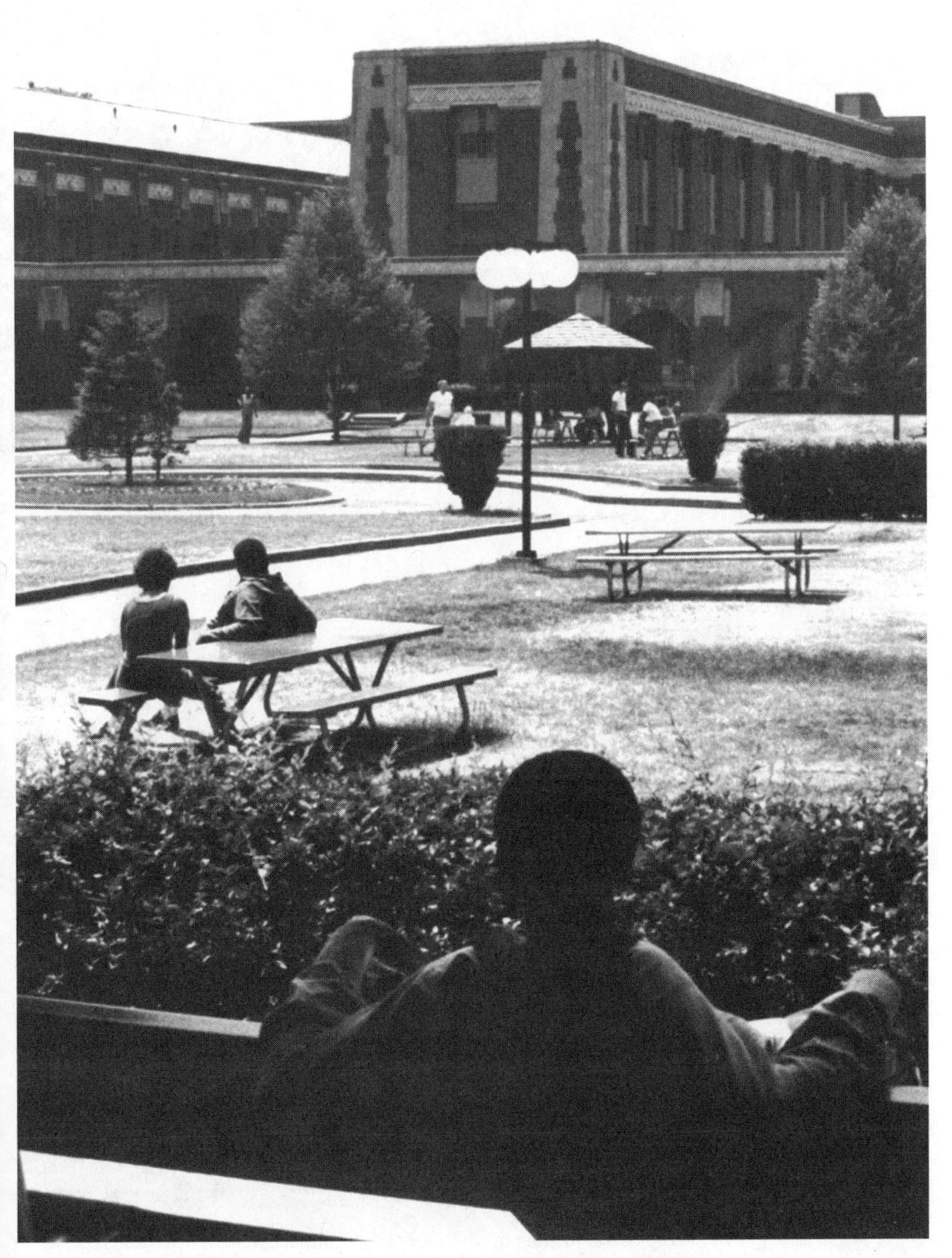

The "relaxed atmosphere" of Lexington in the 1970s during the short-lived civil commitment regime. (Courtesy of the National Archives.)

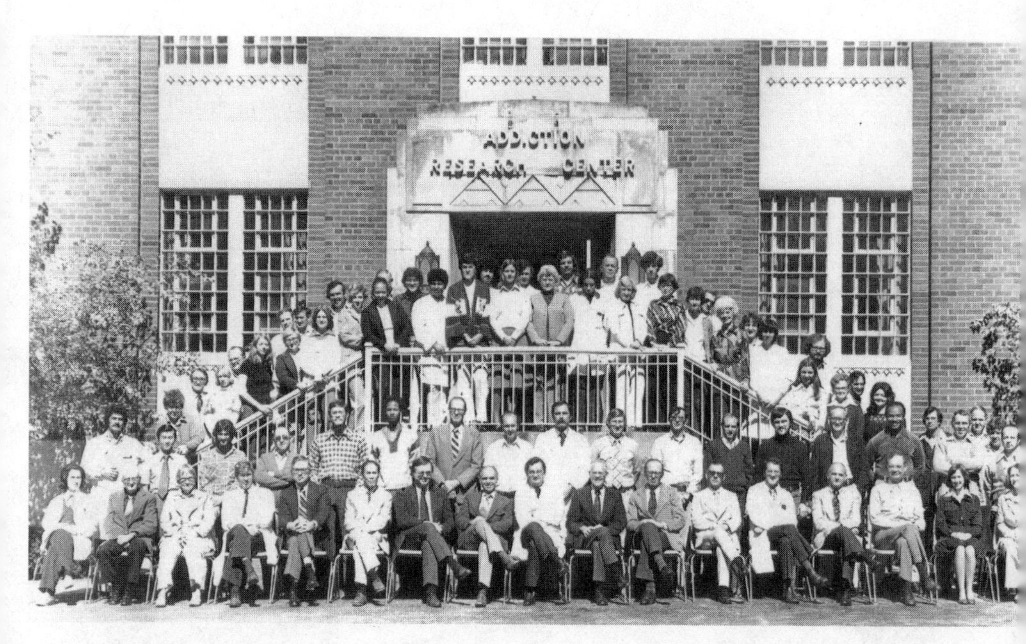

The Addiction Research Center staff still at Lexington on October 4, 1977. (Courtesy of Charles Gorodetzky.)

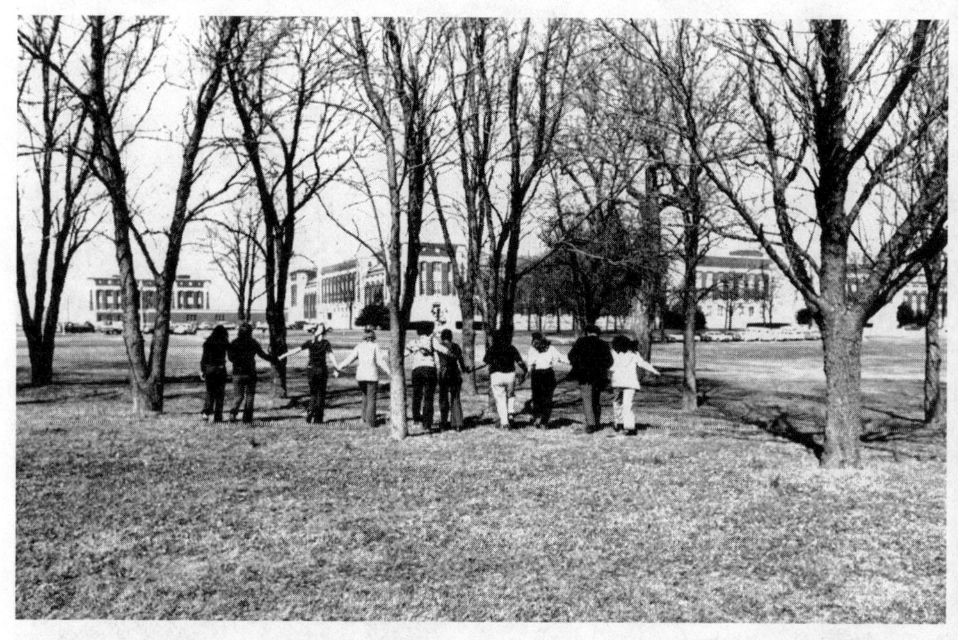

Open-air group therapy session outside the Lexington Clinical Research Center (ca. 1970s). Self-help groups, or "therapeutic communities," were run at Lexington with minimal presence of clinical staff. (Courtesy of the National Archives.)

a public health problem for persons whose "emotional need for morphine, or drugs like it, is so strong that it overbalances the personality defenses (i.e., 'super-ego' structure) against addiction" (Wikler 1950, 506). Describing most postaddicts as "extremely infantile, narcissistic individuals," he conceded that results from "psychiatrically inferior" individuals were invalid for "normal" persons. Retrospectively, he described his research trajectory as interrelating "'psychic' and 'organic' factors in the genesis of drug dependence," titling his 1974 Nathan B. Eddy Award lecture (presented to the Committee on Problems of Drug Dependence and published in 1977) "The Search for the Psyche in Drug Dependence." The problem was that the psychic and physical aspects of addiction could not be disentangled in intact animals or humans, and psychic effects could not be verified through observation. Only through Pavlovian methods did Wikler believe the "psyche" could be supplied an "operational definition" (1974, 2).

Awareness of the limitations of animal experimentation stemmed from Wikler's conclusion that personality organization corresponded to individual variations in "feeling tone." He inferred that "in man, the effects of morphine on overt behavior, affect, and phantasies depend to a large extent on the personality organization of the individual" (Wikler 1948b, 330). To explain this, he turned to émigré psychoanalyst Sandor Rado, who believed that individuals used opiates to self-medicate for "tense depression" (see chap. 1 in the present book). Wikler had more than a passing encounter with psychoanalysis: he himself underwent analysis in Cincinnati in preparation for briefly opening a private practice as a psychiatrist in the town of Lexington (Senechal 2004). Seeking to reconcile psychopathy and physiology, he became committed to the conditioning hypothesis and "learned adaptive response," because these explanations were founded on an operational definition of the psyche. For Wikler, personality factors played predisposing roles: psychopathics used drugs to gain a "positive pleasure," and neurotics used them only to reduce anxiety, which he dubbed "negative pleasure." Although he saw the ARC's efforts as confirming—not disconfirming—the validity of Kolb's classification system, he regarded personality studies as necessary but insufficient explanations of addiction.

Wikler argued that personality factors warranted continued human study: "Clinical experience indicates that other dynamic mechanisms, such as the use of a forbidden drug to express hostility and by the same means to acquire an infant dependent relationship, are operant in some individuals. Such specific psychodynamic factors cannot be investigated by animal experimentation" (Wikler 1948b, 331). He turned to Rado's theory of psychodynamics, a science of individual variation explicated in articles and lectures (the latter were collected and published by Rado's students in 1969). On first reading, Wikler's article on this theory (1948b) appears to shift abruptly between experiments on chronic decorticated spinal dogs and speculations on the social milieu and psychic organization of human beings. Wikler argued that the meaning of drug effects differed from individual to individual—that whereas morphine released fantasies of omnipotence and grandiosity in "highly narcissistic, egocentric individuals," who then experienced a "feeling tone" of unusual well-being and overt behaviors (e.g., garrulity, boastfulness, and psychomotor activity), its sedative effects were more attractive than its euphoric effects for "dependent" persons who were depressed or anxious, who resembled "satiated infants" when on the drug (Wikler 1948b, 330).[35] He concluded that the motivation to use morphine differed according to whether it satisfied deep emotional needs or not, how strongly defended an individual was against gratification, and prevailing attitudes in their social milieu. Such heterogeneity preceded the conditioning process in ways that precluded conditioning to all drug effects in all individuals. Conditioning, in other words, worked as an explanation despite individual variation. Conditioning meant that individual variation need not be explained.

Explaining the long-term persistence of physiological changes and subjective experiences associated with conditioning remains a significant scientific problem. Individuals varied in how they responded when threatened with the disappearance of a drug; anxiety about withdrawal did not appear to motivate all relapse. Most postaddicts relapsed soon after leaving Lexington, a phenomenon that was a persistent public relations headache for the institution.[36] Relapse became Wikler's terrain when he found that unconditioned responses might become "conditioned to various situations or memories associated with taking the drug, thereby evoking subjective experiences similar to those associated with morphine withdrawal, namely anxiety with craving for the drug" (1948b, 337). Conditioning—or learned adaptation to drug effects—accounted for relapse long after withdrawal. Conditioning and learning performed integrative work for Wikler, whose abiding desire was to "describe the indivisible organism in terms of many frames of reference." Psychodynamics and neurophysiology were the most developed frames of reference through which to describe drug effects. Although Wikler hoped that biochemical or anatomical frames of reference would be further developed, he believed that "no individual frame of reference is any more 'fundamental' than any other" (1952a, 11). The problem was that psychoanalytic concepts—such as id, ego, superego, or

Oedipus conflict—could not be confirmed or disconfirmed (Wikler 1952a, 11). Thus he preferred the conditioning hypothesis, in which relapse was a response to environmental stimuli or "cues," over explanations based on "pre-addiction impulse[s]" (Wikler in Martin and Isbell 1978). Although he suspected there was a psychogenic basis to addiction, he dismissed psychoanalysis in favor of testable hypotheses modulated through the concept of "conditioning" (1957, 87). To Wikler, conditioning emerged as the most promising integrative concept because of what subjects said and did.

The ARC played a formative role in constituting addiction research as a specialized enterprise because it was the only place where experienced drug users regularly came into contact with clinicians and researchers. Elsewhere, addicts were treated in ways that foreclosed their becoming patients or human subjects. At Lexington, researchers enjoyed close encounters with postaddicts who, they saw, were not unlike themselves in terms of intelligence, resourcefulness, and creativity. The social structure of Lexington drew attention to the range of individual responses to drugs and the diversity of those who had chronic struggles with addiction. Subjects varied in the meanings they attributed to drug use, social and professional backgrounds, and psychological configuration. What scientific sense was to be made of these variations? The ARC was an engine for individualizing and then aggregating drug effects. The exercise of disciplinary power took the institutional form of "objectification" within this vast prison-hospital, the study of which provokes an echo of Foucault's sardonic question, "Is it surprising that prisons resemble factories, schools, barracks, hospitals, which all resemble prisons?" (1979, 226–28). The slippage between the prison, the hospital, and the laboratory at Lexington results from recognizing the impossible necessity of differentiating between them.

Drug addicts, who occupy the social category of unproductive or even antiproductive, were rendered "useful" through the exercise of scientific discipline at the ARC. Perhaps the most succinct and accurate definition of what Foucault meant by discipline was the "unitary technique by which the body is reduced as a 'political' force at the least cost and maximized as a useful force" (1979, 221). As Foucault reminds us, however, "any mechanism of objectification could be used in [the hospital, the school, and later the workshop] as an instrument of subjection" in the course of the "formation and accumulation of new forms of knowledge" (1979, 224). When the disciplines "crossed the technological threshold," Foucault maintained, they converged to augment the "effects of power through the formation and accumulation of new forms of knowledge" (1979, 224). During the decades when the Lexington and Fort Worth hospitals existed, these institutions were the only sites for treatment, rehabilitation, and research on drug addiction in the United States. At the ARC, researchers sought to account for the mystery of individual variation, especially susceptibility to relapse, turning directly to their subjects for insight.

Loss is a recurring theme among those who did research time at Lexington. As a model of federally funded scientific collaboration, the ARC was a specialized enclave cut off from other centers of knowledge production. Social proximity to research subjects made a difference but also imparted a sense of illegitimacy when the ethical questions taken up in later chapters in this book arose. This chapter sought not to avoid such dilemmas and contradictions but to build toward the full-scale inquiry that commences in the next chapter. When the ARC's work is placed alongside that of a peer institution, the Harvard Anesthesiology Laboratory run by Henry K. Beecher at Massachusetts General Hospital, interesting parallels and refractions appear. According to CDAN's design, the laboratories conducted similar work. The committee expected Beecher's lab to mirror the experimental situation set up at the ARC. Yet one laboratory was ultimately disgraced, and the other was upheld as the birthplace of the randomized, controlled clinical trial methodology used to evaluate new drugs today. Given their similar practices, laboratory logics, and attitudes toward human experimentation, what factors made the difference? Was it the "stigma" that accrues to illegitimate research enterprises? Was it presumptions about exploited research populations? Was it the different levels of prestige enjoyed by the larger institutions of which each thought collective was a part? Finally, how different was the performance of ethical subjectivity by scientists who worked in these very different social locations? Science is more of a social privilege for some. As the next chapter shows, scientific discipline is differentially enacted in different social spaces.

CHAPTER 4

"The Man with the Syringe": Pain and Pleasure in the Experimental Situation

Quoting Sigmund Freud's claim "Behind every psychoanalyst stands the man with the syringe,"[1] psychiatrist Nathan S. Kline added, "At long last, the drugs of which Freud spoke are being found to put into the syringe" (1956, 81; Healy 2002, 105–7). Newly minted psychopharmacologists worked hand in hand with the pharmaceutical industry to expand the pharmacopeia in the second half of the twentieth century (Hertzman and Feltner 1997, 6). Tranquilizers promised transcendence in the popular press of the late 1950s (Gerard 1957). A flush of optimism linked advances in psychopharmacology to beliefs in progress, freedom, democracy, and mental health.[2] Beliefs in the potential contributions of pharmaceutical drugs to cold war prosperity and the well-being of democratic citizens brought about the culture of a pill for every ill. Popular texts on neuroscience and psychopharmacology became best sellers—glossing over addiction researchers' preoccupations with the downsides of such drugs.

Addiction was always the skeleton in the closet of "the man with the syringe." Consigned to the public sector, the study of addiction took place against the backdrop of industrial innovation in the area of pain and analgesia. Abraham Wikler wrote: "We are looking for 'good' analgesics—those which relieve pain in a variety of clinical conditions in such doses as do not impair other important functions to a significant degree. In other words, we are searching for drugs which have a certain 'pattern' of effects on patients with pain" (1952b, 227). Because the ARC was bent on elucidating the basic metabolic and neurological mechanisms of addiction, it was marginalized in industry and academia due to its singular focus when a radical cultural separation was drawn between problem-solving pharmaceutical drugs and problem-causing illicit drugs. Inscribed within popular and political culture, this division also took hold in scientific communities. To circumvent being tarred an illegitimate science and to rehabilitate their patients' image, addiction researchers changed the name of their enterprise. The ARC did not drop the term *addiction* from its name, but by the early 1950s, leadership was urging the World Heath Organization to refer to "drug dependence" rather than "addiction." The WHO did so in the 1960s, and in 1965, the NRC Committee on Drug Addiction and Narcotics (CDAN) changed its name to the Committee on Problems of Drug Dependence. The discursive shift reflected an emerging scientific consensus that aimed to destigmatize "addiction" and to abandon it as a relic of past misattributions of physiological phenomena to weak moral character or vice.

Such attempts coincided with a new regulatory consensus expressed in the 1962 Kefauver-Harris amendments to the Food, Drug, and Cosmetic Act (1938). The 1962 amendments, which came about in response to thalidomide, still govern requirements that pharmaceutical companies present substantial evidence of product safety, efficacy, and effectiveness for specific conditions named in the application to market a new legal drug. The vagueness of effectiveness standards propelled an initially reluctant FDA to take a more prominent role in clinical trials (Hertzman and Feltner 1997, 83–84). The 1962 amendments transformed testing from the use of small, carefully preselected samples to large, randomized controlled trials with minimal selection criteria (Rasmussen 2003, 456). Documenting informed consent became standard in clinical trials: the law mandated that "the person involved has legal capacity to give consent, is so situated as to be able to exercise free power of choice, and is provided with a fair explanation of all material information concerning the administration of the investigational drug, or his possible use as a control, as to enable him to make an understanding decision as to his willingness to receive said investigational drug" (*Federal Register* 31 [August 30, 1966]: 11415). Although these new provisions did not substantially change business as usual at the ARC (because studies done there already met the new requirements), the changed regulatory climate led industry to expand in-house research capacity and cultivate ties with academic units. Despite knowing some products might prove addictive, industry introduced many a new wonder drug as "nonaddictive." Following the introduction of the major tranquilizer chlorpromazine and the minor tranquilizer Miltown in the mid-1950s, this was an era of pharmacological optimism about what drugs could do for society. Cautionary notes concerning addiction were trumped by the belief that drugs would solve not only clinical but social problems.

Psychoactive drugs were touted as harbingers of a new era. Far from confining pharmacological optimism to solving problems of addiction, intractable pain, or chronic mental illness, psycho- and neuropharmacologists attended not just to troubled individuals but to the mundane pathologies of "normal" humans. Understanding everyday life as a series of biochemically directed behaviors was the context for the expansion of pharmaceutical markets.[3] Popular writing about psychopharmacology conveyed a utopian sense that the "toxic side of mental processes" would yield to collective assault. Echoing Aldous Huxley's *The Doors of Perception* (1954), Kline's fervent belief psychopharmacology would open a new door was widely shared—except among those who knew addiction best. They were adamantly opposed to the popular position that psychoactive drugs opened the doors of perception. However, they did believe that useful knowledge could be gained from studying the effects of psychoactive drugs. What doors did such studies unlock?

THE FRONTIER OF THE MIND: THE GENRE CONVENTIONS OF POPULAR NEUROSCIENCE AND PSYCHOPHARMACOLOGY

Aldous Huxley published *The Doors of Perception* and *Heaven and Hell* (1955) to advocate democratic access to mind-altering substances. He was often the sole nonscientist addressing scientific congresses, such as the 1955 annual meeting of the American Psychiatric Association or the 1956 meeting of the New York Academy of Science (Huxley 1977, 61). Huxley urged readers of *Esquire, Playboy,* and the *Saturday Evening Post* to exchange "old bad habits for new and less harmful ones," condemning alcohol for causing accidents and tobacco for making "soil sterile and lungs cancerous." He realized that prohibition was ineffective against the "near, felt fact of a craving, here and now, for release and sedation, for a drink or a smoke" (1954, 64). Rather than advocating hedonism, he promoted using drugs other than alcohol and tobacco for relieving poverty, monotony, pain, and limitation (1954, 67). His ideas had distinctly cold war overtones—he urged Americans to keep pace with the Russians' pharmacological enhancements of intelligence and energy.[4]

Popular texts heralded advances on the neuropharmacological frontier by offering accessible accounts of neuroscience. For example, the best-selling paperback *Drugs and the Mind* (1957), authored by biochemist Robert S. De Ropp, was a lyrical speculative fiction about the potential uses of drugs as tools for mind expansion and as routes to knowledge and self-mastery. Although he acknowledged some dangers of using drugs to offset the increasingly tense, unstable, fast-moving, and explosive aspects of midcentury culture, De Ropp believed that well-balanced individuals were unlikely to become addicts in the coming chemopsychiatric era (32). Warning against random or disorganized drug "trips," he interpreted popular interest in mind-affecting drugs as a signal that science and society had reached a state of maturity. According to De Ropp, only immature individuals who used drugs to escape reality risked addiction, and thus the criminalization of sick or weak individuals would be consigned to the "barbaric" past.

Drugs and the Mind emphasized the positive use of drugs to affect identity, health, and social relations. It differentiated modern drug experiences from those of the "primitive" past through associations with psychopharmacological and neurological research. *Drugs and the Mind* evoked such associations for "nonscientific" audiences by centering the brain as a cultural actor in the drama of drug use. It lyrically described the blood-brain barrier, mosaics of nerve impulses, and brain-borne sensations that overrode deleterious effects, such as enslavement. De Ropp's text made "forbidden" knowledge accessible so readers could judge for themselves "whether chemical agents offer real or imitation happiness, genuine peace or mere numbing" (286). Those who achieved adequate self-mastery could avoid becoming "playthings" of chemicals. As a popular science writer, De Ropp attributed a powerful sense of agency to drugs, but he maintained that the strong could resist their power, and he felt sure that new drugs would be invented for the weak, who were "plagued by inward conflicts and unresolved tensions" (157). As a genre, popular pharmacology cast drugs in the utopian light of scientific rationalism: the new frontier lay within the mind.

In *Drugs and the Mind,* psychopharmacological drugs appeared as modern weapons against the "barbaric" practices of the past; drugs appeared as technologies of the self that could overcome the negative effects of human self-consciousness—fear, guilt, shame, anxiety, mental illness, and depression. Yet Nathan Kline's forward to *Drugs and the Mind* warned against erring too far in the use of "happiness pills."

> The picture of the snarling, vicious, and dangerous monkey transformed by a few milligrams of a chemical into a friendly, "tranquil," and "happy" animal fascinates me in an horrendous way. Such a creature is a pleasure to have around the lab, but he would not last ten minutes in his native jungle. Similarly, mankind is perfectly capable of tranquilizing himself into oblivion. (De Ropp 1957, ix)

In this formulation, self-mastery provided a wedge against addiction, allowing benefits to accrue without incurring the downside of addiction. This discourse represented a marked change from the early 1950s representations of drug use as a sinister subversion of democracy.

The disruptions of World War II had loomed large in the early 1950s. Social experience with returning morphine-addicted veterans had converged in the earlier era with fears of rising crime among ungovernable juvenile delinquents. Nelson Algren's *The Man with the Golden Arm* (1951) showed the maladaptive side of addiction.[5] In that book, Frankie, the "man with the golden arm," is a Polish World War II veteran living in an urban milieu of poverty, crime, irregular employment, gambling, and racial mixing. For him, morphine deadens the "projected image of one's own pain when that pain has become too great to be borne" (74). He describes how the figure of the "monkey on your back" embodies a powerful habit against which addicts are powerless: "You let the habit feed you first 'n one mornin' you wake up 'n you're feedin' the habit" (78). Algren wrote:

> Through the streaked and spotted glass a monkey with a jaunty green fedora on his head returned [Frankie's] gaze. Bent in a sort of crouching cunning there on the other side of the pane, it gave Frankie the look which womenish men employ in sharing an obscenity with their own kind. Frankie felt himself struggle to waken, for the monkey was tucking the covers about his feet, still wearing that same lascivious yet somehow tender look. Felt the unclean touch of its paw and saw its lips shyly seeking his own with Sparrow's pointed face. To kiss and be kissed . . . (382)

Addiction was often depicted through the figure of the monkey, a racialized, homoerotic, and sexualized figure that appeared in popular and psychiatric discourse (Haraway 1989, 153).[6] For instance, Robert Chessick reported a patient who had been "depressed for a long time and felt that 'the monkey on my back' was her mother. She felt that shooting the drug meant feeding the monkey, her mother" (1960, 121). Clinicians believed the metaphor itself presented treatment barriers: "The typical individual . . . conceives of his addiction as essentially ego-alien—'a monkey on his back.' With repeated experiences of failure in efforts to rid themselves of the habit, some unknown proportion of cases come to a realization that the habit really reflects some aspect of themselves and not something externally imposed" (Chein 1958, 149). Reinterpreting addiction as a relationship with the self, rather than possession by an "ego-alien" other, was considered a precondition for successful treatment.

Although professional arenas did not display the same ideological maneuvers apparent in popular portrayals that divide the "modern" subjects of psychopharmacology from "primitive" addicts, the split between biological psychiatry and psychoanalytic or psychodynamic psychiatry was acrimonious. Disciplinary conflicts, conceptual and epistemological issues, and methodological disputes underpinned the configuration of the midcentury drug sciences as they do any problem-centered scientific endeavor. Often perceived as repeatedly failing to make good on ambitious promises, psychiatry and pharmacology are both divided between somatic and mental theories of mind and between biochemistry and behavior. These antagonisms have resulted in protracted social conflicts over the "intense interpretability" (Micale and Porter 1994) not only of psychiatry's past but of the history of pharmacology. Psychoanalysis played an ironic role in the 1950s, when the scientific dismissal of psychoanalytic claims was occurring just as psychoanalysis diffused through the culture, especially through the medium of popular film. Psychopharmacologists aligned themselves with the experimental practices of psychologists and behaviorists, rather than the more interpretive and narrative practices of psychoanalysts.

When psychopharmacologists begin textbook overviews, they often survey the historical dimensions of their enterprise. They represent modern psychopharmacology as an objective, biologically oriented behavioral science and date the dawn of psychopharmacology as a distinct endeavor to the discovery of particular drugs or effects. For example, they might claim that lithium in the late 1940s or chlorpromazine in the early 1950s illustrated the proof of concept for psychopharmacology. They might draw attention to the ways in which meprobamate, mass-marketed as a minor tranquilizer under the names Miltown and Equanil, ushered in middle-class enthusiasm for pharmaceuticals in the late 1950s (Spiegel 1989; M. Smith 1991; Tone forthcoming).[7] Psychopharmacologists writing this way rarely mention illicit drug use or credit addiction researchers with contributing to the field's general principles (for exceptions, see Greenshaw and Dourish 1987; Pickens 1977). They more often delimit drug dependence as beyond their purview—which is strange given that many consider the ARC "probably *the* most advanced human psychopharmacological studies unit in the world at that time."[8]

Textbook histories distinguish modern pharmacology from "protopharmacology" practiced by "great static cultures of antiquity" and "indigenous peoples everywhere" (Leake 1975, 30, 55). Such preambles contrast modern drug use to the crude empiricism of "primitive peoples" using premodern pharmacological agents. Yet pharmacologists often turn to the practices of witches or shamans to depict their science as one of the world's oldest codifications of knowledge. The field of ethnopharmacology is engaged in a "salvage paradigm" to preserve indigenous knowledge (Efron, Holmstedt, and Kline 1967; La Barre 1975). This anthropological cousin of psychopharmacology emerged with the explorations of New World hallucinogens by mycologist Gordon Wasson, botanist Richard Evans Schultes, and cultural anthropologist Weston La Barre (Rudgley 2003). The ethnopharmacological enterprise is pervaded by claims to universalism and a primitivizing rhetoric that literally appropriates indigenous knowledge practices (Siegel 1989; Rudgley 1993; Weil 1972).[9] By contrast to this fascination with premodern ingestion of "essential substances," modern pharmacologists represent themselves as a "mongrel breed" that promises to "extend man's understanding of himself and his ability to control and direct behavior by chemical means" (Claridge 1970, 246–47). The science of modern pharmacology is deeply bound up with the dreams of behavioral control that flourish in appeals to scientific modernity.

A few historians evaluate pharmacology's success or failure to meet goals of prediction and control by using as a yardstick the behavioral improvements that supposedly led to a reduced number of institutionalized mental patients (an assumption that ignores the dismantling of the welfare state that began in the 1940s, prior to chlorpromazine's introduction: see Clark and del Guidice 1978; Castel, Castel, and Lovell 1982). Observers attributed a revolutionary effect to pharmacology, consigning psychoanalysis to the status of a baffled custodian of the appalling conditions of "snake pits,"[10] as in the following remarks about differences between the pre- and postdrug eras.

> Each year the population in mental hospitals increased, since patients continued to be admitted but very few were discharged. Typically, patient living areas were crowded and poorly furnished. Schizophrenic patients with paranoid delusions crouched in corners, living in constant fear. Catatonic patients might maintain the same rigid posture for prolonged periods, developing swollen legs and pressure sores. Hallucinating patients would pace the floor, talking to their voices and apparently unaware of their environment. Violent patients might attack staff members or other patients for reasons known only to themselves, leading to hostility and suspicion on both sides.[11]

The preceding passage associates the era of psychoanalysis with uncontrolled squalor in inhumane institutions, a sadly unscientific state of affairs that contrasts to the clean, controlled conditions gained through the application of modern psychopharmacological technology.

Pharmacology takes place in an ambivalent zone between an evil empire of poisons and a Promethean landscape of panaceas. "Happiness pills" were a riper target—with higher social premiums and more chance of profit—than solving the problems of drug addicts. Addiction has long been the evil twin of culturally sanctioned drug use, be it ceremonial or medicinal. For much of the twentieth century, there was a distance between the cultural momentum of pharmacological optimism and the slow progress faced by clinicians who worked directly with drug users. Users were cast as unruly subjects with intractable problems; hence pharmacology is structured around addicts as repressed subjects and objects of knowledge, as some internalist histories acknowledge (Barchas et al. 1977; Leake 1975). At times, the study of addiction is considered a source of knowledge about brains and bodies that is generalizable beyond the ranks of addicts. Joining historians who reveal the actual practices involved in human experimentation,[12] the rest of this chapter asks: To whom were drugs useful experimental tools? To whom were drug addicts useful bodies and reliable subjects? By whom were they ignored as unreliable subjects? The remainder of this chapter concerns how scientists secured and laid claim to these useful bodies—or disclaimed them as useless bodies.

"MAN AS THE ESSENTIAL FINAL TEST SITE": HENRY K. BEECHER AND THE HARVARD ANESTHESIOLOGY LABORATORY

Oddly, the most prestigious node of the addiction research network coordinated by CDAN did not deal with addicts at all. Decorated World War II veteran Henry K. Beecher, director of Harvard Medical School's Anesthesiology Laboratory at Massachusetts General Hospital, set the standard for randomized, placebo-controlled clinical trials of analgesic drugs in the late 1940s and early 1950s (Meldrum 1994).[13] Most good analgesics are addictive: users build up physiological tolerance to such drugs as morphine, heroin, methadone, other opiates, choral hydrate, amphetamines, barbiturates, and sedative-hypnotics and suffer withdrawal when they stop using them.[14] Addicted bodies can thus serve as bioassays for determining the "addiction potential" of a drug. But Beecher, who tested all these drugs and more, considered addicts unreliable subjects. Despite modeling their clinical research on the laboratory logics of the ARC, the Harvard group preferred the populations of human subjects to which they had access—terminally ill patients, postoperative pain patients, and Harvard college students.

Remembered as the "father of informed consent," Beecher is famed for blowing the whistle on the widespread lack of informed consent in clinical research. Beecher was a flamboyant character with something of the gadfly about him. He obscured his Midwestern, working-class origins by changing his name from "Unangst" to "Beecher" when he moved to Boston to attend Harvard Medical School in 1928 (Harkness 1999, 465). After completing his anesthesiology residency, he won a chair at Harvard just as the United States entered World War II. During the war, he conducted research on the handling of battlefield wounds and other injuries in heavy combat zones. Two decades later, he set the stage for a new regime governing clinical research in the United States when he presented a paper titled "Ethics and the Explosion of Human Experimentation" to a science journalism symposium organized by the Upjohn pharmaceutical company at the Brook Lodge Conference Center in Kalamazoo, Michigan, in March 1965 (Harkness 2003, 240n44). In the following year, the *New England Journal of Medicine* published a revised version, "Ethics and Clinical Research," and the popular press propelled the debate beyond the professional enclave at which Beecher took aim.

Historians have been at a loss to explain why Beecher became preoccupied with the ethics of clinical research. He first took an activist role in exposing clinical practices in 1954, when he and D. P. Todd coauthored an article attributing a high mortality rate (3.7 deaths per ten thousand anesthetics) to anesthesia itself.[15] However, a retrospective interview by his onetime research assistant depicted Beecher as almost cavalier toward his experimental subjects in the 1950s—as more concerned with producing results than with his subjects' degree of informed consent (Lasagna 1994, 13–14). Although Beecher wrote a short book about the ethics of human experimentation (1959a), his scientific work merely mentioned that ethics were "too little pondered and too little discussed" (1959b, 59). As a historical figure, he has been constructed as an iconic embodiment of ethicality, in stark contrast to the ARC researchers, who were pilloried for experimenting on human beings. The Harvard Anesthesiology Laboratory and the ARC encode two symbolic extremes on the spectrum ranging from ethical to unethical human experimentation.

From 1947 until the mid-1960s, Beecher worked at the hub of the addiction research enterprise. Both the Harvard Anesthesiology Laboratory and the ARC belonged to overlapping pain and addiction research networks. Both research sites relied on similar laboratory logics and research practices, experimenting on human subjects with similar levels of compassion and curiosity. The rest of this chapter explores interactions between the Harvard and Lexington groups as well as CDAN, the committee that funded them both. The task of the Harvard group was to study analgesics and cough suppressants that had been tested on postaddicts at Lexington by replicating the ARC's experimental designs in never-addicted subjects. The Harvard group organized large-scale, randomized, placebo-controlled trials and relied on statistical methods.[16] Looking closely at how the Harvard group navigated practical problems of research design goes farther toward explaining Beecher's changed orientation toward ethics and his performance of ethicality than moral or psychobiographical characterizations ever could. His preoccupation with ethics was spawned not simply by his "outsider" origins or "contrarian" impulses but by a set of interactions across the separate but overlapping microsocial worlds that comprised the pain and addiction research enterprise. Understanding these interactions requires answering the following questions: What laboratory logics did Beecher practice in the decade prior to his well-known exposé on abuses of human subjects in the United States? How did they inform the ethical ideals he later espoused? To what extent did the clinical logics of the Harvard Anesthesiology Laboratory diverge from the laboratory logics of the ARC? How did researchers decide experimentation on humans should be conducted in the United States after the Nuremberg Code (1949)?

As a physician turned researcher, Beecher was untrained as a pharmacologist. At first, he was unfamiliar with the centralized coordination that I have described in the previous two chapters of this book, but his participation on the committee reinforced his sense that "the crucial study of new techniques and agents must be carried out in man." Beecher explained:

> The extraordinary skill of the organic chemist and the biologist working together in identifying active agents in natural products and the chemist's progress in creating new and promising compounds which ultimately must be tried out in man, all throw an exceptionally heavy load on the experimentalist. Man as the essential final test site has come into adequate prominence only in recent decades. The current development of human biochemistry, human physiology, and human pharmacology has made it plain that man is the "animal of necessity" here. (1959a, 9)[17]

The preceding quotation indicates how Beecher generally thought science should work and is an apt description of how CDAN triangulated between laboratories in different social and geographic locations.

Unlike CDAN, the Harvard Anesthesiology Laboratory privileged actual clinical settings as research sites. Like the Lexington group, the Harvard group was interdisciplinary, comprised of pharmacologist Louis Lasagna, internist Jane Denton, anesthesia resident Arthur Keats, John von Felsinger, and—an extremely important resource for developing clinical trial methodology—statistician Charles Frederick Mosteller.[18] Their experimental model of the randomized, controlled clinical trial ultimately won acceptance from the medical and scientific elite (Meldrum 1994, 267–372). The Beecher group's experimental design took advantage of access to large numbers of naive—but fully informed and voluntarily consenting—subjects. If meaningful data was to be produced on drug-induced mood changes, Beecher believed it was going to come from aggregated response patterns corroborated by large numbers of subjects and carefully constructed control groups. The Harvard group also did pioneering work on the placebo effect, for which Beecher and Lasagna are remembered now that randomized, placebo-controlled clinical trials have become the "gold standard of objectivity in scientific medicine"; its "epistemological status as an objective scientific method" overshadows the randomized clinical trial's socially constructed character (Meldrum 1994, 373). The "objective" status of randomized clinical trials obscures the fact that subjective responses and meaning attribution comprise part of the data set on which trials rest. During the formative moments described in the present chapter, however, the meaning and significance of pain and drugs that relieve it was much debated.

The instruments Beecher's group developed to quantify subjective responses to drugs resembled those of the ARC, yet work at the two sites proceeded differently and garnered completely different public receptions. ARC studies involved small numbers of subjects and were confined to the obscure pages of pharmacology journals, whereas the large-scale trial designs by Beecher and Denton received immediate public acclaim and a great deal of attention in the medical press. The American Medical Association's Council on Pharmacy and Chemistry, whose Therapeutic Trials Committee promoted adoption of clinical trial methodology, praised Denton and Beecher for making "a distinct advance in the methods available for quantitative evaluation of the therapeutic efficacy" of analgesic and narcotic drugs (Van Winkle 1949). Historian Noemi Tousignant explains:

> The Council's support associated Beecher's work to a movement of therapeutic reform to instil specific values, and techniques—particularly those of the randomised clinical trial—in American drug testing. This movement has been described as a current of elite activism for the promotion of a "rational therapeutics" that would be dictated by the norms of scientific evidence and medical professionalism, and protected against the excessive commercial aspirations of the pharmaceutical industry. . . . [T]he AMA's primary interest was in Beecher's methodological innovations rather than in the precise potency of these new analgesics. (2006, chap. 3, 17)

The Harvard group's methodology helped stamp randomized clinical trials with the highest epistemological status for certifying objectivity. The clinical trial model advanced by Beecher's group was based on a set of criticisms that Beecher leveled against contending approaches.

Experimental Limits and the Emergence of Clinical Trials

Deeply critical of behaviorism and techniques for producing experimental pain, Beecher was an eloquent critic of the laboratory's limitations. He reinforced his critique by drawing on a colorful origin myth from his World War II days, when his curiosity about subjective responses to pain and pain relief was piqued. Lasagna recounted of Beecher:

> He made the observation during the war on the Anzio beachhead that soldiers suffering from wounds at least as grievous as those suffered by civilians seemed not to demand as much in the way of analgesic medication as did the civilian patients with whom he had had experience prior to the war, and he concluded that this was because there was a neurophysiological component to pain and then an emotional response to the stimuli being perceived which allowed the meaning of pain, if you will, to get into the act. (Healy 2002, 136)

Beecher believed that the meaning of a wound could change an injured person's felt need for narcotics: "Great wounds with great significance and presumably great reaction are made painless by small doses of morphine, whereas fleeting experimental pains with no serious significance are not blocked by morphine. The difference here in the two situations would seem to be in difference of significance of the two wounds. Morphine acts on the significant pain, not the other" (Beecher 1959b, 164). Beecher concluded that if meaning could modify response, then emotions, attitudes, and other psychological influences could also block pain or heighten it (Beecher 1959b, 150).

Thus did an event that took place far from the controlled setting of the laboratory become the basis for Beecher's critique of experimental pain and methods used to measure it. On the Anzio beachhead, badly wounded soldiers who should have been in great pain were instead euphoric at the prospect of being removed from the battlefield (Beecher 1959b, 165). Beecher explained: "It seems from this that the reaction, or processing, component can dominate the pain experience. It is more potent than the noxious stimuli in determining the presence or absence of suffering. The total situation has, of course, great influence on the reaction that develops in it" (1959b, 164). In a subsequent study of surgical patients, Beecher found that comparable wounds were experienced as depressing, calamitous events. He determined that outside the wartime context, pain was experienced as more severe, and the corresponding need for pain relief was perceived to be higher (1959b, 164–65). The cultural authority that Beecher gained from this seminal wartime event placed him in a position to argue that "true operationism" embraced subjective factors instead of banishing them from experimental settings (1959b, 157).

Incorporating the subjective brought new problems of experimental design and ethics into focus. These problems were exacerbated by behavioral approaches, which Beecher disdained for mistakenly assuming that "for a given stimulus there must be a given response." Beecher used the Anzio incident to argue that the relationship between stimulus and response was far from simple due to the "interposition of conditioning, of the processing component, of the psychic reaction." He explained that some drugs had unexpected effects depending on the "personality make-up and mental state of the individual involved." Consider, he wrote, the sad drunk and the happy drunk, or the narcotics addict for whom morphine was "euphoretic" versus an inexperienced nonaddict for whom the same drug proved unpleasant or "dysphoric" (1959b, x). From Beecher's perspective, drugs were so "strongly laden with meaning and importance" that they changed the "drug-person relationship" (Beecher 1959b, 339). While the laboratory logics of Lexington and Michigan attempted to disqualify meaning, the Harvard group set out to create a science of significance by quantifying subjective effects.

According to Beecher, the value of experimental pain was sharply limited in contrast to "pathological pain" (1959b, 43–46, 114). The most prominent laboratory research aimed at isolating "pure" sensations of pain from reactions to it was a Cornell University Medical College group that consisted of physicist turned physiologist James D. Hardy, neurologist Harold G. Wolff, and research associate Helen Goodell. Best known for their central theoretical claim about "pain thresholds," the Cornell group embarked on experimental pain research in the early 1940s. They invented several methods to produce pain and techniques to measure it; among the latter was an apparatus they called the "dolorimeter."[19] Beecher was critical of Hardy, Wolff, and Goodell, because he felt their methods failed to eliminate bias and learning effects and because they insisted that pain thresholds were uniform enough to be measured. In contrast, clinicians found that variation between individuals was a pronounced practical problem in clinical settings.

The Harvard group was also skeptical of the "dol scale," a pain intensity scale that the Cornell group advanced on the basis of units called "just noticeable differences" (Beecher 1959b, 21–22; Meldrum 1994, 283). The dol scale was supposed to enable comparisons between different subjects and stimuli, thus standardizing evaluations of analgesic effectiveness. Not only was Beecher unconvinced that it did so with any validity, but he held that it was erroneous to assume that an elevated pain threshold correlated with the intensity of analgesic action. Critical of the entire basis on which Hardy, Wolff, and Goodell proposed to measure pain and analgesic action, Beecher became committed to quantitative approaches as the best route to making objective claims on the basis of data on subjective effects.

Beecher severely criticized self-experimentation data, castigating an early double-blind study comparing opiate alkaloids that is typically credited with originating the scientific investigation of the behavioral effects of drugs. Of this study, conducted by David I. Macht, N. B. Herman, and C. S. Levy at Johns Hopkins University (1916), Beecher wrote:

> [S]ince only the three authors were used as subjects and, considering the time required to test the six opium alkaloids studied, they must have become before long sophisticated subjects well able to differentiate between the aura of the narcotics used and a placebo. These facts plus their vested interest in the outcome lead to a less then "crucial corroboration" of their method. Unfortunately, their error in this regard is a common one, indeed, one that threatens much work in this field. The only safeguards known to the writer, and it must be agreed that these are only relatively reassuring, are to minimize the problem by using fresh subjects for only a relatively few observations, to use subjects who know nothing of the purpose of the experiments or the parameters at issue and who care nothing about the outcome. (1959b, 117)

Similarly, Beecher rebuked the Cornell group for using themselves and close associates as subjects. The Cornell group's practice was well known. For instance, Abraham Wikler of the ARC collaborated with the Cornell group on the only self-administration study in which he participated. In that study, the experimenters and three "volunteer subjects" from Lexington self-administered more than two dozen compounds, including morphine, aspirin, alcohol, barbiturates, codeine, placebos, and unknowns, two or three hours after breakfast, then measured their effects on perception thresholds governing response to touch, vibration, smell, and hearing (Wikler, Goodell, and Wolff 1945). Beecher believed that the Cornell group took inadequate precautions to eliminate bias and suggestion (1959b, 115–18). His growing familiarity with the logic of double-blind, placebo-controlled clinical trials led him to fervently oppose the long-accepted practice of self-administration.

For Beecher, using oneself or one's colleagues or students as experimental subjects was problematic not from an ethical standpoint but from a practical one. Believing that drug-experienced subjects differed from inexperienced subjects, Beecher felt that knowledgeable subjects picked up on a narcotic "aura" that enabled them to identify drug effects (1959b, 53). He argued that no subject who once experienced a narcotic could forget it, so subjects could easily surmise whether they had been given drug or placebo. He thus deemed knowledgeable subjects unreliable, in the sense that their knowledge could invalidate results. Beecher argued that knowing too much was also a problem from the experimenter's perspective, for a "knowing operator's" tone of voice or inflection might heighten subjects' suggestibility to drug influences (1959b, 148).

Self-administration studies conflated the experimenter's role with the subject's role, a situation viewed by Beecher as dangerous because experimenters knew too much and were too deeply invested in outcomes. He disapprovingly quoted Carl C. Pfeiffer, chair of pharmacology at the University of Illinois, who stated that no volunteer should be used who was not "at least . . . a graduate student . . . who has investigated for himself the nature and possible dangers of the drug involved" (Carl C. Pfeiffer to Dr. Stormont, secretary of the Council on Pharmacy and Chemistry, Committee on Research, American Medical Association, September 18, 1951, quoted in Beecher 1959a, 17). In a 1957 personal communication to Beecher, Pfeiffer admitted that he no longer abided by that rule and that he was using Atlanta Penitentiary prisoners as experimental subjects (Beecher 1959a, 17). But one of Pfeiffer's graduate students, Edward F. Domino, has confirmed that self-administration was common in graduate pharmacology departments at the time (personal communication with the author, 2006). Beecher believed knowledgeable subjects skewed results because the "essential unknowns" were impossible to maintain with drug-wise subjects (1959b, 54); they simply could not be kept in the state of ignorance that he viewed as necessary for good science.

> Highly trained subjects come to have a vested interest in the outcome, whether scientific or pecuniary (continuance as paid subjects) or egoistic (personal attention); the failure to eliminate their bias can have devastating results. To be sure, learning on the part of the subject is always a hazard to be watched for and minimized with proper controls, but the hazard is far greater with the experienced group. (1959b, 146)

Beecher maintained that experienced subjects knew too much about drugs and might use their knowledge base to ascertain their role in clinical trials and skew results.

Although he considered postaddicts too knowledgeable, Beecher also realized that clinical researchers faced the problem of getting valid observational information from sick and postoperative patients. He also considered the "casual observations of busy doctors or ward nurses" to be "without value," because clinicians could easily confuse drug side effects with common afflictions, such as nausea and vomiting (1959b, 58–59). Beecher argued that even techniques designed to overcome validity problems—"double unknowns," placebo controls, randomization, correlated data, and mathematical validation of differences—could not always overcome observer bias (1959b, 59). Although the Harvard group was set up to observe around the clock, documenting the clinical experience of variation in drug effects, individual response, and variations in individual experiences over time required subjects to be in almost continuous contact with researchers. As Beecher knew, this kind of proximity and casual interchange about drug effects was next to impossible to achieve in a hospital ward or with ambulatory college students. Therefore Beecher and Lasagna performed some of their studies at the ARC and tried to mimic the laboratory logics of Lexington by setting up similar experimental situations in dissimilar material, social, and institutional conditions. Clinical trials were the Harvard group's solution to these dilemmas. They worked on new experimental logics and statistical methodologies that relied on large sample sizes, access to naive subjects, elimination of observer bias, and disqualification of knowledgeable subjects.

Clinical trials took shape in response to an implicit critique of the laboratory logics and practices of the experienced drug researchers at the ARC, who had access to nothing but knowledgeable, drug-experienced subjects. They could not muster more than a handful of "normal" subjects for control groups and had to use themselves and their coworkers. The researchers at the ARC considered drug-wise subjects the most reliable and ethical route to knowledge about drug effects. They could not conform to Beecher's high-turnover solution to these problems, which was to use experimental subjects only for short periods of time and "turn to fresh subjects before the old ones become drug-wise" (1959b, 146). The Harvard group could afford to adopt this practice, whereas the Lexington group could not. None of its subjects were naive.

SUBJECTS WHO KNEW TOO MUCH: THE MEANING OF "EUPHORIA" IN EXPERIMENTAL READDICTION

Tensions between the ARC and the Harvard Anesthesiology Laboratory personnel were evident at the eleventh postwar CDAN meeting, held in Lexington on January 9–10, 1953. After touring the ARC research ward, the committee held a spirited debate during discussion of a pilot study by Beecher and Lasagna titled "Euphoria: A Study of Drug-Induced Mood Changes in Man." There was such disagreement over the term *euphoria* that the landmark study was later published in the *Journal of the American Medical Association* as "Drug-Induced Mood Changes in Man" (Lasagna, Von Felsinger, and Beecher 1955). Responding to the pilot data, Abraham Wikler said:

> By an odd coincidence we have been concerned with the problem of euphoria for many years. Our first definite conclusion is that the term "euphoria" means very different things to different people, to the same person at different times, and also to groups of individuals after administration of different drugs. . . . To interpret what euphoria means is no easy task but we feel we can interpret what the individual means by euphoria by observing how he behaves verbally and non-verbally, by recording his statements and his behavior in a given setting. (Committee on Drug Addiction and Narcotics 1953, 378)

Wikler admitted that behavior and subjective effects could only be the subject of science if they were predictable and that they would become "predictable only if the situation is clearly delineated" (Committee on Drug Addiction and Narcotics 1953, 378). Whether the feelings of unusual well-being designated by such a diffuse and nonspecific term as *euphoria* were experienced by subjects thus depended on how the experimental situation was structured.

Only if they produced euphoria did ARC researchers believe they could accurately measure the abuse liability of an opiate-like drug or learn anything about how addiction worked. Their goal was not to determine low, therapeutically effective doses but to predict whether the drug was liable to abuse. Determining that required getting subjects high, which meant administering "doses in the addict range" (Committee on Drug Addiction and Narcotics 1953, 382). Because their knowing subjects had considerable experiential knowledge of the "addict range," the ARC researchers set up experimental situations to mimic natural addiction. Only these, they thought, would tell them very much of what they wanted to know. ARC researchers justified the use of high experimental doses on the following grounds: "Addicts do not use small therapeutic doses. They increase the dosage of a drug to the limit of their tolerance, so that if the conditions of natural addiction are to be stimulated, high doses must be used experimentally in evaluating the liability of addiction to new drugs" (Isbell, Wikler, et al. 1948, 391). Operationalizing euphoria raised the very basic question of why some individuals experienced it and others did not. What did it mean that terminally ill, postoperative pain patients and "normal" controls did not experience euphoria whereas postaddicts invariably did so? More important for the kind of work being done at the ARC, did that difference invalidate results of studies on postaddicts?

Looking closely at the Harvard group's study, which was conducted at the ARC and Massachusetts General Hospital, reveals that it followed the contours of a pilot study of nine "young, intelligent, healthy male volunteer subjects" (presumably Harvard students). Experiments were repeated on twenty additional male college students; thirty chronically ill, old, hospitalized patients who were "surrounded by dying" (Beecher 1959b, 323); and thirty post-addict prisoners at Lexington. Although each group of subjects responded differently to heroin, morphine, and amphetamines, responses were similar within the group. So-called normal volunteers (the college students) found amphetamine a "more potent euphoretic" than heroin or morphine, which they experienced as unpleasant or inert. Surprised that amphetamine invoked intense euphoria, investigators who found that it relieved pain in the chronically ill suggested that there was a "real place for amphetamine as a euphoretic in the treatment of the hopelessly ill" (Beecher 1959b, 335).

In the Harvard study, postaddicts differed from both the chronically ill group and normal controls in that the former reported stimulation and "improved mentation" after opiates but found amphetamine's effects unpleasant and prolonged (Von Felsinger, Lasagna, and Beecher 1955, 1016). Unlike normal volunteers, they did not report unpleasant side effects of opiates, such as nausea, vomiting, and mental dullness. However, postaddicts indicated that they had once experienced such unpleasant effects when first using narcotics. The question before CDAN was whether such variations formed a pattern that could be explained. The Harvard group appealed to Beecher's concept of the drug-person relationship (1959b, 339), which was based on data generated in this study. The study correlated personality factors and typical versus atypical drug responses: "For example, the most frequent responses to amphetamine were euphoria and alertness; to heroin and morphine, dysphoria and sedation. These reactions were thus called typical. The opposite responses for each drug were labeled atypical" (Von Felsinger, Lasagna, and Beecher 1955, 1113). The Harvard group concluded that the atypical responders who became euphoric on heroin or morphine and dysphoric on stimulants were the least balanced subjects: "Our group with atypical reactions resembled addicts in their preference for opiates; this group was made up of the more maladjusted subjects, a finding in keeping with theories as to the importance of personality deviations in the genesis of drug addiction" (Von Felsinger, Lasagna, and Beecher 1955, 1119).

Ultimately, the Harvard investigators suggested that "differential personality dynamics, primarily in terms of the balance of mature, socially oriented controls over impulsive, egocentric emotionality, were found to be correlated with the type of drug reaction" (Von Felsinger, Lasagna, and Beecher 1955, 1119). The Harvard group found postaddicts atypical and unsuitable for study because data generated by them could not be generalized. This position had nothing to do with ethics. In fact, Beecher agreed with the Lexington group that "ethical considerations dictate the use of post-addicts in assessing the development of tolerance and physical dependence" (1959b, 340). He drew the same line the ARC did between readdicting a onetime addict and addicting someone who had never experienced addiction. However, he warned that conclusions based on results generated through the use of former addicts might lead to underestimates of the potential hazards posed by new analgesics. For this reason, Beecher was often at odds with pharmaceutical industry representatives, whose economic interests were at stake and who therefore minimized the dangers of releasing drugs onto the market in the era before thalidomide. The skeptical pharmaceutical industry representatives of CDAN treated the Harvard group critically and sought to dismiss its work on the grounds that its methods were too subjective. The pharmaceutical representatives thought such large-scale quantitative studies as Beecher's obscured their actual subjective basis, whereas the small-scale studies of the ARC were more objective.

Drug control decisions by the U.S. government, the World Health Organization, and the United Nations were made on the basis of data produced by the ARC that was sent on to the U.S. surgeon general and the international governing bodies. The positions just related informed the drug policy-making process and global drug control regimes of the mid-twentieth century. According to Beecher, both the Lexington and Harvard groups agreed that "you have to examine drugs and drug reactions under the conditions where they are going to be used" (Committee on Drug Addiction and Narcotics 1953, 381). They agreed that drug effects varied by situation: "It is obvious that the subjective effects of drugs, no less than the objective effects, are dependent on the situation in which the drug is administered. It is also likely that the production of a given mental state, even in the same situation, will not prove equally pleasant to all persons" (Beecher 1959b, 322). Furthermore, they agreed that drug effects differed according to the subject's degree of experience with the drug or drugs like it. The "pharmacological sophisticates" of Lexington, as Beecher called them, consistently rated morphine's effects more positively than did drug-naive subjects. What, then, was the value of assessments of analgesia or abuse potential conducted in so-called postaddicts? How valid were comparisons between addicts and nonaddicts? Could any institutional experimental setting be compared to social situations where individuals self-administered drugs?

Disagreement arose between the two research groups because Beecher maintained that a "hint of a difference" led institutionalized postaddicts to experience euphoria when morphine was administered. He could not specify what this difference was, but he believed it to invalidate results of studies in postaddicts (Committee on Drug Addiction and Narcotics 1953, 381). By contrast, ARC researchers saw similarities between those who had been addicted and those who had not. They argued that just about anyone could become addicted, given exposure to the right drug under the right conditions. They set about persuading others that extrapolations from postaddicts to nonaddicts were valid. One difference was especially apparent to the Harvard group because it had implications for research design. Drug-naive subjects did not know how to talk about drugs, so Beecher's team had to "help subjects verbalize their responses" by supplying semantic opposites from which they could select (1959b, 333). By contrast, drug-experienced subjects possessed a rich vernacular vocabulary for expressing the inner states induced by drug experiences and a "long-standing and complex drug-person relationship that does not exist in non-addicts" (Beecher 1959b, 339). This "drug-person relationship" enabled these subjects to convey their innermost sensations with accuracy and gave them a comparative standard by which to measure drug effects. Only with great care could the meanings that former addicts attributed to drugs be disentangled from the effects they experienced in studies. This practical problem contributed to Beecher's wariness about using former addicts far more than did the underrecognized ethical problems posed by experimental readdiction.

Experimental readdiction would now be considered ethically problematic but did not pose an ethical dilemma in the research culture of the time. Ethical guidelines for clinical research were uncertain during the 1950s, despite the Nuremberg Code (1949). Indeed, as the next chapter demonstrates, Beecher lobbied against basing governance of clinical research on the Nuremberg Code, confirming Lasagna's (1994) insistence that Beecher had shown little interest in the ethics of human experimentation when they worked together in the mid-1950s. Certainly, Beecher's publications were quite typical of the time in not reflecting on ethical issues.[20] Beecher did amass a thick file of press coverage on the Nuremberg Medical Trial, most likely because he considered the Nuremberg Code too rigid and was actively seeking alternatives.

By contrast to the Harvard group, the publications emanating from the

ARC exhibited an awareness of research ethics as early as the late 1940s, a discursive practice the larger biomedical research community did not adopt until much later. Although it is difficult to ascertain the level of awareness of the Nuremberg trials among researchers at the ARC, Wikler was himself a Yiddish speaker who remained the linchpin of a family that was directly affected by the Holocaust. His lifelong interest in Judaica led others to portray him as a Talmudic scholar. Not only was he surely aware of the Nuremberg trials, but his writings often anticipated potential criticisms of the participation of human subjects in natural experiments that mimicked the conditions of addiction. The next two chapters of the present book delve further into the indigenous ethical situation at Lexington. This chapter points to the interpretation that it was not ethics but research design that motivated Beecher's arguments against using postaddicts as research subjects, on the grounds that they knew too much about drugs and had formed unusual drug-person relationships.

Following from the laboratory logics on which their research practices built, ARC researchers believed, conversely, that it was only ethical to use postaddicts. They argued that only postaddicts could provide truly informed perspectives on the subjective effects of drugs or compare morphine's effects to those of the new synthetic opiates with any validity (Isbell, Wikler, et al. 1948, 390)—that only they experienced euphoria in ways that yielded predictive information that could prevent the release of drugs liable to be "abused." Still, addiction researchers quibbled with the use of the term *euphoria* as a framing device, because the term did not lend itself to precise definition or measurement. Researchers at Lexington found the concept of euphoria both fruitful and maddening as they sought to replicate "getting high" in a laboratory setting within a prison-hospital.

Euphoria was hard to define because of the counterintuitive variety of its clinical manifestations. Isbell, for example, recounts giving thirty milligrams of morphine to a nontolerant morphine addict "who turns pale, gags, and heaves": "[A]sk him how he feels and he is fine, wonderful. You ask him, 'You are vomiting and all this, but you are fine?' and he replies, 'Yes, it's such a good sick.' Now is that euphoria, or isn't it?" (Committee on Drug Addiction and Narcotics 1953, 382). The difficulty of quantifying euphoria could be compounded by altering the experimental situation. Drug effects would be altered if subjects were anxious, paranoid, or ill at ease. Wikler urged investigators designing an experimental setting to ask themselves, "Under what conditions are these [drugs] administered, to whom, and what for? Let's recognize the fact that the action of a drug depends upon the particular experimental condition under which it is studied" (Committee on Drug Addiction and Narcotics 1953, 379). In mimicking natural addiction, ARC researchers sought to reproduce the subjective effects that accompanied drug administration, despite the difficulty of operationalizing them in the laboratory.

The Problem of Euphoria: Operationalizing the Concept

Laboratory life at the ARC was structured around "operationalism," a concept drawn from Harvard physicist Percy W. Bridgman, who Wikler admired.[21] Bridgman distinguished between "public science" and "private science." The latter involved nonoperational terms, such as *mind, body, forces, tensions, psychic energies, conversion,* or *somatization* (Wikler 1952c, 95). Although conducted in incommunicable terms, private science offered an intuitive basis on which to build "public science" (Wikler 1952c, 96). Taking the operational view was integral to remodeling psychiatry as a descriptive and predictive public science. This scientistic effort raised epistemological questions of the kind posed by Wikler: "How do they know when they know that they have understood the phenomena, to put it another way? And I insist that this answer must be given in terms of public operations, so that others may know how they know, when they know." Wikler's commitment to operationalism stemmed from his belief that public science should make its methods evident "so that others may know how they know, when they know." Far from seeing scientism as impoverished philosophy, Wikler believed that freedom and self-mastery depended on studying the "reconstruction of necessity through man's ingenious scientific activities." This philosophy was infused throughout the ARC's reconstruction of the physiological, neurological, and psychological experience of necessity that drove subjects' everyday lives. Wikler explained that the laboratory logics of Lexington recognized addicts were not "merely automatons" but individuals who experienced "necessities" differently than others (Wikler 1964, 188).[22]

Seeking to unmask the primary needs that drove his subjects, Wikler turned away from "mentalistic" intuitions, ideations, and insights, which he relegated to the realm of private science. He argued that these would have to be operationalized if addiction research was to achieve the status of a public science.[23] Drugs offered psychiatry tools to accomplish this move, but Wikler believed there were therapeutic limits on how far such investigations could or should go (1952c, 97). Predictive public science would always be limited. Wikler modestly suggested: "[L]imited goals are [the only ones] to which any scientist can possibly aspire. We must be able to give up our time-hallowed but useless quest for 'ultimate realities' in exchange for limited, but useful patches of knowledge. But even a patch-work quilt may be beautiful as well as warm" (1952c, 98).

Limited, partial perspectives were circumscribed further by the thorny problem that the "so-called properties of the bodies revealed by our measurements are in fact primarily the reflex of our measuring methods and not concrete facts *in rebus Naturae*" (Wikler 1952c, 90). ARC researchers were committed to multiple frames of reference because the phenomena they studied did not yield to any one approach. They based their explanations solely on what could be reproduced in the laboratory through, as Wikler described, a modest "demonstration of correlations that are useful for particular purposes, and which can be summarized in terms of operational constructs in a variety of frames of reference, each appropriate to the type of technic used in observation." Wikler continued:

> Thus, there are not one, but several kinds of psychological, physiological, biochemical, and anatomical frames of reference, and their number and areas of usefulness vary as new techniques are developed. Furthermore, these frames of reference are not reducible one to the other, for the particular experimental arrangements that define one type of operation usually preclude those that define another. (1952c, 91)

Wikler emphasized that terms had to be defined operationally, a formidable task for a psychiatry that commonly deployed such terms as *excitation, depression, inhibition, release, energy, homeostasis,* or *levels of integration* (1952c, 91). To Wikler's way of thinking, these terms were useless if they were not linked to observable changes (1952c, 95). Rather than rely on narrative constructions, the ARC sought to manipulate the situation in order to block or produce observable drug effects. Contrary to the Harvard group's constant questioning, Isbell cautioned against asking too much of its subjects: "There is no better way to antidote the effects of analgesic drugs, subjective and objective, than to make measurements and ask questions at stated intervals" (Committee on Drug Addiction and Narcotics 1953, 381). ARC researchers felt that continuous questioning offset potential understanding.

In Henry Beecher's view, the Lexington group tipped too far toward operationalizing everything. He portrayed their use of electroencephalograms as "elaborate" but useless. He criticized the ARC's adoption of animal reflex techniques developed in pharmaceutical houses to assess analgesic activity separately from addiction liability (Wikler 1950). When adapted to human beings, particularly postaddicts, these techniques proved so highly variable that the

ARC was forced to innovate. While Beecher recognized the usefulness of animal reflex tests for predicting analgesia (1959b, 93–94), he thought they relayed nothing about subjective responses (1959b, 57). He believed that more useful information could be generated if the "co-operative statement of the subject" could simply be read properly and interpreted as data (1959b, 158). The problem lay in figuring out how to render subjective responses into objective data without pushing operationalism to the point of diminishing the significance of meaning, the very thing that Beecher thought was most important.

> True operationism embraces the use of questions and answers, and the Harvard group's techniques, for example, are operational. Extreme operationists have gone so far as to deny that one can depend upon what the subject says about his pain. To the writer this is a kind of nihilism. If this extreme view is accepted, then even when dealing with man one would have to depend upon [physiological] reactions to pain. (1959b, 158)

For Beecher, it was the mind—not the brain—that subjective responses to drugs revealed. His purpose was not so much to gain knowledge about drugs and their effects but to achieve a basic understanding of human behavior by controlling for sensation, feeling, or mood, so as to isolate the psychic reaction or reaction component.

Despite differences, Beecher and Wikler enjoyed a scientific camaraderie, as Beecher admired the Lexington group's attempt to operationalize "anxiety associated with the anticipation of pain" or the condition of "giving a damn about pain" (1959b, 8).[24] "Our hypothesis," wrote Wikler in a letter to Beecher, "is that how much one 'gives a damn' about pain can be inferred from observation of the extent to which signals heralding nociceptive stimuli *which the subject cannot escape or avoid,* disrupt previously learned responses that are 'adaptive.' After all, is that not actually the basis on which we proceed in assessing 'clinical' pain for purposes of deciding whether or not to intervene?" (quoted in Beecher 1959b, 7–8). Although Wikler joked that he could not yet refute Beecher's conclusion that "[p]ain cannot be satisfactorily defined, except as any man defines it introspectively for himself," Beecher's rejoinder indicated that he thought that if anyone could define pain objectively, it would be the Lexington group. This repartee lay close to the heart of their differences: Could pain be objectively defined, experimentally produced, or scientifically understood without taking into account meaning, personality, or experience? What about the modulation or absence of pain due to the opiates, whether experienced as "euphoria" or relief? Was addiction a path to understanding pain, or was it a dead end? Was "euphoria" a route to understanding addiction, or was it a meaningless effect? If experimental setting, previous events in the life history, personality differences, or level of social experience with a drug could change how a drug affected a subject, what scientific method could possibly yield the kind of data that spoke to these questions? Methodological and epistemological questions underlay the structural tensions involved in coordinating research conducted under very different material and institutional conditions.

Structural Tensions: Coordinating Industry, Government, and Academia

After Beecher and Lasagna presented the results of their study on euphoria, pharmaceutical industry representatives complained to the CDAN leadership behind closed doors, arguing that Beecher's work was "too non-objective" and disparaging it as tangential to the committee's goals (Committee on Drug Addiction and Narcotics 1953, 387). Stating that Beecher's work was precisely what the committee had in mind, Eddy defended continued "support of fundamental studies within its field of interest, which no one firm would feel justified in initiating or supporting, yet which would add materially to our understanding of analgesia and addiction, and would, therefore, be of interest and profit to all" (Committee on Drug Addiction and Narcotics 1953, 387). Because Beecher's funding was more contingent on results than that of Seevers or the ARC, questions such as these struck at the material basis of the Harvard group and Beecher's scientific credibility. Industry representatives found his work on subjective effects too bound up with the messy world of meaning and the mire of mood and argued that it could not count as the objective science they needed to take their drugs to market. In partial defense against these criticisms, the besieged Harvard group invented the crossover trial design and double-blind method for which they are known. Instead of banishing subjective effects for the sake of objectivity, the group deployed statistical methods to render credible claims about them.

These contentious interactions point to structural problems inherent in trying to accomplish basic research through an NRC committee. Industry wanted a drug-testing service from which it could gain a stamp of approval for drugs going onto the market; the ARC wanted to concentrate on basic research rather than applied product testing; and CDAN wanted a coordinated and successful search for a nonaddicting analgesic by whatever route necessary. Far from being an instrument of the pharmaceutical industry or a subsidiary regulatory agency, the committee's autonomy gave it an independent evaluative capacity and a source of oversight. Committee chair Isaac Starr commented:

> It would be easy for our program to degenerate into a simple matter of clinical testing. I have little doubt that we could get plenty of support from various drug houses for such a program and I hope none of them have had in the back of their mind that that is what is eventually going to come of it. We are interested in fundamental research in a way that the drug houses ought to be interested because in the long run, what they make money on is dependent on it. (Committee on Drug Addiction and Narcotics 1953, 388)

He argued that the committee should not become the handmaiden of industry: "If we can't sell this broader program to industry then we ought to let the program drop. We have no intention of setting ourselves up simply as a drug testing service" (Committee on Drug Addiction and Narcotics 1953, 392). The committee remained committed to basic research and wary of close associations with industry—while cultivating the interests of industrial actors in order to channel resources toward the search for a nonaddictive analgesic.

Arguing that investigators should not have direct ties to pharmaceutical companies, Beecher was convinced that investigators' attitudes could unconsciously influence subjects and results (1959b, 43). He also believed that companies should bear the costs associated with investigating the safety and efficacy of drugs they developed.

> Costly and tedious as the methods and controls are when based upon sound practice, they are far less costly and certainly give answers in far shorter time than when drugs are distributed widely and used without any discernible controls. Also, in the method of wide distribution, the public bears the cost; in the sounder approach, the pharmaceutical industry pays. It does not seem unreasonable that the industry bear the cost of such evaluations. (1959b, 43–44)

Although pharmaceutical companies made minimal contributions to CDAN, they did so reluctantly. Indeed, new drugs were released through physicians without controlled trials or the "masses of data that might have protected them from error" (Beecher 1959b, 44). Well before the sedative thalidomide provided a clear-cut example of underscrutiny and a catalyst for a new regime,[25] Beecher argued that lack of a systematic drug review process led to skewed results, casual findings, and misinformation, all of which were inadequate safeguards to public health. The 1953 CDAN meeting exemplified tensions between drug researchers and the pharmaceutical industry representatives, who had attended in full force so as to get a look inside Lexington, where so many of their drugs had been tested (Committee on Drug Addiction and Narcotics 1953, 388).[26] To better acquaint their guests with their laboratory logics and research subjects, the ARC turned to film.

ANIMATING EXPERIMENTATION: THE FILMIC RECORD AT LEXINGTON

Films made at the ARC were screened at CDAN meetings to better acquaint attendees with the outcomes of the methods pursued there. A film made by Wikler followed the progress of a single human subject through tolerance to and withdrawal from morphine. One made by Isbell, *Abstinence from Alcohol,* showed three human subjects undergoing abrupt withdrawal after consuming between four hundred and five hundred milliliters of 95 percent ethyl alcohol daily for three months. One suffered seven grand mal seizures; the second, evident delirium tremens; and the third, mild hallucinations with insight. Of this film, Isbell noted, "The data suggest that abstinence may be one of the precipitating factors in 'rum fits' and *delirium tremens*" (Committee on Drug Addiction and Narcotics 1953, 385). The Lexington group established that alcoholics could experience symptoms of abstinence while still drinking and helped create the scientific consensus that alcohol produced physical dependency (Isbell et al. 1955). Similarly, Isbell made a film in the late 1940s on barbiturates, as part of a six-subject study to determine whether seizures and convulsions were due to intoxication or withdrawal. At the time, no one knew what caused these severe effects, although clinical reports attesting to them and delirium tremens were widely known. To a greater degree than scientific papers could, these amateur films—made on a sixteen-millimeter camera owned by a staff member—captured aspects of the ARC that would otherwise remain invisible.

A number of conclusions can be drawn about the making of such movies. There was little reflection at the ARC about how such films might look to audiences beyond the research community. Like the "monkey movies" described in chapter 2, these data films were made for insiders. Viewing them helps indicate boundaries between interpretive communities. For instance the subject of Wikler's film *Natural and Induced Abstinence in Chronic "Spinal" Man* was a frequent patient at Lexington whose spinal cord had previously been transected by syphilitic meningo-myelitis. The study was made to validate "inferences [for human beings] previously made on the basis of observations in chronic spinal dogs" (Committee on Drug Addiction and Narcotics 1953, 385). The film participated in the laboratory logic of mimicry—a human subject was found who could replicate the conditions of the experimental animals. Much ARC data was based on animal studies, and questions remained about their validity for making claims about humans. The film was part of the process of convincing CDAN members that animal models could be extrapolated to humans. Meant to persuade those within the addiction research network that such comparisons were valid, the films signaled something very different to those outside it.

The films present martyrlike representations of human subjects undergoing profound physiological crises. Clearly, the prisoner participants filmed were aware of what was happening to them even in the throes of suffering. They had experienced withdrawal many times off camera. For the Lexington group, filming patients going through abstinence was a way to record data—a method Wikler had used previously as a successful diagnostic technique in his quest to isolate underlying organic disturbances. However, the films cannot be seen simply as data films: in the barbiturate film, Harris Isbell was portrayed soothing a patient by stroking his arm and supporting a heavily intoxicated patient walking down the hall. Far from being staged, these attitudes of compassion were what Isbell was particularly known for at the institution. When the clinical side of the Lexington Hospital had difficulty with patients, Isbell was called over from the research unit. Patients arrived at Lexington in a variety of states—still on street drugs, beginning to suffer abstinence, or in the full throes of withdrawal—and detoxification often depended on recognizing what they were on and gradually tapering them off (Conan Kornetsky, personal communication with the author, July 28, 2006). This was something that Isbell had a reputation for doing with compassion and competence.

Within the closed world of addiction research, the films conveyed the "clinical manifestations of drug addiction," as a medical education film made by splicing the research films together decades after they were made was titled.[27] To many outside the social worlds of substance abuse research this film seems callous at best, inhumane at worst. It attests to the use of prisoner patients' bodies as inscription devices to record and make evident the pain of withdrawal. It is impossible to watch the visceral effects of withdrawal without attributing aspects of martyrdom to these lone figures engaged in their own "experiment perilous" (Fox 1959/1998). As Donna J. Haraway explains, the film medium "concern[s] the distancing of observations, the structuring of vision"; vision is "mediated by writing technologies"; and the body "becomes an inscription device" (1989, 117–18, citing Latour and Woolgar 1979, 43–54). Indeed, the bodies of the subjects depicted in these films exhibit unrestrained agitation, convulsions, vomiting, and the undisguisable anguish of withdrawal. They relentlessly, realistically inscribe drug withdrawal in ways rarely seen except through the sentimentalizing lens of melodrama.

These films are compelling documents of the physiological processes of drug addiction. Contextualizing them requires understanding the composition and educative goals of CDAN. Many committee members never saw an addict except when they toured the Lexington facility, whereas ARC researchers were in daily contact with addicted persons. The films provided the researchers with a vehicle to humanize their subjects and persuade clinicians that the natural course of alcoholism, addiction, tolerance, and withdrawal was a physiological process, not a psychological one or an indication of moral weakness. The films graphically narrated and illustrated this process, having effects on viewers similar to the effects of the monkey movies. The films sought to register the scientific status of addiction and underline the validity of studies on postaddicts. They captured and conveyed the essential humanity of the subjects, rather than avoiding, denying, or otherwise dehumanizing them. To my knowledge, the films are no longer shown to medical students, pharmaceutical representatives, or anyone else. They counter the pharmacological optimism expressed in the popular texts analyzed at the beginning of this chapter, and they attest to the limits of euphoria by staging addiction as its problematic outcome.

One study on the history of human experimentation claims, "Through medical experimentation, use*less* bodies were rendered use*ful* by being made *usable* in the national project of regeneration, thus gaining a utility they were believed otherwise to lack" (Goodman, McElligott, and Marks 2003, 12). What precisely was the use value of addicted minds and bodies, of their experiences of euphoria or dysphoria? To which scientific communities was the contested term *euphoria* useful? Could valid conclusions be extrapolated from addicts to nonaddicts, from prisoners to nonprisoners, from drug-wise subjects to the drug-naive? The Harvard research group assumed that conclusions generated by studies of former addicts would not be broadly useful; the Lexington group operated on the opposite assumption. Interactions between the two groups were charged but respectful—mediated by CDAN and directed toward the overarching goal of identifying less-dangerous drugs.

Patterns of interaction between committee members indicate that researchers at the ARC occupied the highest rung of the hierarchy of credibility. The Harvard researchers posed almost naive questions about heroin, with which they had little experience. When Beecher and Lasagna asked about geographical variations in drug preferences, Isbell indicated that addicts from the Eastern Seaboard preferred heroin whereas Southerners preferred morphine or Dilaudid. Questioned as to why heroin was "more dangerous than morphine," Isbell answered: "It takes less [heroin]; euphoria appears more rapidly; therefore euphoria is more impressive to the individual. Morphine creeps up on you; the effect of heroin is sudden" (Committee on Drug Addiction and Narcotics 1953, 383). Wikler answered that heroin's "physical-dependence-producing liability" was greater because of the "race to raise the dose fast enough and give the injections often enough so that abstinence signs do not develop between one dose and the next." He concluded, "If physical dependence is in any way related to addiction, I think this greater physical dependence liability makes heroin the more dangerous" (Committee on Drug Addiction and Narcotics 1953, 384).

Heroin was the drug of choice for prisoner patients at Lexington throughout its existence as a narcotics hospital. The ARC grappled with nonintegrated approaches to addiction and analgesia, which were artifacts of the opposition between nonmedical use of heroin and medical use of morphine. CDAN worked to cross this divide but could not overcome the cultural construction of heroin as a dangerous and unnecessary drug about which physicians knew little. Accounting for the enduring strength of the preference for heroin preoccupied researchers at the ARC, who believed that if they could figure out why heroin was so attractive, they would know something generalizable about addiction. They were prescient in this view—although opiate receptors had been hypothesized to exist, they were not visualized until the early 1970s. The preoccupation with heroin, which fully occupies the opiate receptors so that no other drug can compete, was shared by addicts, researchers, and policy makers. The ARC understood there was something special about heroin addicts, and the scientific pursuit of how exactly to discover what the difference was proved central to its work. Key questions remained to be resolved: What natural and social processes did heroin displace? Why did heroin addicts lose appetite and desire for other forms of gratification—namely, food and sex? If heroin was the key, what would studying it unlock?

CHAPTER 5

"The Tightrope between Coercion and Seduction": Characterizing the Ethos of Addiction Research at Lexington

In "The Lesson of the Hospitals," Michel Foucault revealed an implicit contract between rich and poor governing the organization of clinical experience.

> But to look in order to know, to show in order to teach, is not this a tacit form of violence, all the more abusive for its silence, upon a sick body that demands to be comforted, not displayed. Can pain be a spectacle? Not only can it be, but it must be, by virtue of a subtle right that resides in the fact that no one is alone, the poor man less than others, since he can obtain assistance only through the mediation of the rich. . . . [I]t is just that the experiences of some should be transformed into the experiences of others. (1975, 84)

What was the utility of the rich offering help to the hospitalized poor? Foucault answered that the diseases of the poor were transformed into the knowledge of the rich: "[The clinic] is the *interest* paid by the poor on the capital that the rich have consented to invest in the hospital; an interest that must be understood in its heavy surcharge, since it is compensation that is of the order of *objective interest* for science and of *vital interest* for the rich" (1975, 85). The present chapter weighs how heavy that surcharge was for those who participated in the experiments of the ARC—from the perspectives of those who structured the experimental situation and those who paid the price as subjects. What were the lessons of the laboratory housed at the Lexington Hospital? What were the situated ethics, indigenous moralities, and laboratory logics at work there? What lessons does Lexington hold now that research is no longer conducted in federal prisons but is rampant under the far less controlled conditions of large-scale clinical trials?

This chapter takes an in-depth look at the social organization of knowledge production during the heyday of the world's premier addiction research unit. By distinguishing between the ethos of the laboratory logics—the actual practices, protocols, and spirit with which researchers approached human subjects—and the abstract, codified ethics supposed to govern laboratory life, it is possible to characterize the modes of perception organized at the ARC in relation to the prevailing indigenous moralities of the addiction research problem group.[1] Research networks are key sites for exerting formal and informal social controls over research. Members must adjudicate among "moral traditions for handling investigatory risk" (Halpern 2004, 41, 124). The ARC conducted research on human beings from 1935 until 1974, decades when there was both change and continuity in the conduct of human experimentation. How did laboratory logics, knowledge production practices, and ethical stances evolve at the ARC? What was the relationship of indigenous moralities to the practical logics through which scientific work of the kind the ARC conducted was made possible?

TOWARD A SITUATED ETHICS: SPECIFYING THE INDIGENOUS MORALITIES OF THE ADDICTION RESEARCH NETWORK

Some of the technologies pioneered at the ARC found their way into continuing clinical use; others were consigned to the dustbin of history.[2] The laboratory logics of Lexington were based on systematic attempts to mimic the "natural" course of events in which people encounter, use, build up tolerance to or dependence on, and withdraw from mind-altering drugs, so as to expose the underlying basis of the process. These "natural" conditions were, of course, social conditions that exceeded capture in the laboratory setting. The logic of unmasking the underlying conditions was akin to the clinical logic of nineteenth-century heroic medicine, with its high dosages and purgatives. As shown in the preceding chapter, high dosages and intravenous administration were used to mimic the natural course of addiction. Although the physiological process through which subjects progressed blurred the line between mimicry and actuality, "experimental readdiction" reenacted initiation, tolerance/dependence, and withdrawal. Because many addicts avoided the aversive effects of withdrawal, only those willing to endure it "volunteered" for studies. If researchers failed to document highs or lows, they believed their data would be useless for revealing the basic mechanisms of addiction and for applied studies on the abuse liability of new compounds. Answering basic research questions required human subjects to reenact the very physiological and psychological conditions that landed them at Lexington. Experimental readdiction was addiction itself, not mimicry.

Taking seriously the sociological position that drug use varies according to social setting and cultural context—and is modulated by social norms, beliefs, rituals, and meanings—requires not conflating what was happening with experimental readdiction in the laboratory with what was happening on the street. The setting of the research ward, the expectations of researchers and subjects who framed their activities as the investigation of a scientific problem, and the metrics and technologies developed at the ARC worked against any simplistic reenactment of addiction's "natural course." In the research ward, skilled medical personnel who were extraordinarily familiar with opiates were on hand if anything went wrong with dosage or route of administration, and subjects who were ill were treated for their illnesses and never experimented on. Dosage and purity were carefully calibrated at the ARC, things that could not be achieved on the illegal market due to criminalization, prosecution, and the sanctioned ignorance of most physicians in relation to nonmedical use of drugs. No matter how the ARC tried to replicate "natural conditions," its social location mitigated against it doing so.

Unlike the conditions of the street, laboratory conditions required some version of informed consent. Most studies recounted in this chapter were produced during the long prehistory of informed consent, which was a historical product of the late 1960s and early 1970s (Goodman, McElligott, and Marks 2003, 4). Focusing solely on current concepts of informed consent rides roughshod over the many other social controls over human experimentation that evolved in the early to mid-twentieth century from a logic of "lesser harms" (Halpern 2004). During the Progressive period, courts and legislatures considered the issue of informed consent but did not specify its form (Halpern 2004, 97, 102, 117). Prisoners who participated in research were regularly asked to give consent as early as 1915 (Harkness 1996, 3), and parents were asked to sign consent forms when children participated in vaccine trials as early as the 1940s and 1950s (Halpern 2004, 113). However, until research sponsors began to require written consent statements in the 1950s, consent was obtained nonsystematically. Even after sponsors began consulting lawyers on language and sharing this information with each other (Halpern 2004, 100–101, 117), a "disorganized situation" permeated all scientific research on human subjects and lasted well into the 1960s (Moreno 2001, 200). Because there was evidently wide variation between sites, the indigenous morality of the ARC research group can best be glimpsed by looking at actual practices accepted there.

Research at Leavenworth and Lexington involved a high degree of participation by knowledgeable subjects, prisoner patients who appear to have been quite aware of what was happening to them. As interviews with Himmelsbach indicated (1972, 1994), they were not "unwitting" subjects. The indigenous morality of the ARC placed such importance on consent that a brief note on voluntary participation appeared in many of its scientific publications from its inception. Participants volunteered for studies through the same routes they volunteered for work assignments, vocational education, or recreational activities. "There was no dearth of people who wanted to be subjects," Conan Kornetsky recalled of the late 1940s and early 1950s (personal communication with the author, July 28, 2006). However, questions of what motivated people to volunteer and whether true voluntarism is possible in coercive prison or military contexts contribute to the murkiness of the ethos at Lexington.[3]

One factor relevant to addressing questions of voluntary participation at the ARC was that much of the public understood addicts to have already willfully risked drug exposure outside the laboratory. Among American publics, acceptance of voluntary risk is higher than acceptance of involuntary risk (Halpern 2004, 97). The prisoner patients at Lexington could easily avoid taking on experimental risk—most neither participated in experiments nor were recruited to do so. The only known research participant still living, Eddie Flowers, estimated that less than half of residents even knew of the research program (2004). Far fewer participated in it, and those who did volunteer generally appear to have sought out the opportunity. Flowers's six months of research participation came about through word of mouth in the mid-1950s.

> There was a guy there by the name of Red [Rodney] . . . [who] shared with me, 'cause he didn't share that with a lot of other people, about the fact that he was in this drug program in Lexington, Kentucky. He kind of like laid it out to me, that they'd take him out of the main population for two or three weeks, and they'd try different drugs on him, and then they'd pay him off in heroin, 'cause that was his drug of choice. . . . [T]hrough his finagling, I was able to get in. . . . [T]hat's when I began to be a part of that whole experimentation thing. (2004)[4]

Whether or not one should refer to them as volunteers—and I think there is good evidence that they were—subjects became part of the program largely because they sought access to drugs to break their everyday routine. They were self-identified "dope fiends" (so Flowers referred to his younger self), whose short-term goal was to get high regardless of the long-term consequences. Their prime objective dovetailed with the ARC's scientific goals, which could only be met by studying serious, seasoned, long-term opiate addicts with a tendency to relapse. Most of the ARC's subjects had been admitted to the institution multiple times before participating in experiments. Subjects possessed a range of extra-institutional drug experiences, and a range of treatment "failures." The ARC capitalized on subjects' familiarity with drugs from the category under study, and to my knowledge, never subjected drug-naive subjects to the administration of experimental drugs.

Within the indigenous morality of the ARC, knowledgeable former drug users were considered not only the best source of comparative data but the only ethical subjects. I do not mean to suggest that the ARC's laboratory logic of mimicry would be considered ethical today, since elements of it undoubtedly would not pass our era's scrutiny. For example, in a classic, 1948 ARC study that no institutional review board would now approve, Abraham Wikler set up a single-subject study of "self-regulated experimental re-addiction to morphine." The subject could ask for and receive "by any route (administered by an aide or by himself) any drug in any amount (up to a 'ceiling' judged safe by the experimenter) at any time of day or night for an unspecified period of time which, however, would not be less than one month" (Wikler 1972, 9–10). Wikler retrospectively reported on the study, which was published in 1952 (1952d):

> [T]he subject would be informed one month in advance of the termination date of this agreement. It was stressed that the experimenter had no interest in the subject's getting himself "hooked," but if he should, the experimenter would advise on how the subject might withdraw himself from whatever drug he was taking. The subject assured the experimenter that he would not get "hooked," and elected to take 30 mg of morphine i.v. as his first dose. (1972, 11)

Following the natural course of readdiction with this subject, Wikler elicited free associations and recorded the subject's manifest dream content. Morphine's euphoric effects were displaced by its dysphoric effects within a few days. The subject rapidly ascended to extraordinarily high doses of morphine, denied that he feared withdrawal and did not seek to avoid it, and elected to withdraw cold turkey in the end, apparently having done it before.

This study was extremely significant for the formation of Wikler's conditioning theory, which remains a touchstone in neurobiological investigations, which now define addiction as a chronic relapsing brain disorder (see chap. 8

in the present book). Wikler suggested that the social practice of "hustling," defined as "operant behavior directed towards obtaining opioids," was reinforcing in its own right. This conclusion "furnished a basis for construction and testing of a 'conditioning theory of drug dependence and relapse' in animals" (Wikler 1972, 11). Although supplemented by animal studies, Wikler avers that he worked out his conditioning model by observing and interacting with just one subject. From listening closely to his subject's perceived needs and cravings, dreams and desires over an extended period, Wikler gained what he considered a deeply grounded sense of the gratifications and necessities that motivated his subject to "self-regulate." This experimental design was unusual even in the context of Lexington, inasmuch as the subject himself helped conceptualize the study, was extremely articulate about his dreams and experiences, and was able to convey a great deal about the social worlds of "hustling" in a way that Wikler could translate into the language of operant conditioning. Wikler's well-recognized immersion in his work and his ongoing proximity to the subject were among the conditions of possibility that led to the emergence of conditioning theory at Lexington.

Researchers base moral judgments as well as scientific interpretations on local knowledge they derive from their familiarity with the materials and technologies used in their scientific and therapeutic practices. Thus scientific debate tends to take place through disputes over tools, techniques, and research design just as much as disputes over definitions, theories, or ideas. The "technical character of disputes over local knowledge" tends to mask not just the disputes' moral content (Halpern 2004, 124) but the way in which the requirements of political ideology converge with the requirements of medical technology (Foucault 1979, 38). Certainly, the ARC researchers were intimately familiar with the actions and effects of the potent compounds supplied them. The technical character of their published research rarely allowed them to air their moral or political views and obscured any record of scientists' attitudes toward their subjects. Evidently, they viewed their subjects as a means to advancing the understanding of how addiction worked, but they seem also to have appreciated their subjects as individual human beings (something a large fraction of the American public remains unable to do when it comes to drug addicts). Researchers' perspectives and modes of perception diverged from those of their subjects. After all, these researchers literally held the keys to unlock the secrets of their subjects' lives. Invariably, researchers I interviewed insisted that subjects volunteered in order to make their lives meaningful or "give something back" to society. Many researchers recognized that even altruism may be construed as moral coercion, acknowledging that they "walked the tightrope between coercion and seduction" at the ARC. They were, after all, administering drugs to people who liked them and who would do just about anything to get them. Through their performance of ethicality, addiction researchers attempted to distance themselves from accusations that they were enticing, seducing, coercing, or coddling addicts.

Boundaries of social class in particular separated researchers from their subjects; subjects were court-mandated to Lexington and were literally captive there. The researchers were almost entirely white, upper- and middle-class professional men who experimented on poor, lower- and working-class, ethnically and racially diverse addicts. Although most research participants were white, there is no doubt that the poor were exploited for the scientific purposes of the dominant social classes who were identified with the U.S. government. The production of scientific knowledge was an exercise of social power and privilege—it was extractive, however well-intentioned or scientifically "enlightening." Flowers later said: "I began to come to grips with the fact that I was used. Let me put it that particular way. . . . I kinda like got in touch with being taken advantage of . . . because I was a dope fiend. And being a dope fiend, I used dope! . . . They used my ass and took advantage of me. . . . Back then at that time for a while there I was angry, bitter and so forth. A little further down the line, I kind of chalked it up as a bad experience." Uninterested in the consent process, the forms he signed, or the information given, Flowers was focused on the "payoff," the drug rewards that were given to participants as in-kind payment up to 1955. He characterized researchers as exploiting his vulnerability to drugs: "I was very vulnerable, . . . in the sense that if it's about drugs, I wanted drugs, okay? I recognize that not only just myself but some other people were thrown into a situation, was used, was paid off with what we as drug addicts craved—drugs. I see it from the perspective that it was wrong. It should not have happened" (2004).

Flowers's retrospective account was mediated through the lens of his later participation in drug treatment and adoption of recovery as a way of life. A pivotal moment came during his testimony before the congressional investigation that followed on the Tuskegee study, when he first heard allegations that the ARC's research was part of a project of the Central Intelligence Agency and military intelligence. He sustained a lifelong eye condition that he subsequently attributed to a hallucinogen administered at the ARC. He stands as a rare—and highly credible—witness to the perspective of those whose bodies were used, quite literally, in the name of science. Flowers embodies the "fundamental and appalling structural reality of Lexington": that, as one of the anonymous reviewers of this book in manuscript put it, "addicts who were sent to an alleged rehabilitation center for treatment were recruited for experiments that, instead of trying to wean them from their addictions, subjected them to new drug experiences and then rewarded their voluntarism by giving them free samples of the very drugs they were supposed to be giving up." This characterization rests on the assumption that rehabilitation was taking place at the Lexington Hospital, which actually offered little or nothing in the way of what we would call treatment today. Rather than condemn the experimenters, I present readers with the very ethical conundrums uncovered in bringing this laboratory to life, in order to advance historical knowledge about how research on human subjects was actually conducted prior to the emergence of the human subjects regime now in place (see chap. 6).

What seems valid to me in the preceding critique is that researchers at the ARC were insensitive to how unacceptable their work might be perceived to be beyond institutional walls. This can be illustrated by an example drawn from the animal models pioneered at the ARC and the human analogues researchers sought in order to validate their work in animals. As the previous chapter showed, researchers believed that human response to drugs varied according to the social setting, cultural context, or experimental situation.[5] Among the animal models they considered valid were spinal dogs and decorticated cats. In their quest to draw parallels between animal models and human addiction, researchers did not consider the extent to which outsiders would find animal models cruel or revolting. Their goal was to find a human analogue among Lexington residents, and they identified a so-called spinal man who had been rendered paraplegic by syphilis of the spinal cord prior to admission to Lexington. For the professional network of addiction researchers, such a cross-species analogue was an opportunity for focusing on the laboratory logics of readdiction, substitution, and unmasking. Outside the research community, the moral implications of opportunistically using such subjects as decorticated cats, spinal dogs, or the "spinal man" border on horrific. Although the goal of these studies was unmasking the basic mechanisms of addiction so as to develop more generally acceptable and effective therapeutic responses and testing the potential public health threat of new compounds, the question of just how much "interest" individual subjects paid has to be raised if we are to consider the political and moral stakes at the heart of substance abuse research. The next section considers three addiction therapies for which the ARC followed up on clinical reports: methadone, today used in medical maintenance; nalorphine (n-allylnormorphine, also known by its trade name, Nalline), the narcotic antagonist that was a first-line response to opiate overdose prior to the synthesis of naloxone in 1960; and frontal lobotomy, no longer used to treat drug addiction thanks to studies conducted by the ARC.

CALCULATING THE COSTS OF SCIENTIFIC OPPORTUNISM: THE ETHOS OF THE LEXINGTON HOSPITAL

Originally, the laboratory at Lexington was mandated to study how the U.S. government should best deal with drug addicts, a goal apparent in Himmelsbach's initial studies refuting claims of therapeutic efficacy made by nostrum makers. By the early 1950s, the ARC was struggling to preserve its basic research program in the face of industry pressure to become a drug-testing operation.[6] By dividing the workload between Michigan and Lexington, CDAN buffered the ARC, a research site that offered something no one else could—access to otherwise healthy morphine-dependent human subjects. Such clinicians and pharmacologists as, respectively, Beecher and Seevers could not replicate the conditions of everyday life in Lexington. Alone of all research facilities in the country, the ARC had access to drug-experienced subjects and a constant stream of compounds in quantities great enough to test. These were the material conditions necessary for it to mark the scientific milestones it had by the mid-twentieth century.

The ARC's first signal achievement was the initial human testing of methadone in the late 1940s. Not until the ARC established methadone's efficacy in 1947 had an effective pharmacological agent for relieving the abstinence syndrome been identified. The names *methadon* or *amidone* were assigned to a synthetic analgesic compound developed in Germany at I. G. Farben and rediscovered in a Department of Commerce investigation of German wartime industries (Isbell, Wikler, et al. 1948). Because the ARC found that methadone produced a prolonged but mild abstinence syndrome, it was put into clinical use for managing withdrawal at Lexington in the late 1940s.[7] Subjects likened methadone to heroin, displayed euphoria when they were on it, became talkative and boastful, and attempted to get more of it. Former morphine addicts expressed satisfaction with methadone even at low doses, and their satisfaction increased with dosage increases. Judging from typical responses to the injection of methadone, the ARC concluded that "narcotic drug addicts would abuse methadone and would become habituated to it if it were freely available and not controlled" (Isbell et al. 1947, 892). They concluded that methadone was a dangerously addictive drug that would become a potentially serious public health problem if not controlled.

When researchers delved into subjects' responses to single doses of methadone, they found that their respondents could differentiate what they were told was a "new synthetic drug" from other opiate drugs along an axis they called "drive," defined as the "ability of an opiate drug to produce ambition to work, to engage in games, listen to music, etc." (Isbell, Eisenman, et al. 1948, 86). When researchers pointed out that subjects actually exhibited decreased activity when on methadone, the "puzzled" subjects stated that they felt ambitious after morphine but "knew they were not" after administration of methadone (Isbell, Eisenman, et al. 1948, 86). Obviously experienced and well informed, the subjects agreed that if opiates were unavailable, they would prefer the new synthetic drug to alcohol, barbiturates, marijuana, or Demerol (Isbell, Eisenman, et al. 1948, 86). An "uninformed" control group was then formed out of a group of subjects who had participated in a study on pain thresholds. The controls could not differentiate between the effects of methadone, morphine, or other synthetic opiates, such as Dilaudid. One subject said: "That was great stuff. I wouldn't have believed it was possible for a synthetic drug to be so like morphine. Can you get it outside? Will it be put under the narcotic law? I wish I could get some to kick my next habit" (Isbell, Eisenman, et al. 1948, 88; Isbell et al. 1947, 892). This statement convinced the researchers they had an abusable substance on their hands. They sounded the alarm in the publications that introduced medical professionals to methadone.

Methadone is a long-acting opiate that can be dangerous in cumulative doses. This danger was unknown until the ARC responded to accidental "methadone poisoning" (overdose) in two subjects of a large methadone study consisting of 110 white men and 15 African American men. Two African American men went into comas after being administered cumulative doses of twenty milligrams of intravenous methadone. Both subjects were particularly susceptible to methadone, since others had received similar doses without getting into trouble. Having become cyanotic, they were on the brink of death after failure of the standard responses, artificial resuscitation and Nikethemide. Realizing opiate overdose might be reversed by a narcotic antagonist, researchers reached for a bottle of Nalline (nalorphine or n-allylnormorphine) supplied to them by Merck. University of Illinois pharmacologist Klaus Unna had discovered in 1943 that nalorphine antagonized most of morphine's actions in experimental animals. Two previous attempts to use nalorphine as an antidote had been reported in the clinical literature with equivocal results: one case reported death due to shock; the other patient revived. Thus the question of whether or not clinicians should employ the drug in cases of overdose was still open (Addiction Research Center 1978, 42). In the ARC cases, the researchers reported that the administration of nalorphine "apparently induced spectacular and, possibly, life-saving effects." They explained: "Unless N-allyl-normorphine had been given, one would have expected that both patients would have remained in coma, with depressed respiration, for at least several hours. In fact, if N-allyl-normorphine had not been available, both patients might have died" (Fraser et al. 1952, 1206). Once safe and effective dosages were worked out, methadone was put into clinical use at the Lexington Hospital to ease withdrawal, and there was never, to my knowledge, another overdose incident involving it.

The streak of opportunism that characterizes the will to knowledge was in healthy evidence at the ARC. After the overdose incident, the researchers followed up by studying nalorphine in spinal dogs (Wikler and Carter 1953). At a CDAN meeting on January 22–23, 1954, Isbell stated his intent to "get some patients pretty depressed with morphine and then come in with the Nalline" (Committee on Drug Addiction and Narcotics 1954a, 852).[8] Once it was found useful to combat opiate-induced respiratory depression in newborns and diagnose active addiction, Nalline was used as a rapid diagnostic tool for determining if a person was in fact addicted to opiates (Isbell 1953, 1954). The compound antagonized narcotic effects and unmasked the underlying physical dependence that Wikler, Fraser, and Isbell (1953) believed appeared early in the process of addiction. The nalorphine story illustrates the ARC's resourceful use of whatever substances, situations, and subjects were ready to hand. However, the press of the time represented such resourcefulness not as heroism but as barbarism.

Journalistic accounts of the ARC portrayed "guinea pig volunteers" rewarded in drugs. For example, a 1951 account by reporter Edward Mowery that appeared in a *New York World-Telegram and Sun* series on heroin in Harlem showcased Lexington: "We headed for the research unit of Narco, where gruesome experiments on voluntary guinea pig patients are conducted around the clock by scientists charged with establishing the addiction propensities of new drugs. In this 12-bed laboratory was discovered the potency of Demerol and methadone and the established fact that large doses of barbiturates cause withdrawal convulsions and hallucinations."[9] Mowery described the readdiction of "confirmed addicts beyond rational help" in an experiment with n-allylnormorphine, which he identified as "the best antidote yet developed in treating poisoning by morphine and other opiates." Although addicts "get no bang from it," a doctor explained to Mowery, they begged for more even after "doses which pharmacologists regard as astronomical." The doctor continued: "[T]heir reward for undergoing this unspeakable agony and possible death, is a grain of morphine for each month of the test or days off their sentence. These souls never waver in their choice. It's morphine." Such portrayals sensationalized the science and dealt with human subjects in a cavalier manner.

Even if such stories badly distorted the scientific work of the ARC, selected instances of scientific opportunism verged on preying on the vulnerable. It is important to distinguish between such instances rather than issuing a blanket condemnation from a presentist point of view. There is debate among historians about how to characterize such treatments as frontal lobotomy, which was considered therapeutic for schizophrenia and intractable pain in the 1950s (Dynes and Poppen 1959; Hamilton and Haynes 1949; Mason and Hamby 1947). Lobotomy was adopted partly because it solved certain problems of social control faced by asylum superintendents (Pressman 1998). A handful of clinical observers maintained that lobotomized addicts no longer suffered the pain of narcotic withdrawal but were in no position to measure the abstinence syndrome or to establish controls (Mason and Hamby 1948, 1039). The ARC researchers feared clinicians would come to invalid conclusions and start lobotomizing addicts out of ignorance.

Skeptical that lobotomy was therapeutic, the ARC conducted a study on whether or not it prevented the pain of withdrawal, using the tried-and-true methods through which they had studied the typical progress of the abstinence syndrome (Andrews and Himmelsbach 1944). The ARC researchers knew that predictable signs of the abstinence syndrome were "fairly reproducible in any given person," although their intensity might vary (Wikler, Pescor, et al. 1952, 515). When they learned that four subjects from Kolb Hall, the neuropsychiatric facility for nonaddicts that was also located on the grounds at Lexington, had been recommended for therapeutic frontal lobotomy, they decided to undertake an experiment.[10] Three schizophrenics and one sufferer of phantom limb pain whose arm had been amputated in a childhood accident underwent the procedure (Wikler et al. 1952). Injured in a railroad accident as a child, the latter was a forty-eight-year-old white man who had used morphine, heroin, and Dilaudid for decades. He also had undergone electroshock treatments and methadone substitution therapy in vain attempts to relieve phantom limb pain. Some of these worked for short periods, during which he was aware of the missing limb but not of the pain; but he always returned to Lexington readdicted. The three schizophrenic subjects had no previous history of drug addiction but had been unresponsive to any previous treatment.

Before the surgery, the three schizophrenic subjects were stabilized on morphine and put through a "test withdrawal," to establish a baseline against which the same procedure, repeated after the lobotomy, could be compared. After the lobotomies were performed, the same withdrawal procedure was performed on each subject. The subject suffering phantom limb pain was treated differently: he failed to show any effects from his first lobotomy, so a second was performed. He then resumed work as a railroad payroll clerk, and nine months later, he was reportedly no longer asking for narcotics or exhibiting "concern over his condition" (Wikler et al. 1952, 3). Still, Wikler wrote, "[F]rontal lobotomy should not be considered as a generally desirable treatment for drug addiction per se, since it is not yet clear that the deficits consequent to frontal lobotomy are to be preferred to the problems associated with narcotic addiction" (1951, 163). The ARC researchers thus attempted to hold clinicians back from adopting frontal lobotomy as a treatment for drug addiction. Although they came to what we would now think of as an enlightened position through the lobotomy study, their use of human subjects in the manner described clearly raises ethical questions: Did they go too far, or were they playing a corrective role in helping base clinical practice on evidence rather than on a speculative surgery that resulted in lifelong low affect for its subjects? Did preventing wider adoption of frontal lobotomy save large numbers of narcotic addicts from the knife? Does that warrant the sacrifice these four subjects ended up making?

Many readers will be appalled on discovering that lobotomies were not only performed at Lexington but systematically and intentionally studied there in the manner described. Ethical lines were blurry in the lobotomy study: the schizophrenics had never been addicted to opiates before they were experimentally addicted (not once, but twice) and forced to undergo withdrawal (not once, but twice). Second, who can say whether or not the requirements of mental competence we recognize as so essential for informed consent today were met? Turning to the sufferer of phantom limb pain, there is the matter of offering more than palliative care to someone who had lived most of his life in intractable pain—perhaps even holding out the hope of "cure," and the possibility of a life free from pain. Finally, there is the question of whether or not the study directly benefited or enhanced the health and well-being of anyone involved. My purpose here is not to pronounce judgment retrospectively but to clarify what the lobotomy study meant in the context of the laboratory logics and indigenous moralities of the ARC.

The lobotomy study enabled investigators to elaborate further on basic mechanisms that otherwise could not be seen. They believed that the morphine abstinence syndrome worked to unmask homeostatic mechanisms developed by the nervous system and the pituitary-adrenal system to adapt to repeated administration of opiates. They observed that former addicts quickly built up tolerance to extremely high doses of morphine-like drugs. By putting these experimental subjects into abrupt abstinence, the researchers attempted to unmask the underlying mechanisms they sought to elucidate. Studying the contrast between the schizophrenics, who had never been "naturally" addicted, and the intractable pain sufferer, who had been a regular user of opiates for decades, was a route to show that physical dependence was not "synonymous with 'addiction,' since none of the schizophrenic patients exhibited interest in, or craving for, morphine at any time during that study" (Addiction Research Center 1978, 50). By differentiating between the "purposive," or symbolic, aspects of craving and abstinence and the "nonpurposive," or nonsymbolic, aspects of it, the investigators established that changes during abstinence were "independent of symbolic significance" (Addiction Research Center 1978, 51). The study showed that although users might be "'conditioned' to meaningful stimuli," drugs were devoid of symbolic value to the lobotomized schizophrenic subjects. The experimental situation was set up to unmask conditioning by stripping away desire and symbolism, leaving only "objective" signs of abstinence. The subjects showed the lack of reactivity, or low affect, that typically followed lobotomy. Subsequently, the ARC did not recommend lobotomy or do further work involving it.

As a thought collective, the ARC played a corrective role relative to clinicians, whose ideas about what might be therapeutic were indicated by individual case reports. A compelling example of how haphazard clinical practice could be was provided by University of Michigan pharmacologist Edward J. Domino, who dramatically described nalorphine as the drug that drew him into neuropsychopharmacology.[11] During Domino's internship, he was on a cancer service where an experimental opiate, Dromoran (levorphenal), was being tested on the terminally ill.[12] When a breast cancer patient went into serious respiratory depression and became comatose after small, therapeutic doses, Domino speculated that he could revive her with nalorphine, which he had used to revive overdosed dogs during demonstrations in the medical school at the University of Illinois, where Klaus Unna had first studied the pharmacology of the drug. Domino recounts: "While [I] ventilated the patient, a nurse called [across town] for the nalorphine to be brought. When it arrived, [I] broke the vial and injected it. I'll never forget it. . . . [I]t was remarkable. She was totally comatose and, then all of a sudden, I gave her the nalorphine and she started to breathe." Learning that the patient's cancer had interfered with her liver processing, Domino realized that cumulative doses of Dromoran had poisoned her. "[B]ut, in addition," he observed, "I saved her life" (1995, 5). This defining moment attests to the casual nature of the social organization of clinical research in the days prior to clinical trials, databases, and registries for adverse drug reactions.

Only the ARC was in a position to do the systematic, controlled studies that built up decades of baseline data by the early 1950s. Methadone's profile of action was established, and it remains integral to treatment today; nalorphine was discovered to work as a lifesaving therapeutic intervention; and frontal lobotomy never came into vogue as a treatment for addiction (when it might easily have). In each case, ARC researchers opportunistically availed themselves of particular subjects whose conditions shed light not only on the particular problem at hand but on the underlying dynamics of drug dependence—tolerance, abstinence, and presence or absence of desire for the drug. They wanted to see what was left once desire was stripped away, and they saw the drugs they studied as tools for doing so. How shall we retrospectively calculate the price that human subjects paid in the methadone, nalorphine, or lobotomy studies? On balance, were the studies beneficial to those very individuals or only to those who have benefited since? As the evidence on which the ARC cautioned clinicians, these studies diverged from the ARC's regulatory role.[13] The studies led to clinicians ending the practice of abrupt withdrawal, for the ARC urged methadone substitution and gradual tapering off across a ten-day period (Fraser and Grinder 1953). Clinicians now had an effective response to overdose, nalorphine and, later, naloxone, each of which were later evaluated as possible therapies for addiction. The calculus of suffering was distinctly weighted toward the greater good for the greatest number. Individuals who suffered lobotomy or overdose endured unspeakable trauma; others benefited from the knowledge thus obtained. Unresolved questions remain: Did the twice-lobotomized amputee live out his life pain-free or "drug-free"? Did the two subjects revived by nalorphine know what their near-death experiences meant? Where should U.S. government responsibility for aftercare in the case of long-term effects from research of this kind begin and end? How shall we calculate the moral and social costs of scientific opportunism?

THE DEMISE OF PATIENT-ORIENTED RESEARCH AND THE RISE OF CLINICAL TRIALS

Most of those who worked at the ARC saw themselves as basic scientists who happened to work in a clinical setting. Aware that drug responses varied in terms of individual susceptibility and psychological effects, they documented the range of individual variation but aimed to specify the common neurophysiological pathways that lay along the road to addiction, withdrawal, and relapse. They did this by working closely with subjects and by designing their studies to take advantage of their relatively unfettered access to subjects. In her study of research on a hospital ward in the 1950s, *Experiment Perilous: Physicians and Patients Facing the Unknown,* medical anthropologist Renee C. Fox tells of the "sort of investigation that entails moving back and forth in both directions, between the clinical bedside and the laboratory bench; that involves patients as subjects; and that is directed toward finding more effective modes of diagnosing, treating, and preventing the diseases and disorders from which its patient-subjects suffer" (1959/1998, 259). Although the Metabolic Group, which Fox studied, operated in a very different experimental setting from the prison-hospital at Lexington, the kind of patient-oriented research Fox described was akin to that of the ARC. Patient-oriented research differed from the pedestrian drug trials organized elsewhere, which really did employ human subjects as little more than guinea pigs.

The clearly demarcated division between the clinical and research units at Lexington was reinforced by institutional routines and practices. Researchers were not responsible for treating patients or delivering medical care, although they did monitor subjects living on the research ward. By contrast, Fox's metabolic researchers separated "laboratory life" from the practice of "real medicine." One of her subjects stated, "If you listen for it, you'll hear one or another of us saying, 'How long can I live this laboratory life anyway? I've just got to get back to *real* medicine'" (1959/1998, 27). At the ARC, the value was reversed; the real action was in the lab, which was buffered from the frustrating realities of the rest of the institution. The futility of standard treatment methods was evident to everyone associated with the place. An oral history given in 1970 by Earl Chestang, a thirty-one-year-old trainee of a Detroit methadone clinic, recounted taking three trips to Lexington, beginning in 1959.

> Most addicts knew Lexington wouldn't work the way it was set up at the time, because that place was exactly what Walter Winchell said it was in the '50s. He had only one thing to say about it, it was a multi-million dollar flophouse for

> junkies. That's what he called it, and that's what it really was, and all the addicts knew it, and it seems like the professional staff must have known it. It really was of no help to a guy unless he was right there in the institution. (1970, 10)

Chestang described encountering among his fellow patients an addicted physician who was "one of the worst addicts I ever saw in my life." The physician patient was at Lexington for the second time, in an attempt to reclaim his medical license. He claimed to have become addicted as part of a self-designed experiment to prove to his patients, who kept begging for narcotics, that they were "just weak, immature individuals" (1970, 45). Physician addicts were a regular feature on the wards of Lexington. They often volunteered for studies, sometimes staying on the research ward to record data or do other low-level tasks related to the studies. A physician patient befriended by Eddie Flowers committed suicide by throwing himself down the spiral staircase at Lexington (2004). These examples point to the overall lack of individually tailored or even appropriately specific treatment at the "multi-million dollar flophouse for junkies."

Many patient-inmates experienced the clinical staff at Lexington as uncaring and nontherapeutic, due to lack of direct contact between staff and patient-inmates. A thirty-eight-year-old African American male from Detroit who went to Lexington voluntarily in 1967 criticized the clinical program: "It lacks the type of atmosphere that would motivate, I think, anybody, any addict." He described staff as "people doing their nine to fives and their eight-to-four-thirties, going about their business" (Hall 1970, 5, 18). He explained: "Periodically, you would go before a doctor, and he would do a sort of in-depth interview with you, find out as much as he could about your background, psychiatric interview or something, but there was no closeness. Everything was done on a sort of vast scale. You never really got the feeling that you were part of a drug program and you were going to be helped with your drug problem" (Hall 1970, 18). Decades later, Flowers affirmed that a similar situation prevailed when he was there in the 1950s: "Nobody got no treatment. We didn't go to no group therapy. We didn't go to no individual therapy. We didn't do nothin'. Worked on the job down there, but [there was] nothing in the way of dealing with the individual and addiction. There was no program" (2004). Living in the general population contrasted to participating in the close-knit research ward, where subjects were paid a good deal more individual attention than clinical staff were able to pay to other patients. The benefits of such consideration must have been considerable for some research subjects, even though they knew that the research unit was not trying to "treat" them.

Basic science—or "nontherapeutic" research—was elevated over treatment at the ARC. That distinction proved the ARC's undoing when it became politically necessary to show how research directly benefited individual subjects. Having staked its claim in the making of science, the ARC research program was defined as "nontherapeutic." Unlike many clinical trials today, there was no pretense that individual subjects were being offered therapy—much less a "cure"—for what ailed them. The sociological effect of this situation was that researchers gained social status while clinicians occupied a lower position within the institutional hierarchy. Addiction was experienced as an "intractable" illness—when hopes that research would find a "cure" were alive, addiction was constructed as an acute condition, rather than a chronic, relapsing one. Administrators and clinicians were to explain relapse rates, while scientists were to study them, in hopes that relapse would reveal what caused addiction in some individuals and not others.

Because the treatment of the time was largely ineffective, relapse rates fell periodically under review. Eighty percent or more of Lexington patients relapsed after release. Thus there was a divorce between "successful" researchers and the "custodial" clinicians. This distinction became more pronounced even as higher-caliber clinicians arrived with hopes of studying treatment efficacy, for they voiced frustrations with lower social status and complained to external reviewers (see chap. 6 in the present book). As with the clinical researchers about whom Fox wrote, distinctions between research and treatment solidified at Lexington for four reasons. First, there was a congeries of uncertainties concerning the underlying biochemical and physiological mechanisms of the disease process, chemical compounds, administrative procedures, methodological techniques, clinical or "nonexperimental" aspects of diagnosis, treatment, and the course of disease. Second, everyone involved in research recognized the limitations of therapy. Third, there was the sheer difficulty of locating, recruiting, and maintaining subjects in the study (by contrast to clinicians being overwhelmed with patients). Fourth, there was social conflict between research and therapy. The social organization of Lexington produced two cultures, and over time those who worked in research and treatment began to see themselves at odds with one another.

The day-to-day corridor talk and staff meetings of the ARC have vanished from the historical record. What strategies did researchers use to maintain clinical distance from their subjects? How did they deal with moral uncertainties generated by the fact that they were administering to human beings unknown drugs of unknown potency with unknown effects? How did they respond to the certain knowledge that they lacked effective treatment or to knowing precisely how agonizing withdrawal can be? These questions must have encroached especially on those who were physicians. As Fox found with the physician researchers of the Metabolic Group, coping mechanisms were "group-patterned," involving a pattern of "ritualized optimism" about the potential that basic research might yield therapeutic innovations (1959/1998, 135, 277). Such optimism was ironically based in social distance between research staff and clinical staff, meaning that researchers did not come into contact with the vast majority of patients—only with the self-selected few who participated in studies. This is similar to what we can infer happened at the ARC. To this day, researchers recall friendships with participants or remember with sadness departures of participants to whom they had grown close. Strangely, an ethic of care seems to have pervaded the ARC researchers despite the barriers of class, creed, and sometimes color between them and their subjects. The differences between the researchers and their subjects were in many ways narrower than they are in the clinical trials of today. Clinical trials now take place at increased social distance among primary investigators, researchers, staff, and participants. The scale of the studies alone works against the formation of an ethic of care and the social bonds that go with it. The latitude for exploitation of vulnerable human subjects in clinical trials is great, a topic to which I turn in the concluding chapter of this book. The next section of this chapter lays the groundwork for understanding human subjects regulation.

REGULATING HUMAN SUBJECTS: THE EMERGENCE OF A NEW REGIME OF GOVERNANCE

Federal human subjects regulation sprang from the military public health apparatus in the early 1950s, when the Armed Forces Medical Council established a policy "for the use of human volunteers (military and civilian employees) in experimental research at Armed Forces facilities" (quoted in Moreno 2001, 172–73). Pentagon policy TS-01188, modeled on the Nuremberg Code, was signed by Secretary of Defense Charles E. Wilson on February 26, 1953, but its top secret classification limited its impact. The U.S. Army's Office of the Surgeon General also adopted the Wilson policy in 1954 (Moreno 2001, 243). The policy supposedly applied to extramural clinical research contractors, but there was actually no education, enforcement, or follow-up. When Army Regulation 70–25 restated the policy in 1962 and the U.S. Army inserted the "Principles, Policies, and Rules of the Surgeon General" into its contracts, contractors seemed to have no knowledge of the previous version (Moreno 2001, 179, 243).

Resistance to the army's attempt to impose a set of "rigid rules" based on the Nuremberg Code was especially strong at Harvard University, where Henry K. Beecher drafted alternative rules that became known as the Beecher-Army Compromise (Moreno 2001, 243). Although it is now accepted as the ethical basis for governing human subjects research, the Nuremberg Code was contested by Beecher and others throughout the 1950s, due to perceptions that it was so rigid as to prevent human experimentation altogether and severely restrict investigators' autonomy. Beecher doubted that most subjects understood science well enough to give truly informed consent, and he did not believe that a priori rules could be laid down to govern clinical research. Drug researchers considered full disclosure of the drug under study counterproductive due to the placebo effect. An example of a study in which full disclosure would be counterproductive was suggested by Isaac Starr, who chaired the 1954 CDAN meeting: "Since many people in this country had been taking small amounts of sedatives over long periods of time, [I] would like to see studies initiated on the withdrawal of barbiturates. Would these individuals develop abnormal behaviors as soon as the barbiturates were stopped?" Starr cautioned the committee that valid results would be obtained only if the sedatives were withdrawn without patients' knowledge (Committee on Drug Addiction and Narcotics 1954a, 693). Other participants at the first 1954 CDAN meeting expressed similar concerns about the validity of studies where subjects knew what was happening to them. As shown in previous chapters, Beecher's laboratory and the ARC favored making subjects aware in most situations but cautioned that results could be affected by the experimental setting, the observer's presence, and the questions asked. Theirs was a contention over how to interpret the meaning of awareness for the experimental subject. This was an ongoing contention over whether knowledgeable or naive subjects were best suited for the types of studies undertaken in these research sites.

Better placed than those at the ARC to inscribe views in public policy, Beecher traveled to the Pentagon with a delegation from Harvard Medical School in 1962. There, he offered a compromise that avoided the strict language of the Nuremberg Code and instead established flexible guidelines that retained the cultural authority of biomedical and clinical researchers. The academicians left assured that the new regulations were simply suggested guidelines. No one from the ARC was personally involved in the tussle over the form that human subjects regulation was to take. However, the ARC was implicated in the debate because the Army Chemical Corps was then widely involved in drug research on LSD, mescaline, and other substances that were also studied at Lexington. Army Regulation 70-25 contained exemptions that enabled military researchers and contractors to avoid full disclosure if they thought it would invalidate experiments (Moreno 2001, 244). Disclosure exemptions also applied to "ethical medical and clinical investigations" that were of potential benefit to subjects—as Moreno points out, a tautology at best (2001, 244). The exemptions allowed investigators to decide how much to tell subjects when they assumed the research directly benefited subjects, but it forced full disclosure in instances of indirect benefit. While today's process of informed consent vests the power to discern benefit in the subjects, the nascent regime offered in the Beecher-Army Compromise placed it in the hands of researchers. This compromise over how fully informed subjects had to be in order to meet standards of informed consent was reinterpreted in due course during the events discussed in chapter 6 of the present book, particularly the 1975 congressional investigation of research conducted by the Department of Defense and the Central Intelligence Agency.

Scholars who have brought the historical sociology of bioethics into being have skipped over Beecher's scientific work as a source of his preoccupation with ethics (cf. Moreno 2001, 242). As shown in chapter 4 of the present book, Beecher's clinical logics and his concern with securing high social status and continued funding played a role in his performance of ethical subjectivity. When, in 1966, Beecher published the landmark papers that brought attention to what Moreno has dubbed the "'homegrown' American ethics scandals" (2001, 247), Beecher's involvement with military and intelligence contracts went unmentioned. Deeply invested in guaranteeing that the virtues of the individual investigator would secure ethical practice, Beecher served his own interests by emphasizing the need for continued professional autonomy and the prerogative power of professionalism.

The military was the first source of human subjects regulation, but in 1966, a second stream of regulation issued from the NIH, then and now the main U.S. government sponsor of health-related research. NIH director James Shannon pushed for standards of informed consent and for review committees that consisted of not just professionals but members of the public. Although a uniform policy to protect human subjects went into effect in 1966 (Mishkin 1993), site visits revealed uneven compliance and widespread disarray about what it meant among the research community. Consent declarations were used at many sites, but they effectively allowed even hazardous research to proceed

(Halpern 2004, 119). For the entire time that the ARC operated at Lexington, the legal climate was gray, and the rules, ethics, and customs governing use of human subjects were murky.

A series of public scandals involving unethical human subjects research catapulted human subjects research policy into public view.[14] Prison research programs were implicated in exposés of military and intelligence testing, such as those of the Army Chemical Corps research contracts on the effects of hallucinogens (Moreno 2001, 195). Contractors were supposed to include training lectures so subjects knew what to expect from LSD, but concerns that the power of suggestion would influence outcomes led to noncompliance at most sites (Moreno 2001, 256). In Army Chemical Corps studies of LSD at Holmesburg Prison in Pennsylvania, inmates and scientists quickly found themselves in over their heads: "The researchers at Holmesburg didn't know what to make of LSD's effects, and the inmates were familiar with street drugs but not hallucinogens. They also couldn't be told much about the drug, including its name, because at the time the research was classified" (Moreno 2001, 228). This clandestine LSD research network was funded by the U.S. Army and the Central Intelligence Agency through the Geschickter Foundation and the Josiah Macy, Jr. Foundation.[15] The ARC had no need of foundation support and never conducted research on "unwitting" subjects. The ARC studied development of tolerance to LSD, as well as whether tranquilizers could ameliorate the effects of "bad trips."

Also spurring stronger protection of human subjects were social movements for civil rights, prisoners' rights, and patients' rights, which changed the very nature of clinical care and medical research. Indeed, Halpern attributes the emergence of research abuse as a public problem to clashing historical sensibilities. Shaped by the experience of World War II, an older sensibility justified human experimentation as a sacrifice for the common good. Shaped by the social movements of the 1960s, a newer ethos represented human experimentation as exploitation of the powerless by the powerful. Lexington was a casualty of that clash. The rest of this chapter introduces the policy context that changed Lexington's clinical side in ways that altered both its therapeutic and research missions.

DEVOLUTION AND REVOLUTION: THE ROAD TO CIVIL COMMITMENT AND THERAPEUTIC COMMUNITIES

Ethical concerns were not solely responsible for ending human subjects research at Lexington. Two broad policy shifts in the administration of criminal justice and mental health profoundly altered institutional routines at Lexington. These changed the material conditions of the ARC well before prison research became a national issue. The first policy shift was the Kennedy administration's commitment to community mental health, which encouraged federal hospitals to concentrate on research and devolve treatment to "communities"—states, counties, and municipalities.[16] Even more consequential for Lexington was federal passage of a civil commitment policy, which responded to the evolving social consensus that drug addicts be treated more humanely than they were in jails. The U.S. Supreme Court interpreted addiction as a condition akin to illness in *Robinson v. California* (1962), opining that "even one day in prison would be a cruel and unusual punishment for the 'crime' of having a common cold."[17] Deeming it "unlikely that any State at this moment in history would attempt to make it a criminal offense for a person to be mentally ill, or a leper, or to be afflicted with a venereal disease" (*Robinson v. California,* 666–67), the Court held that the state of California could not criminalize a condition, status, or "affliction." While declaring itself to be "not unmindful of the vicious evils of the narcotics traffic," the Court found that states already possessed sufficient means to attack them (*Robinson v. California,* 665). Indeed, the Court argued that "prosecution for addiction, with its resulting stigma and irreparable damage to the good name of the accused, cannot be justified as a means of protecting society, where civil commitment would do as well" (*Robinson v. California,* 677).

Despite the equivocal results of civil commitment in California and New York, the federal Narcotic Addict Rehabilitation Act (NARA) passed on November 8, 1966.[18] Faced with the daunting task of scaling up civil commitment, the U.S. surgeon general saw Lexington and its sister narcotics farm in Fort Worth, Texas, as quick and dirty solutions and renamed each a "National Institute of Mental Health Clinical Research Center" in 1967. The bars came down at Lexington, which stopped admitting convicts and voluntary patients in favor of those committed under Titles I and III of NARA.[19] Problems surfaced in immediate response to NARA's new disciplinary approach. Implementation difficulties were the strongest contributing factor to the closure of Fort Worth in October 1971 and to the demise, in February 1974, of Lexington as an institution singularly devoted to drug addicts.

NARA introduced changes that put the ARC into a double bind. To quell fears that Lexington was releasing actively addicted individuals, research protocols had long stated that subjects would not be treated with experimental drugs within six months of release. Civil commitment shortened sentences to six months or less, so after 1968, the ARC had to recruit subjects from the smaller pool of those serving longer sentences at federal penitentiaries, such as Leavenworth or Atlanta. Faced with a sudden disappearance of research subjects, the research unit acted to secure new sources through a memorandum of understanding (dated February 15, 1968) between the BOP and NIMH, concerning eligibility criteria for the transfer of prisoners to the ARC (National Commission 1976a). When they volunteered to transfer to Lexington, prisoners had to be at least twenty-five years old and have eighteen months more to serve.

Civil commitment brought minimum security to most of Lexington, but placed the ARC in the position of having to import federal prisoners to serve as test subjects.. By the summer of 1970, the only federal prisoners left at Lexington were the ARC's research subjects. Since most people housed at Lexington were civilly committed under NARA, security was relaxed, and unauthorized departures and increased trafficking in "contraband chemicals" became common. Maximum security was maintained at the ARC to prevent such problems from tainting the research. Ironically, those who had long advocated for treating drug addicts less like prisoners and more like patients were thrust into the role of running a miniprison. Meanwhile, the rest of the institution morphed into the more open environment of a model "federal correctional institute." The difference was palpable to those working at the ARC: "What I didn't like about it was that I had to carry these keys and every morning I got locked in. The guards were friendly to me, but I didn't like all those locked doors. I went down there with bell-bottomed trousers on, a beard, octagonal clear glasses, just after seeing *Easy Rider*" (Mansky 2006). This shift in organizational culture exacerbated existing tensions between the ARC and the treatment side of Lexington, called the Clinical Research Center (CRC) after 1968 despite the fact that little research was done on the clinical side. Treatment evaluation research was widely perceived as scientifically weak, a perception that led to social antagonisms and substantive conflicts between the larger institution of Lexington and the ARC.

Despite its new name, the CRC remained engaged primarily in treatment and occasional rehabilitation, whereas the ARC was solely a research operation. Although interviewees differed about the politics of the CRC and its research potential, most mentioned antagonism due to the very different missions of the two units. An ARC researcher at the time, Peter Mansky, said:

> They were separate entities, run separately. We had locked doors and prisoner patients, or prisoner subjects. It was a very, very different experience in the

> CRC. Since I was young, I wandered around both and didn't have a problem dealing with both. But the clinical people over there weren't as welcome at the research center. Bill Martin wanted people there who were very seriously interested in research. . . . The ARC under Bill Martin was more questioning and challenging every aspect of treatment in the field, whereas the CRC had to accept some treatments as effective in order to be operative. . . . The CRC's task was to treat the people that were there and to help them stay off of substances. The ARC's task was to question all the treatments to find which were effective and which weren't, and to hopefully get better treatments over time. (2006)

This tension between the thoroughgoing skepticism of the research enterprise and the pragmatic orientation on the treatment side was structural, ideological, and enduring. It came from an unresolved contradiction between the will to know the Other and the therapeutic processes that supposedly work to "normalize" so-called deviant behavior.

Lexington administrators and NIMH officials made several moves designed to strengthen or modernize both treatment and the kind of clinical research that was conducted at the CRC. Proposals were floated in the summer of 1970 to import the Overholser Division of Clinical Research from St. Elizabeth's Hospital in Washington, D.C., so as to make the CRC a true clinical research center. The ARC supported the plan to overhaul the CRC, but it was never realized. The CRC nevertheless explored new treatment approaches, most notably so-called therapeutic communities, modeled on Synanon in California and Daytop in New York City. In January 1969, Stanley Yolles, then director of NIMH, recommended implementing self-help approaches at the CRC, and transforming Lexington from a security-oriented institution to a modern therapeutic community. The resulting self-organized and self-governed therapeutic communities—with such names as Numen House, Excelsior House, or Ascension House (for women)—were regionally or racially homogenous.

The most notorious of these experiments was the short-lived Matrix House, which opened in January 1970. Later that year, when the *Lexington Herald* declared, "Narco Dead: Clinical Research Center Revamped to Replace 'Terror Prison' of Past" (October 13, 1970), it used Matrix House to exemplify the change. Reporter Bill Powell favorably noted a "cheerful" visage and a staff ratio of almost one-to-one. By July 1971, administrators had phased out Matrix House because it appealed "only [to] a limited and atypical segment of the addict population."[20] Subsequent accusations of misconduct by the ex-addicts who ran Matrix House led to a civil suit in which a federal grand jury criticized NIMH management of the CRC and, on November 10, 1972, indicted two ex-addict former staff members and two patients involved in Matrix House.

Social change came late to Lexington, arriving in forms that many local staff members found threatening or unsettling. Given the racialization of narcotics problems and drug law enforcement in the United States, a substantial cultural divide between clinical staff and the patients they treated had been growing. In the fall of 1970, a committee for equal employment opportunity investigated allegations made by one of the only African American staff at the CRC of "an ideology that keeps the Negro at the bottom rung of the authorative [*sic*] and economic ladder."[21] Although an internal investigation determined this allegation was unfounded, the incident indicates rising institutional awareness of the changing political climate regarding civil rights.

Researchers at the ARC constantly negotiated boundaries between acceptable and unacceptable risk, justifiable and unjustifiable research. On balance, they did so in ways that were ethical within the parameters of their time. Researchers who began careers there recall a reverence for human life, an appreciation for addicts as human beings, and a research culture based on relationships of mutual respect and social intermingling. Most had come to Lexington knowing little about addiction or research. The social meaning of an "addict" was not the same at Lexington as elsewhere, due to the pervasive familiarity between "addicts" and "nonaddicts" and the lack of any sense of threat from addicts or judgments toward them. Researchers also remember discussions about how to ensure that consent was truly informed, how to design studies so as to safeguard subjects from harm, and how to guarantee the integrity of results. Charles Gorodetzky, a twenty-year Lexington veteran put it:

> I can never think of any time at ARC when the ethics of informed consent research were not impressed on me. I think there was every bit as much concern for the rights of people, the rights of privacy, the dictums of do-no-harm, the dictums of doing beneficial research that was well-constructed that did not harm, the issues of risks versus benefits. (2003)

While at Lexington, Gorodetzky learned to walk what he called "the tightrope between coercion and seduction," without tipping toward either extreme.

> You can't coerce people into research—it has to be free informed consent. I think we went out of our way to get free informed consent. Of course, we were getting informed consent from prisoners, and that's where the ethical climate was different. Because after it developed in 1977, by definition it was agreed that a prisoner could not give free informed consent, because they were in prison. I

> thought that was a very narrow point of view. I thought they did give free informed consent. I think we went out of our way to make sure that they could give their consent freely.

Coercion was not, however, the main situation to which the indigenous ethics of the ARC was structured to reply. The main concern, as Gorodetzky explained, was "seduction," the principled avoidance of enticements or compensation that would be considered disproportionate in the institutional context.

> The other thing we could not do is try to seduce them into research. Seduction had the very practical operational definition of not being able to offer them money or extra time off their sentences. What we were able to offer was exactly the same as they could earn by working in prison industry. We could not offer them anything more. Now they did get more personal attention. Obviously, there were people paying attention to them all the time. They probably got somewhat better medical care when they were with us, because we were concerned with doing frequent physicals and keeping track of vital signs and all the things you would do especially in a chronic study. [But] those were never offered to them in that way, it was never presented to them in that way. (2003)

A shared ethical discourse concerning the need to avoid unethical coercion or seduction was indigenous to the ARC. This ethical discourse was a narrowly technical discourse that evolved far from the political currents of civil rights, prisoners' rights, and patients' rights that subsequently came to pose a serious challenge to the ARC (see chap. 6 of the present book). The indigenous morality of the ARC never extended to the broader question that would be posed in the mid-1970s: Are prisoners free to give uncoerced consent from a position of structural coercion? This question did not arise within the laboratory logics of the ARC but instead arose forcefully from a political space beyond them.

By documenting what scientists who worked at the ARC said and did to contribute to public science and public health, this chapter has shown how they enacted what they strongly believed to be ethical research. The next chapter contrasts the ARC's standards for informed consent with those of the military and intelligence "drug research programs" to which the research program at Lexington was publicly compared during the prison research debates. A new governing bioethics regime emerged from the political struggle between the performative politics of congressional hearings and the "modest witnessing" of scientific expertise (Haraway 1997). This clash changed the meaning of "expertise" and "ethical science" by painting scientists, particularly those who worked for the Public Health Service, as needing congressional oversight and regulatory discipline. Those responsible for the ARC—namely, Isbell and Martin—became subjects of ad hominem attacks, and their careers were essentially sacrificed to the political process. Martin retired from the PHS in 1977 but, like his predecessors Isbell and Wikler, stayed on in Lexington, where he worked at the University of Kentucky until his premature death in 1986. The tragedy of this moment was that there was so little room for careful deliberation about how research on drug addiction could further involve multiple publics.

Much of the ARC research took place beyond the public gaze, and administrators there were proud of their ability to buffer researchers from the political currents that flowed from Washington, D.C. Thus the ARC's relationship with its congressional sponsors was tenuous. Few elected representatives understood the nature of the research well enough to have a sense of the stakes involved in ending it. The data-driven nature of the ARC made the pharmaceutical industry an undependable ally, because new products often turned out to be addictive according to the ARC. Such findings did not earn the laboratory friends among Big Pharma. Nor did ARC scientists have academic counterparts or peers among state-run prison research programs, including industry testing programs, which engaged in neither the kind of basic research nor the kind of public health research and regulatory science conducted in Lexington. For decades, social isolation had protected the research programs; reviews of both the clinical and the research programs cast them as essential to the public health.[22] However, the frequency of program reviews increased in the early 1970s. Growing tensions between the ARC and the CRC became evident as Lexington began to come apart at the seams.[23]

The very isolation of the ARC became a liability in the 1970s, when activist groups fueled several rounds of congressional scrutiny relevant to the laboratory. Congressional hearings are performative arenas that display conflict for political purposes; they are not structured to provide a forum for negotiating in a deliberative or judicious fashion. Various task forces, advisory committees, and congressional investigations were set up to evaluate the research program. According to Gorodetzky, each of them concluded "what we were doing at the ARC was really state-of-the-art in terms of ethical considerations," but "they still threw out federal prisoner research in '76, and they still gave Harris Isbell a hard time . . . for the things that occurred in the '50s" (2003). Although I am persuaded that there was an indigenous ethics at the ARC, it is clear that ethics were conceptualized as of an individualistic, rather than a systemic, character.

Researchers there had a relatively narrow repertoire of collective ethical positions. Gorodetzky put it:

> I think all of us who were involved with the ARC always felt that we were doing things really with the highest ethical and moral standards. And I don't think any of us ever really felt personally that we were stretching the lines, doing things that were dangerous, doing things that were not scientifically justified. Because everything was reviewed and rereviewed. We were under very stringent regulations on what we could reward and not reward. . . . I never remember any treatment of a prisoner that was less than humane. (2003)

One need not question the sincerity of researchers' ethical commitments to recognize that they did not focus on the kinds of questions that came to the fore when prisoner research was politicized: whether it is possible to volunteer in structurally coercive contexts, how to safeguard privacy and confidentiality in a situation devoted to observation and surveillance, or whether access to health care should be conditioned upon participation in research. Such concerns evidently did not arise at the ARC, despite its precocious attention to informed consent and experimental design with knowing subjects.

Why should one expect such questions to have been raised in the terms that came to prevail in the 1970s? To impose such expectations retrospectively is to commit the error historians refer to as "presentism"—viewing the past through the lens of the present. The scientific ethical imaginary that prevailed at Lexington prohibited coercion or seduction of subjects. Lack of seduction—under the rule that subjects could be compensated no differently from work in the laundry, kitchen, grounds, morgue, or "needle works" (the sewing room)—was taken to signal that coercion was not taking place. Coercion was defined not as structural coercion (the kind that is inevitable in the prison environment or in any highly unequal situation) but as individual coercion. Negotiating "the tightrope between coercion and seduction" was an everyday matter at the ARC. Readers may think that there was less reflection than there should have been on power relations between researcher and researched, white and black, rich and poor. But that does not mean that observers in our era can reasonably expect people in the historical situation to have behaved according to standards that evolved in the political crucible of the mid- to late 1970s.

This chapter has broadened the range of questions concerning the calculus of suffering with which it began. Did lack of ethical reflection place subjects in situations of harm? Were the risks that accrued to the laboratory logics of substitution and mimicry too high? Or were the risks so great that no one could knowingly consent to them? Conversely, might there not have been unseen or incalculable benefits for participants? How should we weigh the fact that narcotic addicts regularly subjected themselves to high risk outside the laboratory? Ultimately, should the scientific experiments described in this chapter not have been done? The outcomes of these studies—modulating the pain of withdrawal with methadone, responding effectively to opiate overdose, or saving narcotics addicts from frontal lobotomy—did not simply benefit the rich. We must then ask whether participation in this kind of research can be reduced to a form of "interest" paid by the poor. My analysis has shown how essential these studies were to establishing a knowledge base. Far from being unethical, the research program yielded broadly distributed benefits to persons from the addicted classes.

CHAPTER 6

"The Great Hue and Cry": Prison Reform and the Ethics of Human Subjects Research

"The Panopticon is a privileged space for experiments on men, and for analysing with complete certainty the transformations that may be obtained from them" (Foucault 1979, 204). The Panopticon was not only a surveillance mechanism but a "laboratory of power," which "could be used as a machine to carry out experiments, to alter behavior, to train and correct individuals." It could be used "[t]o experiment with medicines and monitor their effects" and "[t]o try out different punishments on prisoners, according to their crimes and character, and to seek the most effective ones" (Foucault 1979, 203). Foucault drew the dilemma starkly: there was room for neither individual nor collective motive within the Panopticon. The callous could do nothing different from the compassionate. Measured according to this nihilistic yardstick, clinical research amounts to nothing more than an inquisitorial procedure. The metaphor situates the Panopticon as an engine for disindividualizing power, which rendered inconsequential the motives of any individual involved in operating the machine: "It does not matter what motive animates him: the curiosity of the indiscreet, the malice of a child, the thirst for knowledge of a philosopher who wishes to visit this museum of human nature, or the perversity of those who take pleasure in spying and punishing" (Foucault 1979, 204).

Do the motives that animate research matter? I have contended that the motives of the researchers at the ARC shaped the research process and its outcomes in mostly laudable directions. Many people have asked me whether the ARC should be characterized along the same lines of the Public Health Service study of the natural course of untreated syphilis in African American men (Jones 1981/1992; Reverby 2000). The Tuskegee Study of Untreated Syphilis in the Negro Male continued even after effective treatment became available, and the more I learned about Lexington, the less appropriate such comparisons seemed.

Research ethics must be situated within the social conditions, material constraints, and commitments that prevail in specific institutional contexts. Research at the ARC took place within a federal narcotics hospital set up to deliver drug treatment on a massive scale. Treatment at Lexington was not "cure" but gradual withdrawal, detoxification, and abstinence, mixed with psychotherapy and vocational rehabilitation.[1] The Lexington and Fort Worth hospitals set a humane standard of care in contrast to the abrupt withdrawal cold turkey practiced in jails without medical supervision. Unlike the Tuskegee study, treatment was not withheld at Lexington, where the primary goal was achieving a sustained period of abstinence before release. One of the troubling features of the ARC was the administration of drugs that undermined abstinence; research participants were, at least in the early days, rewarded in their drug of choice; some, no doubt, were enticed by the prisoner grapevine's promise of drugs in a "drug-free" setting. A second problematic feature was the racial profile of Lexington admissions in the post–World War II era, when the general population was increasingly composed of poor, young, racial-ethnic minorities. However, it turned out not to be the case that they ever became the majority of research participants. Research subjects tended to be older, more affluent, and white. Written informed consent was obtained; after the summer of 1949, formal written consent forms were read aloud to participants who could not read.[2] Himmelsbach also indicated that consent was obtained from the program's earliest days (1972, 1994).

Despite the fact that African American inmates were not disproportionately experimented on, there remains something unsettling to present sensibilities about systematic research programs housed within structurally coercive institutions. Should research oriented toward understanding addiction and relapse not have been undertaken? Could any research be conducted ethically in any prison? Such questions came to a head in the struggles related in this chapter. The laboratory logics, experimental practices, and ethical norms at Lexington varied over time, which should make us reluctant to issue a blanket condemnation or to measure the ARC by today's standards. We should also be cautious about uncritically adopting the frames that the 1970s prison rights movement used to cast aspersion on all prison research in order to better advance the case for reforms. Such frameworks were not designed to differentiate between greater goods, lesser harms, and necessary evils. Ending prison research became a symbolic terrain on which reformers portrayed themselves as upholding the rights of the disenfranchised. Key Democratic congressional leaders sponsored the hearings that were the mechanism by which the scientific work of the ARC was discredited and its conduit to research subjects cut off. Negative publicity was one means by which the reformers secured their own good name as guardians or protectors of the rights of prisoners. This was, however, a contest over whose constructions of "rights" and "protections" would win out.

HOW LEXINGTON BECAME AN OLD-FASHIONED PRISON

A banner year in the outcry over prison reform and human experimentation, 1973 caught the reluctant jailers at the ARC by surprise. By then, they held the keys to the only federal facility where prisoners still served as subjects. The research staff was responsible for order and discipline among the between forty and sixty federal prisoners who elected to transfer to the ARC. The laboratory became a "miniprison" just when prison research was brought to crisis. Never nuanced, the politics of crisis created the impression that unconstrained biomedical researchers badly needed external oversight and that legislators needed to provide it.[3] The American Correctional Association (ACA), the national accreditation body for U.S. prisons, created its first informed consent protocol for correctional institutions in 1972. The ACA was inspired by a scandal involving Southern Food and Drug Research Incorporated, a "Phase I drug-testing empire" headed by Austin R. Stough, MD, a physician untrained in pharmacology (Harkness 2003, 218–30). Jessica Mitford exposed Stough in a highly publicized *Atlantic Monthly* article in January 1973.[4] She drew favorable attention to the American Civil Liberties Union's National Prison Project, which had begun litigating prison abuse cases six months before, when Alvin Bronstein became the executive director.[5] The ACA then reversed course and disallowed prison research entirely by withholding accreditation from any facility where it was conducted. That move reconfigured the terrain on which prison research took place, just before several controversies came to public notice.

News of the Tuskegee scandal broke in the summer of 1972. Senator Edward Kennedy's Committee on Labor and Public Welfare moved quickly into investigative hearings, to which were invited former ARC director Harris Isbell and ex-Lexington inmates Eddie Flowers and James Henderson Childs.[6] The hearings led to formation in 1974 of the National Commission for the Protection of Human Subjects of Biomedical and Behavioral Research.[7] This commission provided a conduit for new forms of bioethical expertise. Over the next several years, the commission documented the scope of prison research through site visits to the ARC and other drug-testing operations in state prisons. Anticipating an election year, Senator Robert Kastenmeier held hearings in the fall of 1975 on a bill to end prisoner experimentation. Witnesses included three ex-research participants and the current ARC research director, William R. Martin, who had assumed the reins at the ARC after Isbell's departure.[8] Finally, to investigate a project dubbed MKULTRA, conducted under the umbrella of the Central Intelligence Agency (CIA), Senator Frank Church held hearings in 1975, with a follow-on hearing in 1977.[9] Church sought the Democratic presidential nomination in 1976, eventually conceding it to Ford. All of the hearings previously mentioned were convened by Democrats seeking reelection.

The National Commission for the Protection of Human Subjects never banned federal prisoner research outright. However, a new political consensus placed prisoners in the category of subjects most vulnerable to disrespect, lack of benefit, and unfairness in the conduct of research. Given their circumstances, prisoners might be selected for "administrative convenience" or because they were "cheaper than chimpanzees," as Mitford put it (1973b, 138). Three principles—respect for persons, beneficence, and distributive justice—appeared in the commission's culminating document, *The Belmont Report* (National Commission 1978).[10] Each principle was to be applied to informed consent, determination of risk and benefit, and subject selection. Fearing that "social undesirables" might be subjected to exceptional risk, the commission stated a preference that "dependent" or "vulnerable" subjects not participate in research at all.

> One special instance of injustice results from the involvement of vulnerable subjects. Certain groups, such as racial minorities, the economically disadvantaged, the very sick, and the institutionalized may continually be sought as research subjects, owing to their ready availability in settings where research is conducted. Given their dependent status and their frequently compromised capacity for free consent, they should be protected against the danger of being involved in research solely for administrative convenience, or because they are easy to manipulate as a result of their illness or socioeconomic condition. (National Commission 1978)

Drug users have historically been constructed as unreliable subjects because they are easily manipulated and are seen as themselves manipulative (Campbell 2000). Aspects of long-term, chronic drug use and the criminalization of drug use has compounded this public perception. Although addiction went unmentioned in *The Belmont Report,* both illness and imprisonment were found to undermine the capacity for free consent. When the commission required experimenters to guarantee that consent was informed, selection unbiased, and benefit direct, those conducting research with convicted drug-using felons faced insurmountable challenges in continuing their work.

When ARC researchers first told me that they were surprised at the official decision to fold the human research program at Lexington, I was skeptical, until I uncovered considerable evidence that the ARC had been exempt from the generalized political critique of prison research by everyone other than congressional staff. For instance, staff of the National Commission for the Protection of Human Subjects were dispatched to Lexington on May 3, 1976, for a site visit. According to Jasinski, who became director of the ARC after Martin retired in 1977, the commission "found that we had already been doing informed consent [with] all the safeguards." Jasinski continued:

> They didn't say you couldn't do prisoner research, but that you needed some extra safeguards. [W]e had a system which had multiple safeguards. . . . [T]here hadn't been an injury or death in forty years doing this type of research. The Presidential Commission was going to say that, to find that what we were doing was okay. (2003)

In contrast to most commercial Phase 1 studies in state prisons, many of the oversight bodies recognized that the ARC research was essential for providing data for domestic and international drug policy and considered it to be ethically aboveboard.

Nevertheless, the Bureau of Prisons (BOP) cut the ARC adrift from the literally captive population of postaddicts on whom it had relied for almost forty years.

> This became a decision by the administration. We had been receiving cooperation from the Bureau of Prisons. One day Norm Carlson, who had been the director of the Bureau of Prisons, called and said that he was going to end the prisoner program. (Jasinski 2003)

Carlson's reversal changed the definition of what counted as addiction research, who conducted it, how and where they went about it, and how they felt about it. Personally uncomfortable with prisoner research,[11] Carlson had been pressured to broker a phaseout deal with the National Institute on Drug Abuse (NIDA) in the wake of the Kastenmeier hearings, during which Lexington ex-inmates had given damaging and dramatic testimony about their participation in ARC studies.[12] Meanwhile, the broader institution of Lexington shifted away from being a destination solely for drug addicts. Under Nixonian drug policy, responsibility for drug treatment continued to devolve (today, it often resides at the county level). Although access issues remain, treatment is far more available than it was when Lexington and Fort Worth were the only providers. By 1973, Lexington had become an obsolete and "rather expensive anachronism," in the words of Jerome H. Jaffe, director of Nixon's White House Special Action Office for Drug Abuse Prevention (Walsh 1973a, 1004). The institution was transferred completely to the BOP in 1974, and the ARC was then absorbed into NIDA.[13] After 1974, the broader institution at Lexington became what its founders insisted it should never be—an old-fashioned prison that had nothing to do with treatment, rehabilitation, or research.[14] Although the ARC program continued until the end of 1976, it had become clear that change was in the offing.

RACE AND THE CONSTRUCTION OF VULNERABILITY: THE POLITICS OF REFORM AND RESEARCH

Since the first mandatory minimum sentences (instituted by the 1951 Boggs Act), incarceration has been the main plank of U.S. drug policy. Criminalization can be pegged to changing patterns in the racialization of drug-using populations and to drug law enforcement in urban settings. Enormous numbers of African Americans have been imprisoned on drug charges since the mid-1950s. By 1955, two-thirds of the eleven hundred drug offenders housed at Lexington were African Americans addicted to heroin.[15] Only seven years prior, two-thirds had been white. Although the heroin-addicted population grew disproportionately poor, urban, and black, racial conflict rarely rose to administrative attention at Lexington until the late 1960s, when the discourse of civil rights was mobilized within the institution. Racial difference was certainly a practical matter of lived experience at Lexington, where there was a flourishing African American jazz culture. Ex-inmate Eddie Flowers differentiated the racial dynamics of Lexington in the 1950s from those of northern penitentiaries, noting that membership in drug subcultures superseded racial conflict between inmates at Lexington. Racial disparities in drug conviction rates have widened since Lexington closed its doors; they are best attributed not to consumption patterns but to law enforcement patterns, the political economy of global drug trafficking networks, and the cultural geography of drug markets. The racial politics of the U.S. wars on drugs have rendered drug laws "the new Jim Crow" (Boyd 2001).

Prison research became a civil rights target in the 1970s, when some movement leaders charged that research subjugated black bodies. At the 1976 National Minority Conference on Human Experimentation, held by the National Commission for the Protection of Human Subjects, concerns that African Americans bore a disproportionate share of the risks of prison research arose. Such allegations had previously cropped up in a highly publicized case involving a University of Maryland research program (studying infectious disease) conducted at the Maryland House of Corrections in Jessup, Maryland—despite the fact that civil rights leaders became aware that most research subjects were white early in the conflict (Gilchrist 1974). The commission's national fact-finding mission also revealed that research subjects were mainly white, better educated, and employed at the "better" jobs even in predominantly white institutions (National Commission 1976b, 9). Research participants at the State Prison of Southern Michigan in Jackson, Michigan, were also disproportionately white, older, and more experienced with prison life (National Commission 1976b, 36). At Jackson, they were overwhelmingly from the "honor block." The commission determined that African Americans comprised less than one-third of research subjects nationally. Black prisoners actually complained to the commission that there was a selection bias against their participation.

Lexington reflected this national trend. Never did blacks outnumber whites in the research ward. Entirely white study populations were not uncommon prior to when the Narcotic Addict Rehabilitation Act (NARA) went into effect in 1968. After that, the BOP supplied between forty and sixty subjects to the ARC at any given time, dividing them so that the research population would be approximately one-third white, one-third black, and one-third Hispanic. Always in search of seasoned subjects, the ARC upped its age eligibility from twenty-one to twenty-five years old in 1968, to ensure that it did not exploit adolescents. Although it failed to find that the risks of research tilted unevenly toward blacks, the National Commission for the Protection of Human Subjects certainly recognized that the benefits of research tilted toward the affluent. Adopting a language of redistribution, the commission wrote:

> Some populations, especially institutionalized ones, are already burdened in many ways by their infirmities and environments. When research is proposed that involves risks and does not include a therapeutic component, other less burdened classes of persons should be called upon first to accept these risks of research, except where the research is directly related to the specific conditions of the class involved. Also, even though public funds for research may often flow in the same directions as public funds for health care, it seems unfair that populations dependent on public health care constitute a pool of preferred research subjects if more advantaged populations are likely to be the recipients of the benefits. (National Commission 1978)

The commission allowed research to continue if it was "directly related to the specific conditions of the class involved." The category "addicts" was not a named class and in fact had multiple strikes against counting as a "class" in the calculus of vulnerability. Most drug-addicted prisoners were black, ill, or indigent, and all were institutionalized. Under the terms set by the commission, they were multiply vulnerable subjects. The fact that most participants in prison drug research had historically been white did not assure that the vulnerable would be screened out in the future.

The charge that prison researchers exploited subjects was made forcefully by the American Bar Association, which formed the Correctional Economics Center (CEC) in early 1973 to apply economics—the "science of choice" (Meyer 1975, 7)—to prisoner experimentation.[16] In early 1975, the CEC issued a report titled *Medical Experimentation on Prisoners: Some Economic Considerations.* Authored by Peter B. Meyer, the report rendered a highly politicized and emotional question as a logical and analytical matter of the fair distribution of benefits and burdens. According to Meyer, pharmaceutical manufacturers won an "implicit subsidy" when prisoners agreed to bear risks that their "outside counterparts" refused (1975, 7).[17] Pharmaceutical companies were deeply dependent on prisoners for Phase 1 testing.[18] However, the ARC was uninterested in organizing risky Phase 1 clinical trials, which often involved screening drugs that would never make it to market because of toxicity or low tolerability (Meyer 1975, 9). The unit was uninterested in testing drugs that no one was likely to take, focusing primarily on drugs that not only made it to market but remain widely used today and on illicit drugs. Moreover, the ARC was not set up to do the kind of pharmacokinetic studies of safety required in Phase 1 testing and thus never performed "first man" studies (first trials in human beings). Finally, the ARC did not profit from direct relationships with pharmaceutical companies, although it worked closely with Merck and others. Its work cannot be said to represent an "implicit subsidy," because it was basically a form of specialized government oversight.

Although elucidating the neurophysiology of addiction was the ARC's raison d'être, experimentees often misremember the role they played in studies. Sociological studies show that participants attach significance to their role by attributing more risk to it. When social scientists sought to determine the impact of pharmacological testing programs on prisoners, they found inmates "readily report[ed] their consent to be informed" even when it was not. Like their unincarcerated counterparts, prisoners "affirmed informed consent without really possessing it," for reasons including low literacy levels, poor memory, or cognitive issues attributed to power differentials between researchers and themselves (Wells et al. 1975, 49). Two-thirds of those who signed forms listing side effects that clearly stated, "This drug has been previously given to man by mouth in doses up to 2000 mg/day," could not recall reading that statement. After two weeks, participants "claimed . . . the drug had never previously been tested on human subjects." Wells et al. took this to mean that the subjects "wanted to believe, took pride in believing, that they were the initial volunteers, the pioneers performing an act requiring courage and one which marked them for some, if not great, distinction" (1975, 52). Recommending that prison officials not only tolerate researchers inside prison walls but welcome them, Wells et al. viewed pharmacological research as a highly positive and beneficial activity that enhanced prisoners' self-esteem and productivity and reduced their "aggression": "Opportunities for the inmate to interact favorably with well-disposed individuals from the society outside the prison walls, to experience the meaningful satisfaction of having been of service, to feel an often lacking sense of importance and to supplement his often intensely frustrating lack of financial resources may be absent elsewhere in the prison environment" (Wells et al. 1975, 53).

Widening inmates' research participation would not have been the advice of three former ARC subjects—Kenneth Matthews, Richard Alexander, and Otis Clay—who testified on September 29, 1975, the first day of the Kastenmeier hearings. These witnesses presented themselves as vulnerable and exploited, recounting having been lured to Lexington by the promise of drugs, better food, and easier living. Jon Harkness reports: "They also conveyed to the House Subcommittee a perception that, once in the research facility, they had not received adequate explanations of proposed research projects from ARC scientists. And they alleged that ARC researchers had not treated them with kindness and respect" (2003, 278). Two days later, William R. Martin refuted these allegations in a formal rebuttal to Kastenmeier that relied on experimental data and remained almost entirely within the discursive restraints of scientific discourse.

Under court order, Martin refrained from mentioning that Otis Clay was personally motivated to portray the ARC in a negative light because Clay had filed an "inartistically drafted" pro se lawsuit in 1971 against Martin, Carlson, Jasinski, and other high U.S. government officials.[19] The lawsuit was ultimately dismissed, but at the time of the Kastenmeier hearings, an appellate court had just reinstated Clay's complaint and reversed a lower court's dismissal.[20] Clay's case was reopened when the U.S. Court of Appeals for the Second Circuit permitted him to amend his complaint in April 1975. Martin's response to Clay's congressional testimony revealed that Clay's answers in the drug study were at odds with his testimony. While Clay told the congressional committee that he left an experimental pain study because he could not stand it, Martin contended that Clay had characterized the electroshocks he received as not painful, weak, slightly painful, or average. Whereas Clay had testified to having been physically restrained, Martin insisted that subjects were not restrained. Martin stuck close to the facts as he saw them and studiously avoided the far more important question—restrained or not, why were human beings being subjected to electroshock while on drugs?

Failing to communicate the scientific rationale for the studies, much less deliver a defense of them, Martin was unable to counter the ex-inmates' testimony. Nor did he marshal the relevant scientific communities that later rallied around the ARC when it was, to all appearances, too late. The ex-inmates won a discursive and political victory that provided the nails in the coffin of the ARC at Lexington. Although the information in Clay's court documents is limited, it is also instructive in terms of the construction of vulnerability then under way. Claiming he had been treated inhumanely and had suffered a heart attack a week after participating in a two-dose naltrexone study, Clay sought two million dollars in damages. Fifty-one years old when, in 1968, he requested a transfer to the ARC from the Atlanta Penitentiary, where he was serving a ten-year sentence on federal narcotics charges, Clay stated that he was "attracted by the better living conditions at the ARC and the possibility of receiving narcotics under the experimentation program" (*Otis Clay, Plaintiff-Appellant v. Dr. William R. Martin et al. and The United States Surgeon General et al. The United States Defendants-Appellees* 509 F.2d 109–14 (2d Cir. 1975)). During his two-year stay, Clay consented to studies involving morphine, pentazocine, naltrexone, and chlorpromazine. His lawsuit claimed that he had participated involuntarily, and he charged the researchers with having a conflict of interest between their research, administrative, and custodial roles. His testimony played up his personal vulnerability and the structural conditions within which the ARC experiments were conducted.

Following the hearing, in a letter written on November 11, 1975, Kastenmeier urged Carlson to end his "continuing commitment" to supplying research subjects for research conducted at Lexington for the Department of Health, Education, and Welfare (DHEW).[21] Carlson then appointed a task force to determine what the conditions of true voluntarism for biomedical research should be. That body came up with five conditions.[22] First, rewards could not include "meritorious good time" off a sentence. Second, volunteers had to come from "less restrictive circumstances" at the time the choice to participate in research was made. These two conditions alone would have created an entirely new set of administrative circumstances and recruitment logistics for the ARC, by giving prisoners little incentive to transfer. Third, a general fund into which research sponsors were to place supplementary monies for the well-being of prisoners was required, so that prisoners would cost researchers the same amount as free-living volunteers. Unlike the terms on which commercially sponsored prison research was conducted, the ARC had always "borrowed" subjects, paying them nothing beyond the wages they would have received for sewing uniforms, woodworking, or doing agricultural, custodial, or food service work elsewhere in the institution. Given that pharmaceutical companies did not pay the ARC but instead funneled paltry, voluntary donations to the NRC committee that coordinated communication between industry and the ARC, the proposed fee structure would have prohibited the ARC from relying on prisoners even if the BOP continued supplying them. Fourth, the task force required establishment of a "subject advisory group" consisting of prisoners themselves. Lastly, subjects were to be compensated for "all lasting injury or loss of earnings suffered as a result of participation in a research project," a stipulation that would open the ARC to litigation.

Although it set the bar high, the BOP task force unanimously agreed that "the Bureau [should] continue to participate in the valuable research being done at the Addiction Research Center" (Harkness 2003, 286). But Carlson discontinued sending federal prisoners to the ARC and quietly worked out a deal with Robert DuPont, the director of the new NIDA, to end research by the end of 1976.[23] On March 1, 1976, Carlson justified this incremental approach to Kastenmeier as showing respect for the "significant research that has resulted in the past from this program" and permitting the researchers "to continue with the programs they have already initiated at that facility." Attempting to gain some political capital by hurrying things along, Kastenmeier leaked Carlson's letter to the *Washington Post* before dropping the bill. DuPont placed an "irate" call to Carlson to complain that the BOP was "reneging" on its commitment to a gradual phaseout.[24] In the end, political expediency, rather than "abstract arguments concerning the ethical validity of experimentation with prisoners," ended biomedical research in federal prisons (Harkness 2003, 304). The political spectacle displayed in the congressional hearings also played a part in ending the practice, by embarrassing the scientific community and overshadowing its reasoned responses.

Clearly, Carlson believed that continued medical experimentation on federal prisoners was unwise. In a letter of October 2, 1975, to Harold R. Tyler, Deputy Attorney General Carlson conveyed the gist of his testimony before the Kastenmeier committee. Stating that he had "serious doubts about the ability of prisoners to volunteer," Carlson noted that he supported the bill's "general thrust" to ban medical research on prisoners altogether. Dutifully, he explained that the ARC used federal prisoners "to test abuse potentialities of opiate-like drugs" and search for "antagonistic drugs to counteract the effects of addictive drugs," while he distanced the BOP from the project, evidently considering it NIDA's problem. Like Kastenmeier, Carlson had become convinced that most biomedical research then being conducted with prisoners could be conducted more ethically on nonprisoner populations. Diametrically opposed, the scientific community considered the turn to other populations neither feasible nor ethical.

SCIENCE STEPS IN: RESPONSES FROM RELEVANT SCIENTIFIC COMMUNITIES

A deluge of letters praising the ARC research program as essential to the global drug policy regime and to the growth of scientific knowledge on the effects of drugs on brain and body came from the scientific community. An NIMH research task force gave this evaluation in its report "Program of the Addiction Research Center, 1935–Present":

> By any measure, the program of the ARC has been an outstanding success for 38 years and is currently as vigorous as any time in its illustrious history. There have over the years been natural changes in programs and goals of the ARC and changes in emphasis, which were due to changes in either the staff or interests of the principle [*sic*] investigators. Without any reservation, I believe that the

> drug assessment program of the ARC has been, from every point of view, one of the most outstanding and effective public health endeavors in preventing drug abuse. No drug that has been evaluated at the ARC and has been judged to have a low abuse potentiality has given rise to any significant abuse problem. There have been a very large number of drugs, however, where pharmacologic properties are closely similar to those of heroin and morphine and dilaudid, which if they had been uncontrolled most certainly had the potential for creating major problems of abuse. (29–30)[25]

This report is typical: it lauded the ARC for playing a positive role in public health. By contrast the Clinical Research Center (CRC)—as the therapeutic and custodial side of Lexington was called after 1968—did not enjoy such esteem. Its reputation was low within the addiction research enterprise. On January 30, 1973, director Harold Conrad's memo to all ARC and CRC employees assured them that there were no plans to close the ARC but indicated that the CRC might close down. Why, then, was the internationally known, venerable human research program of the ARC shut down in 1976?

Scientists expressed considerable resistance to ending research not only at Lexington but in prisons more generally. For them, a major factor was the regulatory climate set up by the 1962 amendments to the Food, Drug, and Cosmetics Act (1938), which made large-scale clinical trials mandatory. Not only did the amendments require proof of a drug's safety and efficacy, but the particular disease or condition for which it was effective had to be named. This regulatory requirement presented a dilemma to which moral repugnance and prisoner rights could only partly reply: large-scale drug testing of the type that was then largely carried out in state prisons was required for the regulatory process. What would happen if prison research was banned? Some members of the National Commission for the Protection of Human Subjects believed that prisoners should be allowed to participate if trials were conducted off prison grounds—as long as nonprisoners also joined the study for the same compensation. Others felt prisoners would then participate just to get off-site. The commission encouraged researchers to develop "alternative populations" for Phase 1 trials (National Commission 1976b, 11). Although the commission recognized that FDA regulatory requirements triggered pharmacologists' involvement in prisoner research, they provided no guidance as to how the mandates would be met once prisoners were no longer eligible.

Regulatory requirements were a side issue for the ARC, which had far more at stake. Scientific associations flooded the commission with letters of support. Rather than write to the commission chair, Martin appealed directly to fellow pharmacologist and commissioner Joseph V. Brady several times in late 1975. In a letter of September 3, 1975, Martin tried to reframe the ACLU's interpretation of individual civil liberties, warning, "Those who wish to preserve liberty and freedom of the individual by curtailing therapeutic research on psychopaths may find that their efforts will have quite the opposite long-term impact." Pointing out how the "disease process" of "prisoner psychopaths" overtaxed national resources by increasing mortality and morbidity from alcoholism and addiction, Martin warned that repressive laws were likely to be put into place if further research on the disease of addiction and its treatment was hindered. Emphasizing the therapeutic nature of research, Martin urged "sensible reform," rather than outright abolition.[26]

Martin wrote another letter to Brady on December 5, 1975, listing specific ways that skilled clinical investigators could "minimize harm" to participants: "Our society should recognize that participation in human experimentation is an altruistic act for the good of society and should be rewarded as other socially constructive acts." Reframing the question of whether prisoners were capable of informed consent, Martin replayed the ongoing discussion as to whether naive or drug-wise subjects were best for research. Not surprisingly, he favored knowledgeable subjects: "It is my opinion that narcotic addicts who have been the major participants in drug studies of the Addiction Research Center probably give a more knowledgeable consent than do most other patients. From their practical experience they have much more knowledge about what the drugs will do than most other subjects and they understand much of the pharmacologic jargon." No longer referring to subjects as "postaddicts," Martin played on public fears of "addict recidivists," calling them the best research tools because they were uninterested in rehabilitation or perhaps even beyond its reach. Commenting on the idea of finding alternative populations, he wrote, "I cannot think of another population of participants in which the potentiality of inducing an increase in or worsening drug-using behavior would be less."[27] Martin predicted that without studies on addicts, pharmaceutical companies would be freer to place new, uncontrolled drugs on the market, thereby increasing the magnitude of the drug abuse problem.

Dense and closely argued, Martin's letters conveyed a tone of desperation. On January 9, 1976, he traveled to a public hearing held by the National Commission for the Protection of Human Subjects, where he warned that ending prisoner research would "retard development of therapy for addicts and . . . prohibit the evaluation of the addictive properties of analgesics." Martin portrayed participation in the ARC studies as individually beneficial, arguing it was a "safe and constructive experience" that "often improves health" and serves as a "source of pride." Although he agreed that practical measures could reduce the "seductiveness" of the research environment and so reduce subtle coercion, he felt that prisoners and nonprisoners were "equally knowledgeable" about the conduct of research. Citing evidence that prisoners made "informed judgments," Martin stated that prisoner participants should be compensated for their altruism as well as in cases of harm (National Commission 1976b, 45). His position was not paternalistic, and he did not portray prisoners as vulnerable or exploited. Instead, he represented them as adults who could make their own decisions, despite the prison setting.

The spring of 1976 brought a chorus of similar letters from pharmacologists' professional associations, including the Committee on Problems of Drug Dependence (CPDD), the American College of Neuropsychopharmacology, the American Society for Clinical Pharmacology and Therapeutics, and the American Society for Pharmacology and Experimental Therapeutics. Modeled on each other, these associations targeted the chair of the National Commission for the Protection of Human Subjects, Kenneth John Ryan, MD, chair of obstetrics and gynecology at Harvard University. For example, Eddie Leong Way, chair of the Department of Pharmacology of the University of California at San Francisco, stated in a letter dated March 24, 1976, that the phaseout of the ARC was a "devastating blow to progress." Praising the ARC as the "best facility in existence in the world for conducting drug abuse research," he claimed that "studies there have abided by every ethical principle established with respect to human subjects."[28] Given the high public visibility of drug abuse, pharmacologists cast themselves as apprehensive that the bulwark or backbone of drug abuse research was to be eliminated.

The National Academy of Sciences relayed a letter from the chairman of the CPDD, Leo Hollister, who wrote on April 9, 1976, that closing the ARC would present a "major handicap" to the fight against drug abuse.[29] Hollister defended the scientific value and reputation of the ARC, placing the very honor of pharmacology at stake in this struggle. In a letter dated March 26, 1976, Keith F. Killam, Jr., president of the honorary society the American College of Neuropsychopharmacology, depicted the ARC as a "model coupling excellence of research with impeccable regard for the welfare of the subjects."[30] His letter detailed the workings of the CPDD, pointing out that "in practice, the CPDD has acted as a buffer between pharmaceutical companies proposing new narcotic analgesics and those who evaluate them for dependence liability." He argued, "Without the facility at Lexington, this valuable program, which protects the public against the commercial introduction of new drugs with high abuse potential, would be completely devastated." Yet this important argument for protection of the public good was buried in a paragraph on his letter's second page, where it garnered little attention.

These letters were responsible for the decision of the National Commission for the Protection of Human Subjects not to ban biomedical and behavioral research in U.S. prisons. Some members still favored a ban but agreed to allow prisoner research if strict guidelines were met: adequate living conditions, separation of research participation from parole considerations, effective grievance procedures, public scrutiny, the significance or importance of the research, compelling reasons to involve prisoners, and overall fairness (National Commission 1976b, 13). These restrictions would not necessarily have tolled the death knell for prisoner research, for the commission recognized that "in some cases research in prisons is going to be necessary" (Cohn 1976; this article by *Washington Post* reporter Victor Cohn showcased the commission's dismay at the BOP undercutting its authority).

Not wanting to hamper the production of data useful to its reform agenda, the commission encouraged sociological and psychological research into the effects of incarceration or prison conditions if it posed minimal risks. Careful to guard against discrimination resulting from withholding treatment that would directly benefit individual prisoners, the commission distinguished between biomedical research that was related to individual health and well-being and research that was "unrelated to the health or well-being of prisoner-participants" (National Commission 1976b, 15). Interestingly, the ARC served as the commission's prime example of research that was considered "unrelated" to prisoner health and well-being (National Commission 1976b, 23). The commission was equivocal about whether developing new addiction treatments or investigating the nature and causes of addiction to narcotics or alcohol abuse was individually beneficial or not (National Commission 1976b, 26). The lack of clear benefit to the individual, rather than to a class of people, was viewed as problematic given the calculus of risk and benefit put into play at that time.

To document the scope of prisoner research, the commission asked prison administrators and pharmaceutical companies how much drug testing they did on prisoner volunteers. Only sixteen out of fifty-one companies admitted relying on prisoners, yet prisoners still comprised between 85 and 90 percent of subjects in Phase 1 trials overall (Adams and Cowan 1971; National Commission 1976b, 47). Thirty-six hundred prisoners were then participating in one hundred protocols studying seventy-one substances (National Commission 1976b, 31). When the commission made four site visits to prisons where testing occurred, Lexington was not among them. They visited what was then the largest penitentiary in the country, the State Prison of Southern Michigan in Jackson, Michigan, where Upjohn and Parke-Davis, two Michigan-based pharmaceutical companies, had built a research facility on the prison grounds. Prior to the FDA's promulgation of the 1962 amendments, Upjohn had proposed a dedicated facility to the Michigan Corrections Commission; Parke-Davis had gotten involved once the FDA regulations went into effect.[31] For meeting the new FDA requirements, these companies had access to a research pool of about eight hundred subjects who met eligibility criteria (including having an IQ over seventy). The National Commission for the Protection of Human Subjects interviewed eighty Jackson inmates, both participants and nonparticipants, and found that participants "valued the research opportunity" and that nonparticipants did not mind others taking up the opportunity but preferred not to do so themselves (National Commission 1976b, 35).

Prisoners at Jackson apparently valued participating in pharmaceutical drug research. One prisoner participant told Robert J. Levine, a consultant on ethics:

> You tell us you've come here to protect us from the risks of research. But one thing we've noticed is that when you are in those research units, you don't die. . . . But at any moment in the prison yard you could be killed by a fellow inmate for no reason at all that you can identify. You die out here in the yard. If you want to keep us out here in the yard, you are not protecting us. You don't seem to understand that we are living in a place where random death is a way of life. We have noticed that the only place where people don't die here is the research unit. Just what is it you think you're protecting us from? (Levine 1981, 73)

When FDA regulations barring prisoner research were issued in 1980, a group of Jackson prisoners brought suit, and Upjohn soon joined them.[32] Although settled out of court when the FDA issued the indefinite stay of its guidelines that remains in effect, the lawsuit marked some resistance to the de facto moratorium brought about by the correctional community. Even this kind of support from unlikely allies—subjects themselves—could not revive the flagging credibility of the addiction research community. The moral authority of science had been deeply challenged; scientists had been unable to make a politically compelling public case against the charge that they were exploiting prisoners. Disserved by their very modesty, the scientific experts were met by a politicized counterexpertise that contested their motivations, interests, ethics, and findings.

"HUMAN GUINEA PIGS": LIABILITY OF A DIFFERENT KIND

There have been surprisingly few public representations of the ARC's scientific work or the ethical dilemmas crystallized by its laboratory logics. Journalists often devote an obligatory paragraph to condemning research at Lexington, detailing the exploitation of vulnerable subjects at the hands of caricatured "mad scientists." Tarring the ARC with the brush of guilt by association, these accounts link the ARC to the far less systematic drug research conducted by military, law enforcement, and intelligence organizations, notably the CIA, the Army Chemical Corps, and the forerunner of the Drug Enforcement Administration, the Federal Bureau of Narcotics (FBN). Consider this sarcasm:

> One of the first MKULTRA studies conducted was at the National Institute of Mental Health Addiction Research Center in Lexington, Kentucky. At the time it was working hand in hand with the CIA to test and develop new, mind-altering drugs. Young patients, usually drug addicts serving various sentences for drug violations, were offered a chance to volunteer as guinea pigs in exchange for the drug of their addiction. Naturally, the CIA got inundated with eager volunteers jumping at this wonderful opportunity to get free drugs while they were in prison. Each was given a physical examination, administered one of eight hundred or so hallucinogenic drugs, and observed for a few days. They were then given heroin, morphine, or anything else they wanted as payment for their participation. (Goliszek 2003, 158)

Not only does the paragraph just quoted suggest that the CIA ran the ARC, that both organizations developed drugs, and that participants got free rein to decide their rewards, but it fails to acknowledge the ARC's practice of limiting subjects to drug categories with which they had prior experience. It implies that rather than using informed, seasoned felons as participants, the ARC exploited vulnerable youth who would do anything to get drugs.

The Church committee hearings were the source of some of the sensationalistic claims in the paragraph just quoted. Such unsubstantiated and undocumented claims often reappear almost verbatim when the ARC comes up in the hearing documents. Witnesses in the Church hearings described test subjects as "volunteer prisoners who, after taking a brief physical examination and signing a general consent form, were administered hallucinogenic drugs." They explained, "As a reward for participation in the program, the addicts were provided with the drug of their addiction." Yet the next sentence in the hearing documents concerned FBN agents surreptitiously administering LSD to "unwitting nonvolunteer subjects in normal life settings by undercover officials," without concern for dosage or controls (U.S. Congress 1975, 391). Readers of the Church hearing documents could easily mistake all drug research as unethical, rather than sorting out the implications of the very different enterprises in which the FBN and the ARC were engaged.

During the period when the MKULTRA studies were conducted throughout the country, the ARC studied LSD-25 to determine its usefulness as a temporary or "model" psychosis. Well into the 1970s,[33] the ARC studied LSD to discover whether "bad trips" could be cushioned or curtailed by tranquilizers, reserpine, or chlorpromazine and to discuss how its effects compared to psilocybin or mescaline. The laboratory logics of the ARC stood in marked contrast to those of the military and intelligence community, which contracted or conducted LSD research in at least eighteen other sites. However one might define "science," what the CIA and the FBN were doing with hallucinogens was not it. The FBN's drug-testing activities raised "serious questions of command and control within the Bureau," according to the Church committee (U.S. Congress 1975, 421–22). One hesitates to apply the term *studies* to such informal, nonsystematic, and unethical activities.

My initial exposure to the testing program at Lexington came in the form of investigations laced with conspiracy theories, which elided distinctions, erased nuance, and characterized the work in ways that led readers to misinterpret the work of the ARC as science run amok. *The Search for the Manchurian Candidate: The CIA and Mind Control* (1979), by investigative journalist John Marks, delivers a damning judgment for Harris Isbell.

> As Director of the Addiction Research Center at the huge Federal drug hospital in Lexington, Kentucky, he had access to a literally captive population. Inmates heard on the grapevine that if they volunteered for Isbell's program, they would be rewarded either in the drug of their choice or in time off from their sentences. Most of the addicts chose drugs—usually heroin or morphine of a purity seldom seen on the street. The subjects signed an approval form, but they were not told the names of the experimental drugs or the probable effects. This mattered little, since the "volunteers" probably would have granted their informed consent to virtually anything to get hard drugs. (66–67)

Upon first reading this description from Marks, I failed to notice the slippage between witting and unwitting subjects, ethical and unethical practices, and scientific laboratory logics and the amateurish enthusiasms of law enforcement. Representing the ARC studies as "quick and dirty," Marks made it seem as if subjects were in unlimited supply and thus disposable, when few were in fact eligible. Highlighting one "chilling" and "astonishing" study, Marks wrote, "To Dr. Isbell, it was just another experiment, for his 'intense curiosity' and 'relish for the task' shone through his 'dull scientific reports.'" Marks continued: "No corresponding feeling shone through for the inmates, however. In [Isbell's] few recorded personal comments, he complained that his subjects tended to be afraid of the doctors and were not as open in describing their experiences as the experimenters would have wished" (68–69). This description stands in stark contrast to how my interviewees characterized Isbell, who was frequently called on to handle complex cases and had a reputation for being particularly compassionate toward addicted persons (Kornetsky 2003a, 2003b; Mansky 2006).

Testifying before the Kennedy subcommittee in 1975, Isbell described a drug payoff system that had been in place from the institution's founding days (he had first come to Lexington as an intern in 1934–35). "The ethical codes were not so highly developed," he said. Marks made much of this when he located Flowers, one of the ex-inmate research subjects who had testified in the Kennedy hearings. Marks outlined a point system that Flowers claimed had been used to determine drug payoffs: "All he had to do was knock on a little window down the hall. This was the drug bank. The man in charge kept a list of the amount of the hard drug each inmate had in his account" (Marks 1979, 68–69). There is little archival evidence to substantiate the workings of the "drug bank," and my interviewees flatly deny the existence of any payoff scheme during their tenure at Lexington. The drug bank was discontinued in 1955 when the government authorized the ARC to make cash payments as long as they did not exceed what inmates could make when working elsewhere in the institution. Such practices certainly did not exist by 1963, the earliest year for which I can triangulate using multiple interviews of proven veracity.

Investigatory accounts leave open important unanswered questions about the long-term effects of drug exposure, liability, and the need for lifelong aftercare in cases of government experimentation. Unfortunately, such questions were not opened by the social network of prison reform advocates, who were new to the problems of abuse liability testing and pharmaceutical trials. Meanwhile, the social network of addiction researchers who had long labored to find a nonaddictive painkiller became acquainted with questions of legal liability and ethical responsibility. In the clash between politics and scientific expertise that was the prisoner research debate, scientists, lawyers, and prison advocates evidenced little resonance with one another's animating motivations, commitments, goals, or tactics. The National Commission for the Protection of Human Subjects was supposed to resolve this clash but instead left it in limbo.

UNSETTLED ACCOUNTS: THE NATIONAL COMMISSION FOR THE PROTECTION OF HUMAN SUBJECTS OF BIOMEDICAL AND BEHAVIORAL RESEARCH

As a federal intramural research program, the ARC was considered a liability not only because of its geographic isolation in contrast to the other intramural programs but because of the nature of its facility and its subjects. In a report dated April 30, 1976, on NIH intramural research programs, the President's Biomedical Research Panel (under DHEW) offered proposals to overcome both problems.[34] The panel mentioned Lexington only to advise strengthening its clinical and laboratory facilities.

> Location of the intramural program of the NIMH amidst the intramural programs of the NIH appears to have been significant for mutual enrichment. The intramural programs of the other Institutes of the ADAMHA [Alcohol, Drug Abuse, and Mental Health Administration] have not faired [*sic*] as well. The intramural program of the NIDA, located at the Addiction Research Center in Lexington, Kentucky, and the intramural program of the NIAAA [National Institute on Alcohol Abuse and Alcoholism], located at St. Elizabeth's Hospital in Washington, DC, have been relatively isolated and have. . . suffered from inadequate facilities.

The panel advised improving and enlarging NIDA's intramural research program and physically relocating it to the NIH campus (U.S. Department of Health, Education, and Welfare 1976, 31).

In the spring of 1976, William Pollin, director of NIDA's Division of Research, appointed a blue-ribbon subcommittee of the National Advisory Council on Drug Abuse. Headed by eminent Harvard behavioral pharmacologist Peter B. Dews (whose work is discussed in the next chapter of the present book), the subcommittee's main task was reviewing the ARC program and considering a proposal by the Alcohol, Drug Abuse, and Mental Health Administration to combine separate research facilities at one, unnamed location. The NIDA Advisory Council Task Force on Intramural Research met on June 11, 1976.[35] In its hands was a new report from the National Commission for the Protection of Human Subjects on its May 3, 1976, site visit to Lexington.

The report included the operations manual of the Organizational Review Committee at Lexington and illustrated divergent perspectives between researchers and their subjects.

According to the commission, the ARC did not deserve the charge that "administrative convenience" led to the choice of prisoners as research subjects.

> The decision to use prisoners who are ex-addicts for these was not a matter of chance or convenience; rather they were selected because experienced addicts were considered to be the best reporters of the subjective effects of new drugs in comparison with narcotics, and best able to understand what administration of these drugs meant in order to give informed consent. Non-addicts were considered unacceptable for tests involving administration of narcotics. (National Commission 1976a, 4)

The commission explained that ARC researchers considered it ethically acceptable to use "hard-core addicts" with a documented relapse history so that "they are not doing anything to the subjects that the prisoners wouldn't do to themselves if they had a chance" (National Commission 1976a, 5). Although conducted after the BOP stopped transferring prisoners to the ARC, the site visit included interviews with each of the remaining sixteen prisoner volunteers, and the report characterized prevailing perceptions and beliefs of participants. Most of these prisoners had transferred to the ARC to be closer to family members or out of the mistaken belief that participating would positively affect parole eligibility. The commission reported that this belief, "[p]assed by word of mouth in the prisons of origin," was supported not by statistical evidence but by "knowledge of particular men who made parole after returning from the ARC" and was "fed by the men's conviction that participation in research is considered to be a socially beneficial thing to do" (National Commission 1976a, 10). The commission staff attributed the circulation of this mistaken belief not to the ARC but to the prisoner culture.

Participants indicated that they selectively avoided agreeing to studies of drugs or routes of administration they did not like (National Commission 1976a, 11). Many reported having withdrawn from studies without interference from researchers, although they believed that if they withdrew too often, they would be removed from the ARC. Despite being unable to identify any actual cases where refusal to participate had resulted in removal, they argued, "If we all refused, you know they would not keep us here" (National Commission 1976a, 12). This belief led the commission to conclude there was a "significant coercive element in the unit" since "the same people who are responsible for the research are also responsible for decisions regarding the circumstances of the men's incarceration at the ARC, and that decisions to remove a prisoner from the ARC are viewed by prisoners as having a negative impact on chances for parole." Because researchers—not "distant prison officials"—were responsible for discipline, prisoners were "unable to ignore completely the fact of this power when they are asked to participate in a particular study" (National Commission 1976a, 13).

Although commissioners were unable to identify any complaints about particular studies, they turned up four general complaints. The first of these negatively compared the amount of money participants could make at the ARC to what prisoners thought they could have made at their "prison of origin" (National Commission 1976a, 14). The second and third were closely related concerns about the lack of education, training, entertainment, recreation, and therapeutic programs at the ARC as compared to the "model prison," or Federal Correctional Institution (FCI), next door.[36] Implementing NARA had effectively "unlocked" the main entrance to Lexington and brought in "800 male and female young offenders, primarily serving short terms for relatively minor offenses," setting up a situation in which the ARC was perceived as unfairly restrictive relative to the rest of the institution. The commission report pointed out: "The FCI next to the ARC is a facility run for a very different population, so much so that during daylight hours, there is no locked door between many inmates there and the outside world. To allow the ARC greater access to the FCI would require special security for which funds are not available, and which would be counter to the concept of the FCI" (National Commission 1976a, 15). ARC researchers were concerned that their subjects might gain access to contraband drugs through contact with individuals at the FCI. This would not only compromise the scientific value of their studies but pose to participants a risk that the researchers could not control.

A fourth general complaint was the failure to provide aftercare or follow-up to former participants. Couched within a legal climate of increased liability and litigiousness, this concern took on new weight in relation to studies on hallucinogens that might cause "flashbacks" or have unknown effects (National Commission 1976a, 15). The commission staff conveyed the fears underlying participants' arguments for continuing aftercare, which researchers cynically attributed to inmates' desires to transfer to hospital facilities viewed as more desirable than prisons (National Commission 1976a, 16). Health concerns of subjects were sometimes viewed by researchers as faked leverage to gain privileges. Although conducted in the program's waning days, the site visit turned up differing perspectives that suggest research participants did not uncritically absorb but instead actively resisted or negotiated what they were told by those who studied them. This is significant given their construction as vulnerable and exploited, for it indicates that they retained at least some of the wherewithal to make informed decisions.

Although the National Commission for the Protection of Human Subjects had unusual powers due to its birth in the crucible of controversy, it did not use them to ban prisoner research. Something more confusing happened. Ordinarily, the recommendations of national commissions are not binding, but President Jimmy Carter's secretary of DHEW, Joseph Califano, was legally compelled to respond to this commission's recommendations, which set the bar high but left the door open to continued research in federal prisons. Califano tried to arrange an accreditation program through the American Correctional Association.[37] Recall that the ACA's Ad Hoc Committee on Medical Experimentation and Pharmaceutical Testing had not produced a protocol until 1972 and had reversed its stance in February 1976, when its newly approved "Position Statement on the Use of Prisoners and Detainees as Subjects of Human Experimentation" stated that a prisoner was "incapable of volunteering as a human subject without hope of reward" (Harkness 1999, 289). After that, the ACA denied accreditation altogether for facilities that conducted research. Blocked by this move, Califano tried to broker a deal with the FDA to issue uniform rules in 1980. These were stayed as part of the Jackson prisoners' suit.

Still unsettled, the decision lay neither in the hands of the commission nor in the hands of scientists. There were powerful research proponents at NIH, where director Robert Q. Marsden had established the Study Group for Review of Policies on Protection of Human Subjects in Biomedical Research in 1973, when the issue heated up. The three-member Subcommittee on Prison Volunteers in Biomedical Research included one of the most famous public figures in pharmacology, Frances O. Kelsey (Stephens and Brynner 2001). After considering an outright ban, the subcommittee instead opposed one in March 1973, and the full study group accepted the subcommittee's conclusion (Harkness 1996, 267). But none of the arguments advanced by the expert community achieved the public visibility necessary to reassure those worried about whether addiction researchers should be allowed to experiment as they saw fit on vulnerable subjects.

Despite many compelling examples of their regard for the humanity of their prisoner patients, the ARC researchers simply could not see them as vulnerable subjects. The researchers' indigenous morality predisposed them to see prisoners as capable of making reasonable decisions about participation. They saw subjects as seasoned, drug-wise, and possessing knowledge about drug experiences outside the laboratory that were far riskier than those that were ever conducted inside it. The researchers' perspective meshed poorly with the emerging national consensus. There was simply no public discourse available to make sense of the science and politics of the ARC in the face of a critical mass mobilized against prison research on human subjects. The reform discourse positioned prisoners as the unlikely heroes and surprising beneficiaries of a new degree of public compassion. Researchers I interviewed depicted scientists as the victims of this formative moment. Divergent perspectives are to be expected as long as experts see themselves as speaking for others, rather than collaboratively producing expertise better tailored to the social contexts in which it is generated and used. Social distance between researchers and their subjects has only widened since the closure of the ARC at Lexington.

THE DEMISE OF THE "GOLDEN YEARS": LAMENTING THE LOSS OF LEXINGTON

Arriving fresh from Avram Goldstein's high-status neuropharmacology laboratory at Stanford University,[38] Tsung-Ping Su was called into Bill Martin's office in 1976. The ARC was about to shut down due to the ACLU's attempts to end prisoner research, Martin explained. Su laments:

> The glory of Lexington was that from a description of human pathology could come a pharmacological hypothesis. Lexington was a network of researchers asking very basic questions all the time, totally protected from political factors in ways that allowed us to be free to explore anything. That period has influenced me so much that I always try to link the molecular to the global picture, the global addictive process. (2004)

Martin himself was on the cusp of retiring from the PHS, so it fell to Jasinski to cultivate alternative populations. Jasinski later reported: "There was no way we could do human research in the middle of a prison in Kentucky. Lexington was a relatively small town at that time. You didn't have a huge addict population and there would be a lot of hue and cry if we tried to import addicts into Lexington." Jasinski noted that it was due to the "great hue and cry about clinical research" that the ARC did not relocate to Washington, D.C., or Bethesda.

"The NIH campus didn't have any room, and, secondly, the NIH people didn't want to bring addicts and alcoholics into Bethesda," Jasinski recalled, continuing: "At that time, the deputy director of the division of research was a guy named Dick Belleville, who had started out at Lexington. He was a psychologist who did a lot of the original work on drug reinforcement and conditioning. Dick had gone to NASA [where] he was the project officer on the first monkey in space, . . . and [was friends with] the guy who had been responsible for that, Joe Brady, who was at Hopkins" (2003). Sitting on both the NIDA Advisory Council and the National Commission for the Protection of Human Subjects, Brady prepared the ground for the move to Hopkins.

Several false starts later, Jasinski and a handful of researchers moved to Baltimore on July 1, 1979. There was disagreement within NIDA about whether it was desirable to create and maintain intramural research. The move refocused research priorities: there emerged a new emphasis on the clinical pharmacology of nicotine, which had been underexplored when the ARC was rooted in the heart of tobacco country, where everyone received a standard-issue glass ashtray. Researchers reinvented protocols to accomplish studies with free-living volunteers. Abuse liability studies were no longer the ARC's bread and butter, due to lack of support within NIDA for spending research dollars to benefit private industry. The ARC was absorbed into a vast, decentralized, extramural addiction research enterprise.

Fresh from lobbying for drug policy to stay in the White House, Robert DuPont, first director of NIDA, had instead presided over the devolution of responsibility for the nation's drug abuse treatment and prevention capacity (Musto and Korsmeyer 2002, 153). Back in the throes of the "hue and cry," the ARC had commemorated its fortieth anniversary at Lexington on June 9–11, 1975. DuPont sent Robert C. Petersen, then assistant director of the Division of Research for NIDA, to acknowledge the unit's scientific contributions. At the time, Petersen was gearing up to run the extramural funding mechanism. Although he lauded the ARC cadre, who he designated "a brilliant handful of scientists" who had demonstrated the relevance of science to social problems, he also called for greater balance between basic and applied research than that exhibited by the ARC. He characterized the research unit's commitment to basic research as "what comes most easily or comfortably."

> Before we become too self-congratulatory while wearing our researchers' hats, we might also remember that we too have a tendency to do what comes most easily or comfortably. It is often easier to limit oneself to basic research or to well-controlled laboratory settings than to attempt to cope with the messy

> problems of the real world. . . . Too often the most gifted researchers have scorned practical problems as either inappropriate or poorly suited to the well controlled research conditions their career contingencies lead them to prefer. Nevertheless, it is people who abuse drugs, and not rats. And drug abuse must be prevented not in laboratory animals but in people living in a complex world. (DuPont 1978, 263–64)

DuPont's reminder that it is people, not rats, who abuse drugs, can be taken as indicative of the NIDA leadership's need to distance the new agency from a potential political liability at a time when animal and prisoner research had both come under attack.[39] Although there was clearly continued respect for the ARC among the scientific community, the science side of NIDA was at times portrayed as a mafia by those concerned with education, treatment, prevention, and evaluation research.

Despite the venerable ARC's foundational work, NIDA portrays substance abuse research as moving from infancy to adolescence in the compressed time frame of the mid-1970s. From September 1973 to this day, NIDA estimates it has coordinated 85 percent of the world's scientific research on drug abuse. During this time, degrees of respect for the intramural program have fluctuated.[40] When at Lexington, the ARC had a great deal of autonomy in its research trajectory in coordination with the CPDD. By contrast, NIDA had to be extremely responsive to national priorities, legislative mandates, and external pressures, such as the emerging parents' movement. The agency concentrated on large-scale quantitative surveys, such as the household survey; the emergency-room-based Drug Abuse Warning Network; a treatment unit survey; and, beginning in 1975, the national high school survey "Monitoring the Future," implemented by the University of Michigan. NIDA was national in scope, tightly bound to policy, and interested in epidemiological and applied research. It had less use for the hybrid kind of "basic" and clinical research undertaken by the ARC.[41] Although many within NIDA were aware of the proud tradition of the ARC and its scientific preeminence, this legacy was portrayed as both an asset and a liability after the ARC moved to the site of the old Baltimore City Hospital in the summer of 1979. Animal research continued at Lexington until the early 1980s, when the unit reconsolidated at the Baltimore campus (then called the Francis Scott Key Medical Center and now known as the Bayview Medical Center at Johns Hopkins University). The ARC morphed into NIDA's Intramural Research Program, the official name given to the program under Alan Leshner in the 1990s.

One casualty of the move to Baltimore was the intensity of focus achieved through daily interaction about the conceptual basis of drug addiction. As ARC researcher Charles Gorodetzky describes, the ARC had the ideal "low walls" of problem-based, interdisciplinary knowledge formation.

> I always felt that the whole problem of drug abuse, the whole concept was a multidisciplinary issue. It took in everything from sociology to molecules. . . . [The directors] felt that we should span the entire gamut. My own feeling was that it was the ideal bridge between pharmacology, basic science, and medicine, which was one of the things that attracted me to the field. One of the beauties of the ARC was that interdisciplinary research was so easy to do. (2003)

Despite this, the hierarchy of credibility within the institution owed something to disciplinary formation. Tensions between social science and basic research seem to have increased over time; my interviewees attributed these to ideological differences. Some sociologists clearly felt pressured by "bench scientists," as did John Ball, who says he left Lexington because his publications were delayed or censored by "biomedical scientists believing that social science is not scientific enough" (Ball 2002, 31–32).

Contrary to the image of unproductive government scientists, those whose laboratory lives began at the ARC recalled their time at Lexington as highly productive. They were shielded from administration, fund-raising, and advocacy, and they inhabited a research culture that was completely devoted to the problem at hand. Gorodetzky recalls:

> [T]here was some sadness that what we knew had been really golden years of research. There were times when Don and I used to agitate with Bill [Martin], "Let us go up to Washington more with you, we want to mix with those folks" and he said, "Forget it, stay where you are, you don't know how good you've got it, stay a thousand miles away." He was right. We were unbothered, we were not really bogged down with all the kinds of committee work and administrative work that we would have had if we were at headquarters. . . . [and] we were a very, very productive group. (2003)

The loss of the prisoner research program meant that researchers had to adapt to outpatient populations, which changed the nature of their scientific inquiry. "[B]ecause we had prisoners who were institutionalized, and the government was already paying for their upkeep, we could do more complex and long-term studies that you couldn't do in other types of units" (Jasinski 2003).

The research suffered when researchers lost daily contact with subjects. Of his time at the Lexington ARC in its heyday, Conan Kornetsky remarked: "We knew all the subjects by name, we interacted with them daily. We drank coffee with them. We were concerned about their pain" (personal communication with the author, August 3, 2006). With the Lexington ARC's shutdown, close observation, once central to this basic research facility, was displaced. The interactive process of interpreting clinical phenomena, inner sensations, and subjective effects was gone. With the exception of profoundly literate artists who have translated their inner sensations into communicable form, the words of drug users have rarely been listened to, recorded, or taken as seriously by anyone as they were at the ARC. This irony was apparent to Charles R. "Bob" Schuster, a NIDA director who recognized Lexington's value: "I understand [the ethical concerns that ended the Lexington research] but I really do believe that the research that came out of Lexington was some of the most important research on addiction and it could not have taken place anywhere else" (2004). The pharmacist who compounded medications at the ARC, Rolley E. "Ed" Johnson, felt, like other Lexington veterans, that the move to "protect" prisoners took something away from them.

> I think it's appropriate to make sure you have a prisoner advocate on an IRB [institutional review board], but to just say outright that no prisoner should be allowed to volunteer is taking away a right instead of protecting a right. There are different sides to the question. How free are you to volunteer? How much coercion or how much seduction can be used? You can look at those private rooms, or other things that subjects got, and say "that's seduction." Nobody put a gun to anybody's head and said do it, but if you knew you were going to get a private room, even though it may only be three feet wide and six feet long, but you're not sharing it with four people, that certainly could be looked at as seduction. If you have a private TV and can watch any station you want instead of what everybody else is watching, that certainly can be looked at as seduction. There's seduction in everything we do if you stop and think about it. In the real marketplace you're trying to seduce people into buying what you've got all the time. It's hard to reconcile that in a prison situation, so the easiest thing was to just say they can't do it. (2005)

The last drug-addicted prisoner was transferred out of the ARC on December 31, 1976. By then, the broader institution had become the ordinary prison that James Bennett, Walter Treadway, and Lawrence Kolb had insisted it never become. Portrayed as the "guys who did research on prisoners," ARC researchers faced the dispiriting loss of their laboratory at Lexington, which created a vacuum into which the new science of behavioral pharmacology stepped with a new set of laboratory logics.

MAKING SENSE OF THE DEMISE OF PHARMACOLOGICAL TESTING AND PRISONER RESEARCH

Resistance to the emerging form of the new human subjects regime issued from pharmaceutical manufacturers, scientists, clinicians, and even prisoners themselves, some of the last of whom protested the removal of their rights to participate in research. Social scientists, legal scholars, and corrections professionals debated professional practices and ethical conduct. Civil rights organizations, consumer groups, the women's health movement, and, later, the HIV/AIDS movement engaged in concrete struggles for and against access to particular drugs and therapies. Yet philosophical abstractions predominate in public deliberation of complex ethicopolitical issues in the United States. In retrospect, the prison research episode was a struggle over whose expertise would prevail in a moment of political turmoil over the proper connections between science and governance.

A report dramatizing the ethical dilemmas of prison research appeared in 1980 to restage the struggle between proponents of continued prison research: namely, William R. Martin, still in Lexington but by then at the University of Kentucky; Robert J. Levine, chair of the Yale University Human Investigation Committee and consultant to the National Commission for the Protection of Human Subjects; Henry K. Beecher's onetime coauthor Louis Lasagna of the University of Rochester; and Alvin J. Bronstein, the ACLU National Prison Project's chief litigator. Commissioned by the Center for the Study of Drug Development at the University of Rochester, the report was authored by Seymour Shubin. It traced the contours of an epic clash between a certain kind of scientific expertise and a certain kind of politics, neither of which recognized the nuances of a socially situated ethics.

Research proponents barely gained a moral toehold against those arguing against continued federal prison research. Marshaling research-promoting arguments, Shubin framed the report with a loaded rhetorical question: "Should prisoners be permitted to volunteer as subjects in scrupulously-run, carefully-reviewed research projects that require their informed consent and permit them to withdraw at any time?" Scattered throughout the report were dire discursive flags: medical research in prisons was said to be in its "death throes," "killed" by DHEW and the FDA; its quiet death "without headlines" was expected to "cripple" pharmaceutical companies (Shubin 1980, 1–4). Shubin's report was structured to showcase research programs that did not deserve to die, instead of the "few widely publicized cases of thoughtless or unscrupulous prison research" (1980, 4). It offered two exemplars: the Malaria Project at the Stateville Penitentiary in Joliet, Illinois, phased out in 1975; and the ARC in Lexington, Kentucky, phased out in 1976.

Casting Martin as an exemplary scientific proponent of prison research, Shubin depicted Bronstein as disrespecting the very prisoners whose rights he supposedly championed. Highlighting Levine's claim that most prison research was not unduly risky, Shubin cited actuarial calculations indicating that risk levels were as minimal as those of office secretaries—much lower than risks faced by window washers or coal miners (1980, 16). Minimization of harm and risk did not play well in the climate of the 1970s. However, what historical sense is to be made of the ethos at the ARC depends on some calculus of the risks to which participants were exposed. By limiting studies to small groups of subjects, the ARC reduced exposure to drugs known to be risky. They rarely exceeded one hundred subjects and did not randomize; nor did they often use placebos, which would have been recognized by the drug-wise subjects who comprised their pool of eligible subjects.

The indigenous morality by which ARC researchers worked calculated risk in the laboratory by comparing it to the much higher risks encountered by those who used illegal drugs of unknown provenance in unknown dosages on the streets. The ARC emphasized the lack of mortality and morbidity associated with its research, because dosage was precise and drug supplies unadulterated: "In over 40 years of using human subjects we had had no mortality at all and virtually no morbidity" (Shubin 1980, 5). Foregrounded was the indigenous morality against coercion or seduction at the ARC, a frame often echoed by my interviewees. Martin conceded that prisoners were more vulnerable to coercion and seduction because almost anything could be used as an incentive. He argued against using parole as the sole incentive if research were the only way a prisoner could shorten his sentence. But he contended:

> [I]f it's just one of many ways, I see nothing wrong with it. In fact, I think that by denying [prisoners] the opportunity to volunteer for research, we're denying them still another freedom. And I also think that if a prisoner wants to provide a very useful service to society, he shouldn't be denied it. (Quoted in Shubin 1980, 7)

Laying out a different ethical yardstick for prison research, Martin argued that captivity was itself an important safeguard: [I]f we were to make someone dependent on morphine or a new analgesic that turns out to be addicting, and the subject has the right to leave the unit any time he wished, he could of course cause harm to himself and to other people. If he left the Center, say, and he was dependent on drugs and became sick and robbed a drugstore, I think the investigator would have to bear the responsibility. . . . I would never conduct an experiment in which I chronically administered a potentially addicting drug to a patient who could leave the setting at will" (quoted in Shubin 1980, 7). This statement replied to the pivotal question of whether or not clinical trials could be conducted on free-living volunteers, as maintained in the Katzenmeier hearings by John D. Arnold, once a proponent of prisoner research until he discovered he could gain participation from college students.

The existence of populations of free-living volunteers willing to participate in clinical trials was not just a matter of logistics but a scientific issue haunting the halls of Lexington. Were prisoners physiologically and psychologically similar to those living outside prison walls? Bronstein argued that differences invalidated prisoner research on scientific grounds: "There is a lot of data now which suggests that much of the testing that's been done on prisoners is not scientifically valid for free world people because of the physiological changes that take place in prisoners—blood changes, metabolism changes, as a result of the kind of life you are living in a closed institution" (quoted in Shubin 1980, 15). Portraying prisoners as unreliable witnesses, Bronstein said:

> We also know that prisoners are the greatest con artists in the world. They have to do it to survive—and they were doing it, many of them, before they got to prison. They are screwing around with placebos and things. We have documentation of some tests at Connecticut State Prison. We've got affidavits from prisoners that, with only 24 prisoners in the test, only two were taking the pills each week; the others were hiding them or getting rid of them. And the two shared their urine specimens for the week with the other 22. (Quoted in Shubin 1980, 15)

Kornetsky counters: "Bad research is done in non-prisons, as well as prisons. In fact, there has been badly designed human experimentation done and sponsored by some of our most prestigious universities. Generalizing from that example is logically absurd. It is obvious that the experiments were poorly designed and poorly supervised" (personal communication with the author, August 3, 2006). However, deciding if prisoners were physiologically or psychologically different from nonprisoners was a political question. By the early 1980s, the social stakes involved had changed due to the ACLU Prison Project, which was at heart a reform movement focused on prison research as a vehicle to change prison conditions and expand prisoners' civil liberties.

The sociology of bioethics that emerged in the 1970s lent credence to the prison reform movement by representing biomedical researchers as collectively conservative and resistant to scrutiny. In the book *Research on Human Subjects,* Bernard Barber explained:

> Just as powerful businessmen in the past resisted, and still do, the "encroachments" of governance on their autonomy and self-defined expertise, so the medical research community today feels itself beleaguered by an excessively intrusive general public and the government as well. Even small requests for change, for more effective self-regulation, are viewed by the "powerful profession" as fundamental threats. (Barber et al. 1979, xiv)

Soon after *Research on Human Subjects* initially appeared, the Tuskegee scandal broke, and Barber testified in the Kennedy hearings.[42] Because they emphasized systemwide effects, the sociologists saw themselves as separate from the bioethicists (Barber et al. 1979, xv). Still, the National Commission for the Protection of Human Subjects modeled its survey research on Barber's methodology and identified a similar overall pattern: ward and clinic patients were "differentially poor, less educated, and members of minority groups"; most likely to be involved in studies with the least favorable risk-benefit ratios; and less likely to be able to "give a free and informed consent" (Barber et al. 1979, viii). Contra Barber et al., the commission did not find that "children, women, minority, or low income persons were more likely than others to participate in projects that were above average in risk" (Cooke, Tannenbaum, and Gray 1977, ix).

Barber et al. identified a faulty assumption made by many biomedical researchers: "[I]n order for medical knowledge to grow, some people have to serve as subjects for risky but important research. These people, it is assumed, should rightly be the ward and clinic patients who receive their medical care either free or at reduced charge. In return for cheaper care they will provide the crucial ingredient for medical knowledge to grow" (1979, 57). The ethical problem of this assumption bears a precise resemblance to Foucault's insight into the implicit contract governing clinical research (quoted at the beginning of the present chapter). Overcoming this structural unfairness required the new social role of an "informed outsider" who could represent the stakes of current patient-subjects, future subjects, and researchers (Barber et al. 1979, 196). Informed outsiders would ideally know more than the man in the street about biomedical research, as well as understanding the laws, codes, and social norms relevant to effective and ethical use of human subjects and social-psychological techniques for discovering the feelings and values of representative publics.

> The uninformed man-in-the-street cannot know what "the community" thinks about catheterization of the heart, or the use of levodopa in the treatment of parkinsonianism, or the transplantation of vital organs, or the injection of live cancer cells into terminal cancer patients. The informed outsider would have access to the techniques and resources that could provide such information from the community. (Barber et al. 1979, 196)

The lack of informed intermediaries in the prison research debates was responsible for their discursive and political impoverishment. The moral compass of the time inscribed only two, starkly drawn positions: those who were for it and those who were against it.

Social location and social status played a role in determining positions within the debate. The ARC researchers held high social status within scientific communities close to them, because they were extremely competitive in terms of productivity and placement of their research. They enjoyed preeminent status in the pharmacological sciences and among psychiatrists and clinicians. Their institution was the mecca of substance abuse research. This position rendered them unused to explaining themselves, for they had received little external scrutiny or challenge from any quarter. Misunderstanding the playing field, they pitched their responses within the narrow parameters of the scientific terrain they sought to defend. If anything can be learned about the political contestation of knowledge and expertise issuing from this turbulent moment, it is that science and scientific research are inevitably political acts taking place on social terrain. They are as much about the performative enactment of ethical science as they are about the content of scientific claims or the logics of laboratories.

In conclusion, this chapter has sought not to defend the overall practice of prison research but to distinguish among widely varying research practices and laboratory logics that prevailed in different research settings. Under no circumstances would I now turn back the clock to the "bad old days" of federal prisoner research, for abundant unethical experimentation occurred both before and after the ARC was quietly phased out.[43] No one should be given free rein to conduct research in total institutions. However, the state of suspended animation that federal prison research entered in the early 1980s effectively did away with public scrutiny over private research conducted in state prisons. The issues raised in this chapter hence remain unresolved. While free-living volunteers are the human subjects of clinical trials and scientific studies today, this situation creates new risks that may someday be considered unethical.

Addiction research took new forms in the post-Lexington era, and the trajectories it took remind us that a concept like "addiction" comes into being only through a confluence of several lines of collective thought (Fleck 1979, 23). Some of these will be privileged over others in ways that lead them to become the dominant frame that renders all contending systems of thought "alien."

> Whatever is known has always seemed systematic, proven, applicable, and evident to the knower. Every alien system of knowledge has likewise seemed contradictory, unproven, inapplicable, fanciful, or mystical. May not the time have come to assume a less egocentric, more general point of view and speak of comparative epistemology? (Fleck 1979, 22)

Leaving Lexington, the ARC lost some of its privilege to channel the conceptual confluence that is "addiction," and new streams of thought became dominant tributaries. The "great hue and cry" over prisoner research ultimately shut down the research program at Lexington but opened the floodgates to new laboratory logics for substance abuse research and new practices in the social organization of clinical trials.

CHAPTER 7

"The Behavior Is Always Right": Behavioral Pharmacology Comes of Age

Popular drug experimentation in the late 1960s stimulated interest in the difference between use and abuse. Behavioral scientists took up this challenge, placing themselves on the frontier staked out by the once-pioneering ARC. Sites for drug abuse research diversified as the research establishment that had labored for more than thirty years in Lexington lost its virtual monopoly. Through CPDD, established researchers welcomed some newcomers but shut others out. This conflict is best seen not as a generation gap, paradigm shift, or zeitgeist but as a struggle over which hierarchy of credibility would prevail and whose voices would count as the voice of scientific authority. Differences between enunciative communities became evident in the multiple conceptual practices and laboratory logics that developed in the 1960s.[1] Behavioral pharmacologists formed a tiny but cohesive scientific community that moved from margin to center in the economy of drug abuse research.

The newcomers whose pathways I chart in this chapter either had personal drug experience or had witnessed drug use in friends or family. Macrosocial changes increased the range of available legal and illegal drugs while relaxing popular attitudes toward taking them. This fact alone differentiated newcomers from the previous generation, most of whom had never seen an addict before ending up at Lexington. Newcomers had different scientific vocabularies, logics, and techniques at their disposal, most notably those of behaviorism. Long concerned with "habit," behaviorism evolved in the United States in response to urbanization and mechanization (Bakan 1966). Although early behaviorists—such as John Watson, Clark L. Hull, and B. F. Skinner—attributed psychoanalysis with more cultural authority than it actually exercised, they used the scientific power of behaviorism as a "new psychological claimant" to displace psychoanalysis during a time of considerable change in social relations, sexual mores, and the organization of work in the United States (Bakan 1966, 22).

Asserting the potency of physiological responses while recasting "habit" and "habit strength" as a set of measurable physiological changes, behaviorists carved out a nonjudgmental position in a field they perceived to be dominated by moralism and bias. Ironically, Kolb's K-classification system, an early attempt to place addiction on a scientific footing and so destigmatize it, stood for "prescientific" moralism. Despite Kolb's goal to wrest from U.S. marshals their power over addicts' fates, the founding medical officer in charge of Lexington relied on the psychiatric terminology of the mid-1920s and so became an enduring emblem of what behaviorists were using science to overcome. The orderly framework of behaviorism was well suited to explaining the persistence of the "irrational" behaviors associated with drug abuse.

Behavioral pharmacologists encountered the field with tools, techniques, and, as Roland Griffiths observed, the confidence that "Skinnerian behaviorism seemed to explain everything about the way the world worked." Griffiths continued:

> We came into graduate school and were given an understanding, almost a philosophy of life, the key to the nature of the way behavior occurs. We were radical behaviorists at the time. We wanted to explain everything in terms of stimulus response interactions, partly Skinnerian, but also Pavlovian or classical conditioning and operant reinforcement. It gave us a paradigm and a methodology in which to work. . . . [We were] ready to explain everything about drug behavior interactions using this paradigm and methodology. It gave us the chutzpah to attack problems that might otherwise overwhelm other people that didn't have "the answer."

Radical behaviorists were typically graduate students in experimental psychology or "behavior engineering," who studied what they called "drug-seeking behavior" or "drug self-administration." Griffiths, who saw his personal sense of humility emerging only in retrospect, noted of his cohort: "We knew everything we needed to know about the field. It was with great zeal, but complete naïveté, that we stepped into this" (2005).

Although youthful confidence in the power of behaviorism has waned, many still speak of the explanatory power, conceptual force, strength, and rigor of the concept that drugs are reinforcers, which is central to this epistemic community.[2] The idea that drugs work to reinforce certain behaviors and extinguish others is no longer restricted to the tightly coupled network of behavioral pharmacologists but has diffused throughout the field. The diffusion process has not gone unremarked by those who enjoyed scientific careers in the heyday of behavioral pharmacology. Behavioral pharmacology remade the laboratory logics of addiction research. Ironically, those who stormed the citadel of the ARC are now one of few sources of collective memory about it.

The behavioral laboratory logic of drug self-administration diverged from the logics of classical pharmacology. Griffiths explained:

> [Behavioral pharmacology was] characterized by intensive single-subject designs and parametric manipulations using the kinds of methods that come straight out of the experimental analysis of behavior. It was a new paradigm. The Lexington folks had been doing drug abuse research for years, but they were using classical clinical pharmacology methods, group designs, statistical analyses, and classical pharmacology approaches that are very powerful—and about which we were completely ignorant. Undoubtedly we thought that our methods were better and much more interesting because we were going to get to the core of the drug abuse problem, so there was [a] sense of glee and naïveté. (2005)

Almost universally, behavioral pharmacologists convey this zeitgeist in their origin stories about the hotbeds of behavioral pharmacology.

Derived from the work of B. F. Skinner, who originated the terms *respondent* and *operant* in 1937 to differentiate between behavior elicited in response to environmental conditions and behavior emitted to operate on the environment (Morris and Smith 2004), operant conditioning offered a new set of laboratory logics that aligned with but was different from Wikler's work on so-called classical (Pavlovian) conditioning. The vocabulary and methodology of operant conditioning, once called "behavioral engineering" or "social engineering," attracted newcomers who were less interested in drugs per se than in using drugs as tools for studying the persistence of behavior despite negative consequences. Substance abuse attracted behavioral pharmacologists because it was a socially pressing problem that had not yielded to previous approaches. Oblivious to the vast accumulation of human and animal data amassed by the ARC, adherents of behavioral pharmacology rarely crossed paths with the existing addiction research network until each social network began using the other's techniques to produce and render data (Brady 2004). As references to "addiction" and "drug dependence" were replaced by references to "drug and alcohol abuse," behaviorism and pharmacology united to change how sustained drug use was viewed more generally.

MAKING THE WORLD OF DRUG ABUSE A PLACE WHERE BEHAVIORAL SCIENCE WORKS

As quoted at the beginning of chapter 2 of this book, sociologist Howard S. Becker observed: "Science works when you make the world into the kind of place where that kind of science will work. That's the purpose of creating laboratories."[3] The two primary origins of behavioral pharmacology were Pavlov's Institute for Experimental Medicine in Saint Petersburg, Russia, and the Psychobiology Laboratory at Harvard Medical School, where B. F. Skinner joined the faculty in 1948 and British pharmacologist Peter Dews joined shortly thereafter.[4] Previous laboratory stirrings occurred at the University of Minnesota, where Skinner was from 1936 to 1945, during which time he trained Kenneth MacCorquodale; at the University of Chicago when Joseph V. Brady was in graduate school; and in the "military industrial academic complex at Walter Reed, the University of Maryland, and at Johns Hopkins University," to which Brady emigrated (Brady 2004). Individuals central to the history of behavioral pharmacology share a delightfully self-reflexive streak, using the field's lexicon to describe their own behaviors and the powerful reinforcements afforded by their scientific method. Brady wrote: "[T]wo laboratories (Harvard and University of Maryland) potentiated the methodological and conceptual interplay by increasing the baseline rate at which drug behavior experiments were undertaken in laboratory settings. Clearly they raised the operant level" (2004). At Maryland, Brady trained Travis Thompson and Charles R. (Bob) Schuster, who cowrote the field's first textbook after Thompson departed for the University of Minnesota and Schuster was lured to the University of Michigan by Maurice Seevers. Once in Ann Arbor, Schuster pioneered primate self-administration using the platform built by Jim Weeks and Tomoji Yanagita described in chapter 2. The striking observation that nonhuman primates could be induced to self-administer the same drugs that human primates use to modulate their emotional and physiological states undergirded the institutionalization of behavioral pharmacology in industry and academia.

Drug self-administration marked both a turning point and a zenith in the long history of the behavioral enclave, which enjoyed ascendant status in the 1970s. Although they knew relatively little about addiction (having been trained primarily as experimental psychologists and incidentally as pharmacologists), behavioral pharmacologists experienced their entry into the field as an intellectual and technical insurgency that displaced and invalidated all previous approaches to substance abuse. The problems of substance abuse—including techniques to measure drug abuse liability—became one of the main arenas in which behaviorism enjoyed enduring preeminence. Like all seeming scientific revolutions, this one came about gradually and was preceded by acolytes who were not accepted by more established scientists. Behavioral pharmacologists' feelings of marginalization were so intense that they formed a CPDD satellite, named the International Study Group for Investigating Drugs as Reinforcers, in the early 1970s.

Behavioral pharmacology emerged as both experimental and observational. Over time, behavioral researchers played an increasingly large role in pharmacology, as evidenced by their growing presence in the American Society for Pharmacology and Experimental Therapeutics. Alexandra Rutherford (2003) argues that behaviorism was institutionalized by the research undertaken by B. F. Skinner and Peter B. Dews at the Harvard Psychobiological Laboratory and by Brady's consultations. The framing of drug abuse as a social problem that behavioral pharmacology might help control led to expanded funding and institutional support for conducting abuse liability assessment on behavioral terms. In turn, evaluation of pharmacological effects helped make human (and animal) behavior accessible to the research techniques developed by behaviorists, turning the attention of pharmaceutical companies to side effects.

The founding fathers of the first generation of behavioral pharmacologists, Dews and Brady, credited the 1954 discovery of chlorpromazine (CPZ) as the triggering event that led to the differentiation of behavioral pharmacology from behavioral analysis and pharmacology.[5] They disputed the view that serendipity led to the discovery of CPZ/Thorazine, credited with creating the conditions for deinstitutionalization in the United States (Caldwell 1970; Healy 2002).[6] Assuring readers that he did not mean to discredit the pioneering work of Macht, Skinner, and others who worked the field prior to 1954, Dews foregrounded the significance of CPZ, which he called "one of the half dozen most important drugs in the history of mankind, . . . achieved by the systematic use of methods of behavioral pharmacology: not by serendipity or by molecular biology" (1985, 3).[7] This statement, made at a conference in 1984, indicated the extent to which behavioral pharmacologists already felt pushed aside by psychologists, pharmacologists, and, especially, molecular biologists. Only in the halls of NIMH,

Dews wrote, were behavioral pharmacologists appreciated and rewarded. To drive home his point, Dews used an extended parenting metaphor, in which behavioral pharmacology was the "offspring of pharmacology and psychology with the paternal genes of pharmacology predominating."

> Unfortunately when behavioral pharmacology was born, father was beginning a long infatuation with molecular biology which still continues, in spite of the fact that most of the major achievements in pharmacology since that time . . . are by no means achievements of molecular biology. Behavioral pharmacology has tended to be judged by its molecular relevance, which has been, and still is, modest to say the least. Psychology has been an even more unsympathetic parent. Living in halls of ornate theory, psychology has asked what behavioral pharmacology had to offer in the way of additional embellishment. Behavioral pharmacology is close to earthy reality, so the answer has been again, precious little. Indeed heavy-footed behavioral pharmacology has caused tremors that have jeopardized the whole filmy fabric of theories. (1985, 4)

Acknowledging that behavioral pharmacology was not yet a mature science by the mid-1980s, Dews urged his colleagues not to wait for neurobiologists or molecular biologists to provide the impetus for further discoveries (1985, 5). Although Dews's reproductive metaphor was especially colorful, behavioral pharmacology is often depicted as a flat-footed, descriptive science in contrast to other, more fanciful sciences.

Behaviorism and pharmacology were coconstitutive, a quality projected through the parenting and marriage metaphors of its participant-historians. The field's first textbook, *Behavioral Pharmacology* (1968) by Thompson and Schuster, offered a companionate marriage metaphor: "As is true in any marriage, the two partners, while sharing common conceptions and goals, must settle certain differences before a harmonious working relationship can be established" (ix). Steering clear of neural, mental, or emotional events in favor of observable changes in behavior, Thompson and Schuster cited a debt to B. F. Skinner for the assumptions, technologies, and techniques on which the new science rested (x). Laying bare the fundamentals of the two disciplines, Thompson and Schuster did not promise a "new synthesis" but, rather, mapped the "remaining chasm separating the two domains" (6). They also conveyed a felt sense of the "limited popularity" of the tactics and methods to which they subscribed, which they attributed to their empirical emphasis: "The overall advantage of the descriptive approach lies in the empirical soundness of the entire structure of scientific knowledge, from the microstructural foundation to the molar behavioral superstructure" (7). This degree of integration was unprecedented, despite the best efforts of the collaborative team approach tried at Lexington.

When Smith Kline and French Laboratories bought the rights to CPZ from Rhône Poulenc in France, a new set of behavioral laboratory logics for finding specific uses for drugs through behavioral techniques was elaborated in the U.S. pharmaceutical industry, which built an infrastructure of psychopharmacology laboratories in hopes of finding another CPZ-like drug. This was reverse engineering, the systematic use of behavioral responses to predict drug effects. Rather than agreeing that drugs affect behavior, behavioral pharmacologists see the behavior itself as "a predeterminant of the quality of the drug effect" (Cook 1991, 2).

Despite their commitment to what seems like an applied science, Thompson and Schuster conceptualized behavioral pharmacology as a basic science of behavior that utilized drugs as tools. Differentiated from clinical research, their work used behavior to study the mechanisms of drug action. Criticizing those who studied drug effects on "unlearned reflexes," they focused on learning as a form of "conditioned response" (1968, 2). Although they cited Wikler (1953), they carved out a different practical terrain by using behavioral techniques to screen clinically desirable compounds and describe effects by drug class. Seeing such popular categories as "tranquilizers," "psychic energizers," or "antidepressants" as false or misleading labels, Thompson and Schuster set out to place classification on a more systematic footing and criticized the ARC's physiological and psychological instruments as unrefined (1968, 5). They extended the study of drug effects beyond the central nervous system, in contrast to pharmacologists, who tended to see the "brain [a]s the primary site of action of most behaviorally active drugs" (1968, 32). Behavioral pharmacologists recognized that drug effects went beyond the central nervous system because behavior had to be understood in intact organisms (Thompson and Schuster 1968, 33; Iversen and Iversen 1981, 52). Contra depictions of behaviorism as simplistic relative to cognitive science, they saw it as a nonreductive science.

Operant conditioning along Skinnerian lines became the cultural currency among psychologists who adopted the vocabulary and techniques of behaviorists. Susan and Leslie Iversen explain:

> The demands of behavioral pharmacology are more consistent with Skinner's approach to behavior [than cognitive theories], which is basically a description of the variables influencing behavior in a particular situation, with no recourse to explanation. This is not to say there are no underlying reasons for behavior, but simply that if behavior can be defined, described, and consistently manipulated, these reasons are irrelevant. (Iversen and Iversen 1981, 12–13)

Behavioral pharmacologists saw the interpretive vocabulary of psychology—such terms as *motivation, emotion, anxiety,* and *neurosis* or attempts to name internal drive states—as misleading (Iversen and Iversen 1981, 12–13, 35–36). "From fish to men," as the Iversens put it, Skinnerians found that schedules of reinforcement were predictive: "There is every reason to think that man's behavior is controlled by the same basic contingencies as is behavior in the pigeon" (1981, 32). This fundamentalist refusal of anthropomorphism sparked antipathy toward behaviorists, who viewed themselves as moving psychology away from softheaded early psychopharmacology to hard-core science. Moving from the soft science of subjective effects into a hard science of objective observables was embraced so fully by converts to the field that it had the quality of a revolutionary call to arms (cf. Fleck 1979, 43).

Second-generation acolytes of behaviorism, such as Thompson and Schuster, emerged as staunch defenders of their science. In their 1968 textbook, Thompson and Schuster concluded: "Critics of this descriptive approach to behavioral effects of drugs find it superficial, 'know nothing,' and grossly oversimplified." They conceded that behavioral pharmacology was "superficial in that it deals exclusively with observables; 'know nothing' to the extent that it does not claim to know anything that can't be replicated by independent observers; and . . . oversimplified to the extent that the world is simple." Calling theirs a "modest approach," they asserted that they were "content to add descriptive links to the body of knowledge relating drugs to behavior" (229). This potent combination of modesty and technique catapulted behavioral pharmacology to the center stage of the drug abuse research enterprise, while molecular, neurobiological, and genetic approaches waited patiently in the wings. The proud but distracted parent disciplines watched the performance. Earlier in their textbook, Thompson and Schuster presented a very different picture of behavioral pharmacology as a "young and complex" science requiring a great deal of imagination and opposed to "oversimplified and premature judgments about the behavioral actions of drugs" (157). Citing numerous paradoxes of action and effect, they made ingenious attempts to control for the complexities and nuances imparted by contingencies in the environment.

Drug abuse research offered an ideal arena in which to work out the basic mechanisms of behavior in complex environments. Behavioral pharmacologists considered the designation "drug-behavior interaction" a misnomer, because they recognized that intact organisms interact not with drugs but with environments. They criticized research that failed to account for environmental factors, arguing that "drug-behavior interaction" should be thought of as "drug-environment interaction" (Thompson and Schuster 1968, 158). Not unlike Beecher, they believed that physiological states and environmental contingencies modified drug effects.[8] However, once complex transactions between drugs, behavior, and environment were recognized, behavioral pharmacologists acted to "strip away uncontrolled conditions" and reveal the lawfulness of behavior and its roots in "causally determined events" (Glick and Goldfarb 1976, 1–2). Steve Goldberg wrote: "Drug addiction is a complex type of behavioral disorder that depends in part on specific biochemical and physiological mechanisms of drug action, as well as the present and past behavior of the individual addict and the environmental conditions under which the behavior occurs." Studies conducted prior to use of operant-conditioning techniques were dismissed by Goldberg as merely biochemical or physiological or as misguided attempts to identify "metabolic aberrations" of addicts or potential addicts, while he defined operant behavior "simply as behavior that is controlled by its consequences" (1976, 283). For a consequence to act as a reinforcer, it must follow the response immediately so as to increase its frequency. For behaviorists, reinforcement depended not only on intrinsic, pharmacological properties of drugs but on individual behavior and environment.

Behavioral pharmacologists walk a thin line between their recognitions of complexity and multiplicity, on the one hand, and their straightforward, hardcore scientific ambitions, on the other. This ambiguity showed up in their assessments of prior work. For instance, Goldberg dismissed "wrongheaded" claims that "psychological disorders" caused addiction, crediting several early works (Tatum, Collins, and Seevers 1929; DuMez and Kolb 1931; Kolb and Himmelsbach 1938; and Seevers 1936b) with establishing the biological basis of physiological dependence. Describing how behavior leading up to morphine injection could be interpreted as "escape behavior" designed to terminate or avert abstinence symptoms, Goldberg traced a genealogy by which addiction researchers realized that physical dependence was "neither a necessary nor sufficient condition for addiction." "Drug dependence," he stated, evolved away from "addiction," "habituation," "abuse," "pleasure," "euphoria," and "craving," due to difficulties involved in quantifying and operationalizing such states (1976, 284). Recalling his forebears' dissatisfaction with terminology, it is difficult not to see behavioral pharmacology as amnesiac. Offering neutral terms, such as *drug self-administration, drug seeking,* or *drug taking,* behavioral scientists sought to operationalize similar concepts to those Abraham Wikler had decades earlier sought to place on the firm ground of public science.

Propelled by the rise of behavioral pharmacology, laboratory sites for evaluating drug effects proliferated and decentralized. The events recounted in the previous chapter of this book created a vacuum into which behavioral pharmacologists were prepared to step. As Chris-Ellyn Johanson put it (personal communication with the author, March 22, 2005), the ARC's hold over human research loosened just as behaviorists invented and adapted the apparatus and recording devices that made their science visible. Pharmacologists had long performed animal research and toxicity testing; they were more experienced in animal care than were behavior analysts (Rowan 1984). The convergence between behaviorism and pharmacology occurred simultaneously at multiple sites.[9] Like other interdisciplinary fields, behavioral pharmacology "maintain[ed] itself through regular and purposeful interaction with other fields and other domains" (Frickel 2004, 5). Yet it also consolidated its own lexicon and laboratory logics, which came to predominate in the field of addiction research by the late 1970s.

Behavioral pharmacology emerged with unusually tight connections between basic and applied research modes. Those who rely on its techniques today to assess the abuse potential of chemical compounds have been deeply involved in developing policy-relevant approaches to drug dependence or addiction. The institutional core of behavioral pharmacology did not initially lie in the federal science system—an "upstart" science issuing outside the ARC, it was perceived to be part of a competing approach. However, in the 1970s, the field of "substance abuse research," as it increasingly was called, became a reliable funding stream for behavioral pharmacologists. Despite Wikler's own previous preoccupation with classical and operant conditioning and his long-standing interest in Pavlovian approaches, behavioral pharmacology was heralded as a new experimental paradigm. Something about it smacked of an assault on the citadel. Behavioral pharmacologists saw the knowledge they produced as relevant not only for understanding drug abuse but also for treating or even preventing it. Going beyond basic research, behavioral pharmacologists threw themselves into the political fray, taking responsibility for policy, treatment, and prevention in ways their forebears had not. An unprecedented chance to affect national drug policy and federal research priorities arose during the Nixon administration. Drug abuse researchers gained influence over drug policy in the early 1970s, when the political opportunity structure enabled them to control the setting of research priorities and to translate basic knowledge into wider use.

Substance abuse offered an opportunity for behavioral pharmacologists to demonstrate innovative animal self-administration and drug-discrimination techniques (Lasagna 1969, 23). Such major figures as Henry K. Beecher understood that bridges between behavioral science and psychopharmacology were being built in the 1950s—despite subscribing to the sense that psychopharmacology was an inescapably "subjective" science (1970, 60). Previous work had focused solely on chemical compounds that had visible, measurable effects on the bodies of monkeys and men.[10] Now behavioral pharmacologists saw drugs as reinforcers of behavior, learning patterns, and conditioned responses. This insight allowed them to invent precision techniques, protocols, and laboratory logics for producing new knowledge about drug self-administration in humans and animals. To discern the patterned sociality of this particular community of scientific practice, the next section of this chapter examines the career trajectories of behavioral pharmacologists who worked out the new laboratory logics.

COMING OF AGE: BEHAVIORISM AS THE KEY TO SOLVING SOCIAL PROBLEMS

Coming of age in Camden, New Jersey, during World War II, Charles R. (Bob) Schuster played jazz underage in local bars and nightclubs, hanging out at the WCAU studios in Philadelphia, where Red Rodney was the featured soloist for a big band that played live every afternoon.[11] Schuster's first close encounter with heroin addiction occurred in 1947, when Rodney, an African American musician who played with Charlie Parker and was a few years older than Schuster, started to use heroin. In a 2004 interview, Schuster said: "I watched Red and others of his friends shoot up heroin. . . . At that period of time I smoked marijuana, jazz musicians did that. I thought, gee, if I'm a jazz musician, that's part of the game."[12] Schuster recounted getting fired for getting high while playing, after others noticed the distorting effect of marijuana on his sense of timing: "Once I got up and played about six notes and sat back down because I thought I had played too long; my friend, who was playing saxophone, realized why and started laughing. We both got fired for that. But I was too neurotic at that point in my life to think about putting a needle in my arm, . . . I was too anxious. Fortunately, I never experimented with it, because, of course, opiates are very good anxiolytics. I was definitely at risk."

Confrontations between drug users and the law shaped his political commitments. Schuster recalled that the "jazz musician's lawyer," Charles RoYceman, would invariably be called when Billie Holiday checked into Philadelphia hotel rooms, and the police found "stuff" up in the ceiling or behind the lamp:

"They wouldn't arrest her, they just didn't want her in town. . . . That was the other thing that got me out of the nightclubs. I was always underage, so I always had false ID. You had to have special permits for working in night clubs . . . I saw that police didn't have much regard for jazz musicians, and I was frightened. I just couldn't see myself at age forty being subject to being pushed around by them." His familiarity on the jazz scene put Schuster in the position to witness racial segregation, police harassment, and red-baiting at a young age: "Philadelphia was segregated at that time. I went to a segregated school as a child in Camden, New Jersey. Black kids went to school fifteen minutes before or after we did, so we wouldn't be on the street at the same time." After moving to Albuquerque, New Mexico, where he frequented a South Fourth Street bar called the Chicken Shack during his junior year of college, Schuster witnessed the arrest of an African American friend for selling marijuana: "The police just couldn't understand why I would go to this place on South Fourth Street if it wasn't for drugs. And it wasn't for drugs. It was because there was good music there" (2004).

Most people imagine a world of difference between the jazz clubs of Philadelphia and the animal models of behavioral pharmacologists, but Schuster drew connections between research, personal observations, and his political commitments: "Back when I was a jazz musician, I had seen people who would sit around and play with needles, even injecting themselves. They were so-called 'needle freaks.' [Y]ou could make a monkey a 'needle freak,' too, by associating stimuli with the drug. After a while those stimuli became conditioned reinforcers. So I looked at 'needle freaks' as an instance of individuals who were engaging in a behavior that was frequently associated with drug use, and therefore the whole act of taking the drug, cooking it up and so forth, had some conditioned reinforcing properties. I was also able to demonstrate that when they went into withdrawal they would work to a much greater extent for opiates. I was surprised that the drugs that animals would take were by and large the same drugs that some humans got into trouble with. It was amazing, the concordance" (2004). Schuster would have been less likely to make such connections working solely in the laboratory. The insights he garnered from social relationships with active drug users lay at the basis of the kind of scientific knowledge he pursued.

Social proximity between the researcher and the research subject is important because researchers are constituted in part by the social process of research, the form of work that is situated within the social context of the laboratory. Schuster said,

> First of all, I have always felt a great deal of compassion for individuals who have become addicted to drugs because I witnessed the transformation from people who were just playing around with drugs to becoming truly addicted and unable to stop despite the fact that they were quite aware of the fact that there were huge deleterious consequences to their continued use. Secondly, I guess I also came out of it with the feeling that to deal with it as a problem of morality didn't make any sense to me either. I didn't think of these people as being immoral, perhaps because I knew them prior to the time they became involved with drugs. By and large most of them were pretty decent individuals who for a variety of reasons became involved with drugs and became addicted.

For this reason, Schuster found it made sense to think of drug abuse as a behavioral disorder in which drugs functioned to reinforce social learning. Setting out to induce animals to self-administer drugs of abuse, Schuster anticipated he would have to "trick" animals into taking drugs. He found that he did not have to make animals physically dependent, however, in order for opiates to serve as positive reinforcers: "All I had to do was make them available and I found very, very few animals who would not learn to emit some sort of operant response when you used drugs as a consequence for that" (2004).

Marching rapidly through the known pharmacopeia, behavioral pharmacologists cataloged drug effects in animals and drew up tables of concordance between human and animal responses. Schuster explained: "Drugs that are aversive in humans, such as phenothiazines—animals would actually learn to avoid injection of them so they served as negative reinforcers. The concordance was striking. I don't know of any other animal model in any area of psychiatry that has both the face validity and construct validity that animal self-administration studies do." Preoccupied with establishing concordance and responding to critics who saw behaviorists as reductionists, behavioral pharmacologists eventually got around to exploring the existing knowledge of the field into which they had blundered so enthusiastically. Now in graduate school at the University of Maryland, Thompson and Schuster made a visit to Nathan Eddy, who they recognized as the leader of the NRC Committee on Drug Addiction and Narcotics. Schuster said: "He was at NIH in this funny building off campus that had to have structural supports because there were so many books in it. He was essentially blind. He invited us to a CPDD meeting in Ann Arbor, Michigan" (2004).[13]

After reporting on his animal self-administration work with Thompson at the 1963 CDAN meeting, Schuster was lured by Seevers to the University of Michigan. Seevers imported behavioral approaches and the devices on which they depended. Because of his early interest in desire for stimulants (see chap.

2 of the present book), Seevers was predisposed to accept the behavioral tenet that drugs acted as positive reinforcers, and he believed that desire signaled something beyond physiological need.[14] Animal self-administration differed from previous drug screening done at the monkey colony, where emphasis lay on describing the toxic consequences of drugs at doses that animals would voluntarily take. Schuster said, "Whereas I was interested in behavior, [they were] interested in describing what happened to animals when allowed free access to drugs. [They were] not necessarily interested so much in their behavior as [their physiology]."[15] The work of the Applied Psychology Laboratory, as Schuster's laboratory at the University of Michigan was called, emphasized behavior and reinforcement. Schuster explained that in the social world of behavioral pharmacology, "the behavior is always right," and "the behavior is the reality" (2004). The work accomplished in the brief time that Schuster worked at Michigan with James Woods—who was hired as a lab assistant but worked his way up to head the lab—is often pointed to as one of the chief origins of the drug self-administration breakthrough.

Behavioral pharmacologists embraced single-subject designs and were skeptical of statistical analysis in ways that led them to focus closely on individual subjects. From his faculty position at the University of Minnesota, Travis Thompson trained individuals who became prominent in the field—among them George Bigelow, Thomas Crowley, Roland Griffiths, and Roy Pickens—before becoming interested in behaviors of self-injury and self-harm. Bigelow and Griffiths migrated to Johns Hopkins University, spending their careers in behavioral biology and neuroscience. Their long-standing scientific collaboration began in the unlikely halls of Faribault State Hospital in Faribault, Minnesota, where they tried to use behavior modification techniques with severely mentally disabled individuals. Griffiths described this first collaboration as follows:

> Here were these grossly deteriorated institutions with profoundly and severely retarded people just being housed under what would have to be described as inhumane conditions. There was no sense that you could do anything for them. They were cleaned up and then they sat in these bare dayrooms and rocked back and forth or were put in restraining rooms when they misbehaved. This whole technology of behavioral control (and this is the power of the experimental analysis of behavior) says, wait a second, these people don't have to sit there, let's teach them something. We have the technology for teaching them something. It's a question of contingencies. Take a look at what contingencies exist in this situation, and no wonder they run around hitting each other. The only time that anyone gets any attention from the staff is if they soil themselves

> or if they get aggressive. Then the staff come over and start interacting with them. From a behavioral paradigm, it was just backwards. (2005)

A palpable enthusiasm for radical behaviorism still shines through in the early work of Bigelow and Griffiths but has been tempered with the awareness of naïveté and with the discovery of the limits of behavioral approaches.

Another early collaboration between Bigelow and Griffiths, a study on a single chronic alcoholic at the Baltimore City Hospital, illustrates an important aspect of research design in behavioral approaches (Bigelow and Griffiths 1973). This study resembled Wikler's experimental readdiction paper and focused on establishing a baseline of how much a chronic alcoholic would drink when allowed to do so. Then Bigelow, Griffiths, and Pickens stabilized the individual and tailored a set of contingencies to which they felt he would respond. This approach presaged today's "individual treatment plans" and derived from a sense of the human costs of a widespread phenomenon. Yet behavioral pharmacologists confronted a broader pharmacological research enterprise that was in the process of becoming hostile to within-subject designs.

Single-subject design contrasts to large-scale clinical trials. "[Behavioral science] is not interested in gathering data that are then described by using inductive or deductive statistical measurements. The interest is in the individual case rather than in the mean of a sample. . . . Much of modern behaviorism also concentrates on detailed work on one individual in preference to the descriptions of groups, on the grounds that an effect, once properly demonstrated by the unique individual, will be found to be true of all" (Candland 1993, 356).[16] The belief in the power of single-subject designs placed behavioral techniques and knowledge at odds with today's drift toward large sample sizes, statistical analysis, and population-wide assessments. Those who entered the field when single-subject designs were still possible lament a loss of precision: "People don't get the power of single-subject analysis anymore. It is the anomalous finding that is most interesting" (Griffiths 2005). Coming of age brought behavioral pharmacology into a more realistic integration with other currents of the addiction research enterprise.

THE USES OF PROXIMITY: PUTTING BEHAVIOR INTO ADDICTION RESEARCH

Establishing cross-species concordance between animal models and findings in humans was an impressive reinforcer for behavioral scientists. It required either proximity between animal and human laboratories that produced data under similar conditions or access to cumulative data sets produced by other researchers. Eventually, behavioral pharmacologists turned to the only existing human data set—that produced by the ARC. They did not do so until they were ready to trust the validity of the ARC's results. This happened only after they matured beyond the enthusiastic, almost religious fervor of the 1960s. That readiness did not emerge until after the ARC's relocation to Johns Hopkins University, a stronghold of behavioral pharmacology. Two members of the Hopkins Behavioral Pharmacology Research Unit, George Bigelow and Roland Griffiths, visited Lexington to talk over the possible move.

> The real issue for the Lexington people was not that we were looking at them but that they wanted information from us about the prospects of their being able to prosper in Baltimore. They were interested in the fact that we had experience doing human drug self-administration research and working with an IRB [institutional review board] for getting approval and could describe the environmental context of being able to recruit substance abuser volunteers from the community. That's something they were unfamiliar with and very afraid of. For forty years they had been dependent on a literally captive population for doing their work. They had a lot of doubts and concerns about whether their methodologies could be transferred over to working with a truly volunteer population who could walk out and choose not to have anything to do with them. The main purpose of [our] mission on that visit was for them to get somewhat reassured by us and from us that you can do human clinical pharmacology work in Baltimore, in this institution and in this urban setting, and both get the regulatory approvals and the volunteer participation and cooperation. (Bigelow 2005)

As members of the behavioral pharmacology enclave, Bigelow and Griffiths were initially oblivious to the work of the ARC. Griffiths remembered giving a paper in the 1960s after which Bill Martin had chided him for not acknowledging work done at Lexington. There were deep conceptual and technical divisions between the classical pharmacology of the ARC—which relied on group design, subjective ratings, and classical (Pavlovian) conditioning—and the operant (Skinnerian) conditioning of the new guard. Griffiths admitted that such divisions mattered: "It didn't occur to me that there was any value in asking people how they felt. I continue to have huge skepticism about what people say" (2005). Divisions of lexicon and training were consequential for research design, development and deployment of instruments, and interpretation of results.

As Griffiths observed, "getting animal and human laboratories to talk to each other" requires material conditions and institutional circumstances that enable such cross talk (2005). Such circumstances align in few places, and the ARC had been one when at Lexington. Intensified scrutiny and the loss of Lexington increased "pressure for methodological adaptations that would permit similar scientific evaluations to be done in other settings and with other [nonprisoner] populations" (Bigelow 1991, 1617–18). A new set of alliances was enabled when the Behavioral Pharmacology Research Unit at Johns Hopkins University gained access to the knowledge base produced by the ARC. Describing his initial exposure to the history of the field while at the University of Minnesota, Bigelow noted: "We had some familiarity with the methods of the Addiction Research Center, but I think it was a pretty superficial understanding. Frankly, their methods were viewed somewhat skeptically by people from a rigorous operant background. They were giving drugs to people and asking them what they thought, not using any operant principles. Not until later, certainly after I moved to Hopkins, did I really develop an appreciation for the quality of that work and the orderliness of those types of measures and that methodology for assessing drug effects" (2005). The relationship between the ARC and the Behavioral Pharmacology Research Unit provides a perfect example of what Ludwik Fleck maintained occurred when "a large group exists long enough [that its] thought style becomes fixed and formal in structure": "Practical performance then dominates over creative mood, which is reduced to a certain fixed level that is disciplined, uniform, and discreet" (1979, 103). As a dominant thought collective, the ARC had reached a position where its ways of going about things were formalized to the point of being stylized. As a stable, specialized group, the ARC was an exclusive enclave that can in some sense be said to have "discovered addiction"—and came to occupy the same space as a thought collective of "true believers."

Behavioral pharmacologists constituted "addiction" anew, rendering it subject to the method of operant conditioning. Bigelow reported that not until operant conditioners ran up against limitations did they "largely but not completely" abandon "the most rigorous operant methods" and adopt "self-report measures as an index of drug effects in humans to a substantial degree" (2005). He explained that prior to the advent of computers in the laboratory, it was cumbersome to collect, store, manage, and analyze qualitative data generated from self-reports or questionnaires.

> In the early seventies when Roland [Griffiths] and I were working together at Baltimore City Hospitals, doing our first human operant work, we started off trying to be rigorous operant conditioners. We had people pull levers and

> ignored, to a large extent, opportunities to ask people to provide self-report information. We didn't have confidence in self-report as a useful measure. When we did try to do things like that, we quickly found ourselves overwhelmed with more pieces of paper than we could conveniently look at and analyze. With the advent of personal computers, all the questionnaires could be put on the computer. Instead of having to sort through and score things, you'd get a nice, orderly spreadsheet of summary data at the end. It suddenly became a domain of data that could be really conveniently collected and managed and analyzed and appreciated. (2005)

Despite instruments designed to elicit and compare the subjective effects of drugs, not until computational resources became commonplace in laboratory settings could the subjective domain really be analyzed and understood.

Surveying the standardization of methodology and instruments for measuring abuse potential, Bigelow credited the ARC with nearly six decades of work forming the "primary foundation for virtually all of our currently available methods for clinical drug abuse liability assessment" (1991, 1615). Crediting the ARC with foundational, seminal, or pioneering contributions to the field is commonplace in the publications of behavioral pharmacologists to a far greater degree than in the other arenas of addiction research. This may be in part a "cohort effect," where today's senior behavioral pharmacologists once found themselves relying on the ARC data as a way to establish concordance and back up their assertions concerning the power of their methodologies. Yet the Addiction Research Center Inventory (ARCI)—consisting of five hundred true-false statements concerning the subject's emotions and perceptions and administered in conjunction with observation and physiological tests (e.g., of pupil diameter) while the subject is on drugs—is far more subjective than behavioral pharmacologists generally get. The ARCI was many years in the making at Lexington, where psychometricians Harris Hill, Richard Belleville, and Charles A. Haertzen developed it in response to Harris Isbell's request for a sophisticated way to measure the subjective effects of drugs and distinguish their profiles of effects from one another. While Isbell intended the project to meet short-term needs, the ARCI became a complex, multiscalar inventory still used to distinguish the subjective profile of each major drug category.

Efforts to standardize the study of subjective effects relied on the use of drug-experienced human subjects—the very postaddicts described in previous chapters—as bioassays. Coupled with intensified scrutiny of human subjects experimentation and the absorption of the ARC into NIDA, the loss of Lexington increased "pressure for methodological adaptations that would permit similar scientific evaluations to be done in other settings and with other [non-prisoner] populations" (Bigelow 1991, 1617–18). Among the collaborations undertaken between the relocated ARC and the Hopkins unit were animal and clinical studies of buprenorphine, a drug approved in 2003 for treatment of opiate addiction. When they moved from Lexington to Baltimore, ARC researchers brought both the drug itself and the idea to use it in this manner.

By the late 1960s, behavioral pharmacologists had invented a new lexicon, in which the process of addiction was one of conditioning, learning, and motivation. As experimentalists, they saw pharmacology as a means to an end for studying the principles by which drugs act as peculiarly powerful reinforcers of behavior. They were critics of physiological functionalism and psychoanalytic constructs alike. From their earliest days, however, some believed that neurobiology would one day be reintegrated with the study of behavior (MacCorquodale and Meehle 1948). Behavioral pharmacologists formed an enunciative community that occupied fertile ground between, on the one hand, such antecedents as Wikler's long-standing interest in classical conditioning and, on the other, harbingers of change in the material, social, and technological conditions of work in the laboratory. When behavioral pharmacologists entered the social worlds of addiction research, a gradual but wholesale transition was under way. This transition was not unlike what the field of substance abuse research is undergoing with the current shift to neuroscience and genetics and the eclipse of behavioral pharmacology. Rather than experience this transition as a negative event, many of my interviewees in behavioral pharmacology used what Renee C. Fox has called "ritualized optimism" to cope with change (1959/1998). They pointed out how integrated and holistic their enterprise was relative to that of reductive, molecular or subcellular approaches. According to Schuster, reductionistic approaches "can only be so successful," because unexplained phenomena emerge at each level of integration. Others argue behavioral pharmacology served as a gateway for neurobiology to enter the field.[17] General acceptance of behavioral pharmacology paved the way for the appropriation of its specific vocabulary and precise concepts—since, as Schuster argued, "everybody thinks they're an expert in behavior" and uses the language of drugs as reinforcers. Schuster explained:

> A lot of the techniques that are used by neurobiologists have been taken from behavioral pharmacologists. Now that we are getting into subcellular events, it's extremely exciting, it's absolutely marvelous. Ultimately, however, I believe that not just in this science [but] in all sciences, . . . a reductionistic approach can only be so successful. As one moves up levels of integration, at these higher

> levels of integration, new phenomena emerge that are not reducible to those that are below. Ultimately, no matter how well we understand the enzymatic and protein pathways of the cell, we've got to explain the behavior of the intact, integrated organism. The behavior is always right. It is ultimately the job of the biologist to be able to predict that behavior because the behavior is the reality. The behavioral effects of drugs are the reality. Understanding them at different levels is fine, and I'm excited about it, but we cannot forget that the end product is that we're trying to change people's behavior. (2004)

Statements such as "the behavior is always right" and "the behavior is the reality" mark both the specificity of behavioral approaches and their singularity. These statements impart the flavor of a mantra that still conveys some of the earlier, almost religious fervor with which behaviorists approached "addiction."

Behavioral pharmacologists themselves go to great lengths to differentiate the range of reinforcers with which they work and have become increasingly refined at doing so. However, they have also been criticized for being "biological determinists" or believing in "universal reinforcers." Both charges obscure the degree to which behavioral pharmacologists try to analyze social complexity, the working of memory in environmental cues, and the divergence between what happens in animals and what happens in humans. A science that shows that subjects being conditioned to experience drugs classed as "stimulants" as depressing, or vice versa, can hardly be accused of making universalist or biologically determinist assumptions. Behaviorists in fact reject universalism and biological determinism, favoring direct observation and objective measurement, in contrast to views that drugs provide inherent biological rewards.

Arising to counter what they viewed as unjust stigmatization of addiction and mental illness, Skinnerian behaviorists applied the principles of operant conditioning as an alternative to moral judgment. They were not particularly modest witnesses—indeed, many were cocksure until the limits of their own philosophy and techniques became clearer over time. They remain an interesting species of practitioners of the experimental life, having been chastened by realities but still successful at translating their science into practical knowledge through the evidence-based practice called "contingency management." Because of them, it is now generally accepted that drugs act as reinforcers and that social or adaptive learning sustains the social structures and neural substrates of addiction. They offered a useful explanatory model of how addiction works that accounted well for a wide variety of phenomena, including the idea that drug addiction can be an inflexible response to negative consequences.

Behavioral pharmacology enjoyed what Helen Longino called the "epistemological success of content" (Longino 2002, 114–21). By experimentally isolating behavior, behavioral pharmacologists recognized social complexity, but their Skinnerian upbringing led them to set up experimental situations according to the laboratory logics of behavioral reasoning. Their laboratory logics depend on observation, a socially organized form of perception: "Observation is not simple sense perception (whatever that might be) but an organized sensory encounter that registers what is perceived in relation to categories, concepts, and classes that are socially produced. Both ordering and organization are (dependent on) social processes" (Longino 2002, 100). Behavioral researchers are more cognizant than many scientists that they slip between what is actually happening and the conceptual categories through which they make sense of what is actually happening. Their discourse is replete with casual and systematic acknowledgment of that gap. However, as sociologists of science show, science depends on producing "intersubjective invariance of observation" by narrowing what counts as a plausible way to produce credible findings and claims (Longino 2002, 103).

Behavioral pharmacologists have built tightly interwoven social networks that enable ongoing social interaction with similarly situated others in order to share tacit and formal knowledge in ways that reduce intersubjective variance. Longino wrote:

> Cognitive processes have a social dimension. Of course, while the sociality of cognitive processes is part of what grants them their warranting status, this social dimension can be a source of difficulty. For example, the invisibility of many background assumptions as assumptions . . . means that a closed community will not be able to exhibit those assumptions for critical scrutiny. (Longino 2002, 107)

The founders of the behavioral pharmacological research enclave set forth its underlying principles and tenets as if they were, in fact, revolutionary.

Typically, the underlying assumptions of a particular mode of knowledge production become most available for scrutiny during shifts in dominant modality. The rise of neuroscience in the mid-1990s pressured behavioral pharmacologists to incorporate new findings concerning the neural substrates of behavior (Blank 1999, 81). Behavioral pharmacologists came to occupy a subordinate position relative to the neuroscientist newcomers, who the behaviorally oriented had once tried to attract to the field in hopes of creating a more socially situated neurobiology. We might analyze this story as one of social succession, paradigm shifts, scientific revolutions, or zeitgeist. The narrative illustrates the social process by which scientists "transform the subjective into the objective, not by canonizing one subjectivity over others, but by assuring that what is ratified as knowledge has survived criticism from multiple points of view" (Longino 2002, 129). By the mid-1970s, there was considerable heterogeneity in drug abuse research, which included the fields of neuroscience and genetics—the second of which had rarely, if ever, been mentioned at Lexington—and even a few scientists beginning to study drug taking as the result of metabolic defects. Far from waiting for the visualization of the opiate receptors in the 1970s for promising leads (Acker 2002, 63), behavioral research had earlier pointed toward the neurochemical and molecular basis of repetitive behaviors, as well as to the social environments in which they occurred and were interpreted to be "addictions." Multiple thought styles were becoming a way of life in the social worlds of the addiction research enterprise.

CHAPTER 8

"The Hijacked Brain": Reimagining Addiction

When President George Bush officially proclaimed the 1990s the Decade of the Brain, he stated the value of brain research for the U.S. war on drugs, "as studies provide greater insight into how people become addicted to drugs and how drugs affect the brain." He explained, "These studies may also help produce effective treatments for chemical dependency and help us to understand and prevent the harm done to the preborn children of pregnant women who abuse drugs and alcohol."[1] Tilting steadily toward neuroscience by the 1990s, the Decade of the Brain raised the public awareness, social status, and cultural capital of the field. As the brain became the "target organ of addiction" (DuPont 1997, 93), drug addiction, dependence, or abuse was redefined as a chronic relapsing brain disorder, a unified framework for a problem-based field in conceptual disarray. The laboratory logics by which addiction was localized to the brain dislocated it from the rest of the physical body and from the social body. These laboratory logics strategically borrowed the technical resources and social authority of neuroscience to garner new conceptual and political resources for the substance abuse research enterprise.[2] Although the borrowing strategy alienated some in the treatment community, it raised the profile of the research enterprise and enabled new forms of scientific learning.

Several preconditions had to be in place for neuroscience to "hijack" the field of substance abuse research. "The Hijacked Brain" was the title of the second part of a series narrated by Bill Moyers called *Moyers on Addiction: Close to Home.* The part aired on March 29, 1998, in the midst of public revelations of the heroin addiction of Moyers's son. The hijacking metaphor conveys how forcefully the brain is held "hostage" to drugs of abuse (Bloom 1997, 15).[3] It was used to characterize what drugs of abuse did to the brain: "We have learned how some drugs and alcohol can disrupt volitional mechanisms by hijacking the brain mechanisms involved in seeking natural reinforcement and weakening brain mechanisms that inhibit these processes" (Volkow and Li 2005, 1429). The travels of the hijacking metaphor—and its staying power—forcefully convey how neuroscience remade the social worlds of substance abuse research with the claim that addiction was a chronic relapsing brain disorder. The implication was that the elusive secrets of this "disease of the will" would now yield to the powerful force of brain science.

Visualization of the long-hypothesized opiate receptors and the technical capacity to image the brain in situ created a new optics that made plausible the neuroscientific claim that addiction results when neurobiology goes awry. Opiate receptors, the molecular sites where drugs accomplish their work in the brain, were quickly mapped according to location and density. Neuropharmacologist Michael Kuhar explained: "A receptor is a place where a drug works. Receptors are all over the brain. You take a drug orally, get it in your stomach, then the blood carries it to the brain, bam, the drug sits in a receptor, and that receptor is activated" (2005). Here, individual cells are represented as actors in the dramas of pleasure and pain that underlie patterns of social interaction and cultural life.

Neuroscience gave substance abuse research the stamp of legitimacy, which was particularly important when NIDA faced becoming an NIH institute in 1992. Attracting neuroscientists raised the social and scientific stature of the enterprise, but it was a double-edged strategy that reduced the recognition that addiction is a complex disorder consisting of socially situated behaviors that occur within the particular cultural and economic geographies that shape which drugs are available to whom for what price. Although neuroscience has made legible "new modes of embodiment" (Wilson 2004), the ascension of neuroscience and genetics has also suppressed behavioral and sociological approaches better attuned to persons living with addictions. However, genetic, neurobiochemical, and behavioral approaches need not be mutually exclusive or opposed to one another. There are differences between, on the one hand, scientists already in the field of addiction research who, to advance knowledge about substance abuse, instrumentally took up new tools and techniques (e.g., positron-emission tomography [PET] scanning; functional, or "fast," magnetic resonance imaging [fMRI]; or cloning) and, on the other hand, scientists who saw the substance abuse arena as yet another arena in which to display what these new tools and techniques can do. The latter have little historical connection to substance abuse research or pharmacology and low regard for both. The former have an instrumental interest in putting new tools in their place without attributing too much power to them or to explanations based solely on their deployment.

Outside the addiction research enterprise, neuroscientists viewed incursions from other fields with cynicism. A developer of PET scanning remarked:

> I have had many people express an interest in using PET, typically established scientists in many fields who may be on a downhill curve of their career. Very overtly they express that PET is such a high road to science that they're willing to get involved now. They kind of held back before, but now they are willing to get involved because it is obviously so easy! They lack an understanding of what is entailed, I think, because the data comes out as pretty pictures. (Quoted in Dumit 2003, 57)

Indeed, many of my pharmacologist interviewees began to use these techniques late in their careers, after other approaches had proved inadequate. They learned how to work with PET scanning, genetic data banks, or microassays as the techniques came on line. Outsiders still construct pharmacology as merely an "acting accountant" of the pharmaceutical industry. Michael Phelps, one of the founding fathers of PET scanning, explained his view of the relationship between pharmacology and neuroscience as follows:

> Pharmacology as a discipline began to fail in many ways. . . . If you go back about three decades ago, [when] pharmacology began, the major activity in pharmacology was neuropharmacology. It was a time of grind and bind, doing assays of neurotransmitter systems. That is how neuropharmacology became very popular and very productive. It was teaching a lot of new things about the brain, and drug companies had focused on the brain and were developing drugs for the brain. And pharmacology became the acting accountant for that. But then neuroscience was born, and neuroscience in a decade went from a group of maybe twenty-five, thirty people to fourteen thousand [by going into other disciplines] and collect[ing] out the neuroscience people. Well, in pharmacology, that was particularly devastating, because the best and the majority of people were neuroscientists. . . . [P]harmacology started to lose its way. . . . The industry was moving a lot faster than pharmacology was. It was lagging behind. (Quoted in Dumit 2003, 183–84)

Haunted by second-class citizenship, the modesty of the pharmacological sciences contrasts to the overpromising hubris of neuroscience, which echoes the optimism described at the beginning of chapter 4 in the present book. Yet neuroscience simply does not explain enough of the complex social phenomenon that is addiction to be completely satisfying. Telling the story of how addiction became a brain disease as one in which neuroscience displaced all other approaches does not quite fit the data or the ethos of scientists who have spent their lives laboring in this field. A more accurate sense of the material conditions and thought constraints within which scientific labor yields scientific claims can be obtained by looking at how particular commitments and logics are embedded in practices, techniques, and technologies. Behind today's neurobiological models lie the shadowy outlines of perennial beliefs about drugs and drug users that shape their innermost experiences, as well as external observations of their behaviors. Neuroscience entered substance abuse research not as a revolution but as a legitimizing force deeply interconnected with behavioral antecedents and with Abraham Wikler's work on conditioning and the role of cues in triggering relapse.

Neuroscientific concepts of addiction emerged as the result of tools and techniques initially developed to visualize opiate receptors and trace their exact locations in the brain. These techniques and the conceptual advances they enabled profoundly changed scientific research on drug dependence. While neuroscientists have moved toward modular theories that "delocalize" capacities and show the diffusion of receptor sites, popular depictions relentlessly "localize" specific functions to particular locations in which the brain is the central actor (Wilson 2004, 93–94). Neurobiological claims are used in public discourse to stabilize a particular set of claims about innate differences and irreversible alterations of brain structure and function. Yet most neuroscientists in the substance abuse field have a considerably more multiple and elastic view of brain structure and function than public discourse admits. Today's neuroscience and molecular genetics are far from the reductionistic or deterministic endeavors of some of their historical antecedents.[4] Yet they are still viewed with some suspicion. Whether neuroscience is depicted as in a state of underdevelopment or arrested development or as on the cutting edge, it is evident that it has not yet reached anything resembling a settled consensus on substance abuse or drug treatment.

REDEFINING ADDICTION AS A CHRONIC RELAPSING BRAIN DISORDER

People interpret their innermost sensations through the dominant lexicons of their time, which are often based on scientific scripts that have diffused through social space. The earliest constructs of addiction as a chronic or relapsing disorder were not neurological. Starting in the 1950s, they were by the Public Relations Office at Lexington to explain high rates of release among those treated at the institution. The 1965 edition of Goodman and Gilman's *Pharmacological Basis of Therapeutics,* the monumental textbook for clinicians on drug action and drug-disease interaction, contained the following words in the chapter on "Drug Addiction and Drug Abuse": "In extreme forms, the behavior [compulsive drug use] exhibits the characteristics of a chronic, relapsing disease" (Jaffe 1965, 285). Having been asked to write the chapter by Alfred Gilman, who chaired the department of pharmacology at Albert Einstein, Jerome H. Jaffe had been a "two-year wonder" at Lexington and was on the cusp of embarking on a career to place science and treatment evaluation at the base of drug policy. Jaffe neither constructed drug addiction or abuse as a "brain disease" nor referred to anything but its most extreme forms as displaying the characteristics of a chronic, relapsing disease. The discursive shift to a "chronic, relapsing *brain* disease" came about in the 1990s. For instance, the now defunct Office of Technology Assessment (OTA) repeatedly asserted throughout a 1990 report, *The Effectiveness of Drug Abuse Treatment,* that drug abuse was a chronic relapsing brain disorder (CRBD) with "patterns of relapses and remissions that resemble other chronic diseases, such as arthritis and chronic depression." Written in the context of the HIV/AIDS epidemic,[5] the report framed the "fatal link between the two epidemics" as fueling the HIV/AIDS epidemic due to the heterogeneous and unmarked population from which drug abusers were drawn (OTA 1990, 1).[6] The OTA report suggested that a lack of rigor, unsophisticated design and analysis, "anecdotal, uncontrolled studies," and "poor study methods" pervaded the addiction research enterprise. Focusing on the need for comparative treatment evaluation, the OTA suggested "dissecting" programs to determine which components were effective for which client groups and custom fitting treatment to individuals: "Ultimately, research on drug abuse treatment should lead to what has been a common practice in medicine, namely a case management approach with an individual tailored plan to maximize the likelihood of treatment effectiveness" (1990, 10). The OTA favorably cited NIDA for embarking on randomized clinical trials, which would gradually displace disparaged forms of social, behavioral, and cultural research.

Translating between the specialized domain of neuroscience and the popular realm required a compelling figure. The "hijacked brain" was a condensed ideogram for the minute biological changes that manifested in the social phenomenon of "compulsive, uncontrollable drug use." Alan Leshner, director of

NIDA from 1994 to 2001 before becoming head of the American Association for the Advancement of Science, was the leading proponent of the discursive move to replace old ideology with the new science of the hijacked brain. A self-described "science guy," Leshner was beloved by audiences mesmerized by his "tough-guy swagger" in the town meetings through which he brought the concept of the CRBD to the field (Kreeger 1995, 12).

Central to the CRBD concept was the idea that neurochemical changes caused fundamental alterations in the brain that, as Peggy Orenstein reported, led to "drug-seeking becom[ing] as biologically driven as hunger, sex, or breathing." Orenstein continued, "Long after the addict quits, some of those brain changes remain, creating vulnerability for relapse" (2002, 6). The claim that vulnerability to addiction is a basic, biological drive to which some are genetically predisposed might be put to a variety of political uses, as could the idea that compulsive drug use fundamentally alters the brain.[7] Defining addiction this way cemented neuroscience as the dominant approach to its study. This problem definition was then translated to a treatment workforce typically described as "backward," scientifically illiterate, or inadequately professional.[8] The result was that those who enrolled neuroscientists in substance abuse research alienated frontline treatment providers, who were, until recently, often drawn from the ranks of addicted persons. However, Leshner was charismatic for treatment providers, who became friendlier to the science he embodied and still recall being transfixed when they listened to him (Bunk 1998, 1–2). The concept of the CRBD helped close gaps between the "science guys," the treatment community, and a public widely subscribed to recovery discourse.

Figuring addiction as a brain disease at the fundamental level finessed myriad differences within the research and treatment enterprise. NIDA could not monologically proclaim neuroscience as the one best way to understand addiction, given the dominance of behavioral pharmacology within substance abuse research at the time. Concessions to the effect that substance abuse is a social and behavioral process still had to be made. As Leshner stated in a 1997 article in *Science*, addiction is "not *just* a brain disease" but the result of a welter of environmental and historical factors. Proclaiming to viewers of Moyers's "The Hijacked Brain" that no singular approach was likely to yield adequate knowledge of the "most complex phenomenon that's facing our society," Leshner declared—and NIDA insiders echo him with little irony—that a thousand flowers would bloom at NIDA. He explained: "We need to bring a multidisciplinary approach to this problem, and that's what I hope the science will give us."

A thousand flowers did not in fact bloom at NIDA. Neurobiological models were pitted against social research and behavioral models, a struggle that took place barely beneath the rhetorical surface of the Decade of the Brain. A well-established drug ethnographer put it: "[T]here's a lot of flowers blooming, but the ones that get cut and placed on the main table are very different. . . . Findings do not get disseminated in the same way. There's all kinds of areas that we could be looking at, like controlled drug use, like harm reduction, like recreational drug use that [I just don't see happening] in the political climate that I've been functioning in since I've been doing this work" (Murphy 2003). Similar complaints arose from geneticists and behavioral pharmacologists who felt cut out of the action by the redefinition. Privately skeptical of the assumptions behind the assertion that addiction was a CRBD, many conceded the usefulness of Leshner's attempt to unify the highly differentiated interdisciplinary field of which he had assumed the helm, especially for raising its social status. The ascendancy of neuroscience, they agreed, was a necessary, if not inevitable, step to maturity.

Concerns about the field's maturity arise periodically. In the mid-1990s, they led to the formation of the National Academy of Sciences Committee to Identify Strategies to Raise the Profile of Substance Abuse and Alcoholism Research, which in 1997 reported that the endeavor was a "mature field that should attract the very best scientists in both basic and translational research" (49), although it was largely failing to do so. The Institute of Medicine's 1996 review of NIDA's research portfolio proposed an agenda to ensure wiser public investment in drug abuse research (30–31). The consensus was clear—the field should court high-status neuroscientists (who were not yet occupying the field in great numbers) and also should perhaps invest further in genetics.

Advanced during the Decade of the Brain, the redefinition of addiction as a matter for neuroscientific investigation was more than a cynical ploy for appropriations. Once the word *brain* had been inserted into the phrase *chronic relapsing disorder*, neuroscience became the chief reference point. Beyond rendering addiction research a neat, tidy, and clean enterprise, the chief stake was the strong differentiation of addicted brains from nonaddicted brains. "The Hijacked Brain" cast neuroscientists as heroic "archeologists of the brain" united in their quest to unravel the "mysteries of the addicted mind," mounting "extraordinary scientific expeditions to explain how some people will sacrifice everything to satisfy their hunger for a chemical fix" by showing exactly "how drugs enter pathways of the brain and how they alter the brain to create something that didn't exist before." The film depicted neuroscientists at

Massachusetts General Hospital using PET scanning technology to get a picture of "Denise," an African American cocaine user. The white-coated researchers complimented their subject—who is not "Denise" but her "nice lookin' brain"—and enacted the careful choreography that went into producing a "map of her feelings" when she is high. Claiming to see exactly "where craving for the drug actually takes place" as the drug was coursing through her veins, Steve Hyman, then the head of the Harvard Interfaculty Initiative on Mind, Brain, and Behavior and later director NIMH, interpreted the resulting image as one of "desire in the brain."

Leaving aside issues of interpretation and lack of standardization in the analysis of these images (issues pointed out in Dumit 2003), Hyman's use of the word *desire* signaled an older lexicon of addiction. At stake in the CRBD construct was the degree to which differences between addicts and nonaddicts could be characterized in terms of neuroanatomical brain signatures, neurochemistry, and neurogenetics and how long such differences endured. Leshner put it tautologically in "The Hijacked Brain": "It's a disease because it's the result of drugs changing the brain in fundamental and long-lasting ways. . . . [I]t's actually a different state." The debate was over the relative permanence of that different state. Leshner offered a haunting characterization of addicts: "Imagine being in a state where the drug has totally taken over their being; what that means clinically is that they're in a condition where they suffer from compulsive uncontrollable drug-seeking and use." Leshner was not in the addiction field; he had to be recruited to it, and reports have it that he was a hard sell because stigma pervaded his own structures of belief. As he did in "The Hijacked Brain," he would publicly say such things as "Stigma is one of the biggest problems for us in dealing scientifically with addiction," "People hate addicts," or "People are nervous that an addict is going to do something to them." The CRBD construct was supposed to banish stigma once and for all, a feat quite unlikely in American society, given the racial, ethnic, and class stratification evident in the history of drug use and drug policy. Instead, a neuroscience of difference is likely to simply become a way to render social and economic distinctions scientific.

There is a similarly repetitive pattern of claiming fundamental differences and asserting their inevitability in the neuroscientific approach to sex differences. Taken together, these beliefs converge on the long-standing notion that women are more biologically vulnerable to addiction and even further gone as a species of addict (Campbell 2000). An African American woman who appeared as a recovered heroin addict in "The Hijacked Brain" took up a common rhetorical role for women when she stated, "You don't feel like a human being when you do drugs because the things you are doing are inhuman—you lie, you cheat, you steal." Those are, of course, relatively human activities, but the point is that racialized female addicts serve as a condensed and potent metaphor for social decline. The figure of the addicted woman encodes compulsion without control, failures of self-governance, and the overwhelming power of illegitimate desires and insatiable needs. Because prevailing views of citizenship include the notion that only those who can govern themselves are fit to govern others, there are huge political stakes embedded in the claim that addicts' brains differ fundamentally from nonaddicts' brains.

Conceptual definitions work as technologies of visibility to channel attention and resource allocation in scientific research. External depictions of addiction science cast it as deeply riven with questionable approaches and results (Institute of Medicine 1996 and National Academy of Sciences Committee to Identify Strategies 1997). Moves to portray the results of addiction research as unequivocally known rather than unknown do not take place in a sociocultural vacuum. Historians have shown that the margin of social tolerance for addicted persons depends on how members of the dominant classes perceive them. Because scientific constructs perform cultural work within institutions, such redefinitions affect the governance of drug use and drug users. A nagging sense remains that addiction is not just a brain disease and that neuroscience is not quite enough to erase the traces of the cultural repository of ideas and images that underlie assumptions about the essential ungovernability of drug addicts.

"THIS IS YOUR BRAIN ON DRUGS": THE BRAIN BECOMES A MATERIAL-SEMIOTIC ACTOR

Claims issuing from behavioral pharmacology and neuroscience differ in the cultural work that they perform. By defining drugs as reinforcers, behavioral pharmacology leveled social distinctions between organisms who use drugs of abuse and those who do not. In the United States, neuroscience, in contrast, has been pursued as a science of difference and used to reinscribe social hierarchies.[9] Relationships between the new old-timers (the self-proclaimed radical behaviorists described in the previous chapter of this book) and neuroscientific newcomers were sometimes tense. Michael Kuhar explained: "Drug self-administration had captured people's imagination very, very much like receptor binding had. The thing about drug self-administration, one of the things that I think people overlook, is that it really was another paradigm shift because it showed that animals will take drugs. There's nothing intrinsically bad about this animal or that animal. That was a very important paradigm shift for treating drug addicts. It was clear that taking drugs and seeking drugs was a capability of everybody's brain" (2005).

When neuroscience became useful in the addiction research enterprise, behavioral pharmacology was the dominant approach. Neuroscientific newcomers remember being treated like "redheaded stepchildren." Coming from physics and mathematics, they had misgivings about whether behavior was "a rigorous science": "Instead of looking at a moving, behaving animal and observing how much drug they were taking, we were looking at the molecular site where that drug acted. We were stepping into a new microscopic realm of drug action and drug taking" (Kuhar 2005). When the opiate receptors, the main nonhuman actors of that microscopic realm, were first visualized, few established addiction researchers were studying the brain, and those doing so used in vitro and in vivo techniques. They were divided over whether receptors or single-molecule binding sites were "real" or not. Among believers, there were those who thought there were multiple opiate receptors and those who did not.

Michael Kuhar's career trajectory provides a sense of what it was like to work in a field going through profound conceptual, technical, and discursive shifts every decade or so. Upon entering the field in 1973, Kuhar was scolded by a professor at a prominent university for "talking about receptors as though they were real": "He said that everybody knows receptors aren't real. They're mental constructs that we use to think about how drugs work." Kuhar's first "NIDA" grant came from ADAMHA in 1972.

> There weren't drug receptors at that point, and we didn't know how drugs worked. There was no cloning. We didn't understand the molecular biology of brain proteins very well. The drug self-administration model, that behavioral model which is very important in the field, had really just become established. There was no PET scanning then. There was very little or no brain imaging then. There were few brain banks. I was one of the first individual investigators to have a brain bank, a repository, actually a freezer, where brains are kept for experimental purposes. . . . The patient from which the brain was taken is well documented in terms of his medical history, whether or not he's an addict or she's an addict. (Kuhar 2005)

Evolution of the technical means for studying the brain without access to postmortem human tissue, a scarce and contentious commodity, expanded capacity for neuroscientific research. Nonradioactive methods expanded that capacity once again.

The highly publicized visualization of opiate receptors, the molecular sites of action often described through the metaphor of a lock and key, ushered in an era of "receptor fever." Long a hypothetical entity, the receptor came into theoretical existence well before it could be visualized. As early as 1913, Paul Ehrlich described how toxins injured cells: "They are absorbed by certain specific component parts of the cell side chains which I have characterized as 'receptors'" (quoted in De Jongh 1964, xiii–xvi).[10] Somewhat later, he wrote: "Only such substances can be anchored at any particular part of the organism, as fit into the molecules of the recipient complex like a piece of a mosaic finds its place in a pattern" (quoted in Ariens 1964, xiv). The 1960s elaboration of a science of molecular pharmacology (the systematic knowledge of interaction between body and drug molecules) stands as a singular example of prescience or—in another, more masculinist lexicon—Nature unveiling herself: "To most of the modern pharmacologists the receptor is like a beautiful but remote lady. He has written her many a letter and quite often she has answered the letter. From these answers the pharmacologist has built himself an image of this fair lady. He cannot, however, truly claim ever to have seen her, although one day he may do so" (Ariens 1964, xvi).[11] The feminization of the receptor is inescapable in this passage, which relies on a courtship metaphor long associated with the discourse of Western science.[12]

Elucidation of the opiates' chemical structure led to postulation of receptors in the mid-1950s. However, technologies for locating, purifying, or visualizing receptors had not yet been developed.[13] In the 1960s, several laboratories made unsuccessful attempts to locate and isolate receptors (Cozzens 1989, 68–69). Unable to purify the receptor in 1969, Avram Goldstein nevertheless demonstrated stereospecific binding at the opiate receptor site in 1971 in the membranes of mouse brains. He is not credited with discovering opiate receptors, since Candace Pert and Solomon Snyder exerted a stronger claim to have shown actual receptors, not just binding sites, in 1972 (Cozzens 1989). Soon after, John Hughes and Hans Kosterlitz discovered the endogenous opioids that they named *enkephalins.* The myriad implications of these multiple discoveries ranged from the popular reconfiguration of ideas about body and brain to the production of a "common language for psychiatry and the pharmaceutical industry," which brought them into alignment rather than competition (Healy 2002, 212–15).

Once visualized, receptors could then be located by using autoradiography, to study their distribution and density in monkey and human brains. Kuhar observed: "At that point, the immediate world started working on receptors.

Very quickly, receptors for all the major drugs of abuse were discovered: there were the serotonin receptors for LSD; there were all the opiate receptors for opiates; [there were] barbiturate binding sites, or GABA receptors" (2005). Among the technical limitations was the need for postmortem brains, until PET scanning enabled noninvasive study in a way that researchers experienced as "almost like Alice in Wonderland." Kuhar put it: "There was an old Chinese mythological figure called Shen-Nung [who] was a physician who had a magical power. He could ingest an herbal medicine, make his body transparent, and then he could point to where the drugs were working. Here we were with PET scanning, showing where drugs were working as if we had made the body transparent, which of course we had! It was an absolute fairy tale come true" (2005).

It is hardly remembered as well that ARC research director William R. Martin had hypothesized the existence of multiple opiate receptors in the mid-1960s, when Lexington was in its heyday. Frank Vocci, head of the NIDA Medications Development Division from 1995 to 2003, explained: "Martin's conclusion was that when you look at the whole body of research on the opiate receptor, it can't just be one receptor. He said there had to be more than one opiate receptor. He was actually the first guy who deduced this from pharmacology data. What happened in the mid-seventies was that you had people who started to look at what these multiple receptors were from the standpoint of radio receptor binding, and to then find endogenous ligands for them. This was during a really exciting basic science explosion that was occurring in terms of the neurochemistry of all this" (Vocci 2005). Propelled by development of neuroimaging technologies, this discovery period was a technique-driven scientific process through which receptor location and density was mapped. Candace Pert wrote, "My method was to develop a technique and then ask all the questions to which the technique could supply an answer" (1997, 128).

The imagery of "photoneurorealism" (Pert 1997, 126) not only yields pretty pictures but has practical applications for drug development and screening. The pharmaceutical industry uses PET scanning to determine exactly which receptors a drug occupies, a relatively noninvasive way to screen compounds by determining the molecular profile of action, predicting likely side effects, and determining clinically effective dosages.[14] As Kuhar explained, substances compete for receptors: "When you inject radioactive morphine, morphine sits in that receptor but it's competing for the endogenous ligand. It's competing for opioid peptide. Another thing that PET scanning of receptors gave us was a way to measure endogenous activity because there would be a competition between endogenous substances and the radioactive drug" (2005). The relative success of one compound over another in this competition provides a high-throughput drug-screening method. But PET scanning also enabled a neuro-scientific rehabilitation of pharmacology and the legitimization of substance abuse research as a domain of neuroscience.

Public sector science sensed that the frontier of drug abuse research was moving, so NIDA inaugurated its Neuroscience Division in 1985, choosing Kuhar to head the overall division and one of the four laboratories in it. The division, which included a genetics laboratory headed by George Uhl, embarked on a quest to find out whether there were structural and/or functional differences between the brains of addicts and nonaddicts. One of the first important breakthroughs was the isolation and cloning of genes for dopamine receptors, which ushered geneticists into the inner sanctum of the substance abuse research enterprise. Another important moment was development of the technical capacity for signal transduction. Kuhar explained: "When a drug binds to a receptor, there's a whole bunch of things that happen inside the cell. That's called 'signal transduction,' changing the signal from a chemical binding to a whole series of biochemical reactions inside the cell, [which] involve[s] changing gene expression, and changing the genes that are turned on" (2005). The convergence between genetics and neuroscience yielded new conceptual and technical approaches that rendered many previous approaches obsolete. For instance, the kind of drug abuse liability studies once done on the monkeys of Michigan or the postaddicts of Lexington are accomplished today by molecular pharmacologists using single-cell preparations onto which cloned opiate receptors are grafted. This technique allows far more accurate measurements of the affinity that a particular compound has for opiate receptors, and researchers who work on intact organisms are free to work on other problems.

Remaining in the problem-based field of addiction research requires disciplinary mobility. As Kuhar explained, neuropharmacologists had to learn much in order to incorporate genetics.

> The actual nuts and bolts of cloning, for example, involved technical things called plasmids, vectors, recombinant enzymes, a whole series of things that existed in other fields, that hadn't been brought into neuropharmacology. These were now being brought into neuropharmacology. We had to learn what the hell they were. How do you handle them? How do you store them? How do you make one? How do you know when you have one? How do you know when it's not working properly? How do you know if it's an artifact? So we had to learn all those things. (2005)

Software programs were among the necessary tools required to access the new gene depositories created by the Human Genome Project. Kuhar recalled: "We had to figure out how to use them. What do the words mean? A lot of that stuff was just coming out. It was clumsy. It was awkward" (2005).

Since departing NIDA in 1995, Kuhar has used the Human Genome Project to study a particular peptide neurotransmitter called the CART gene, a candidate gene involved in behaviors central to addiction. Describing his onetime skepticism toward both behaviorism and genetics, he said: "I didn't think we could ever understand behavior. I thought behavior was so complex that we couldn't really get a good handle on it. I don't think that way anymore. Very, very complex behaviors can be shown to be dependent on a single gene." Potential treatment applications are sought by using genes to blunt or modulate behavioral effects of drugs of abuse. Pharmacotherapies that work by blocking drug effects have found little popular acceptance among the addicted, despite their seeming elegance at the molecular level. Neurogeneticists explain lack of social acceptance by appealing to the idea that the "brain-reward system" is basic to survival. Kuhar said, "If you're dealing with a system so fundamental as appetite and addiction, and they're intertwined, blocking something so vital to our survival is not going to get so far" (2005). The construction of the brain as the central coordinator of this reward system comes out of James Olds's work on electrical brain stimulation during the 1950s, which helped inaugurate behavioral approaches to self-stimulation and drug self-administration. The construction of the brain-reward system as crucial to the survival of the species has come about rather more recently. Substance abuse researchers construct their enterprise as fundamentally concerned with human evolution and ultimately useful in unmasking responses to pain and pleasure, mechanisms that regulate appetite and satisfaction, and the compulsion to repeat drug experiences.

As a central organizing metaphor, the brain-reward system transformed the old addiction research enterprise into the current substance abuse research enterprise by expanding the behaviors and substances—endogenous and exogenous—under consideration. Kuhar observed:

> Just think about how many different kinds of medical morbidity are associated with the reward system. There's not only drugs of abuse. There's cancer because of smoking, liver disease because of alcohol, Type II diabetes because of overeating, cardiovascular disease because of body weight and food intake and all. While we think of the reward system as specifically related to drug addiction, it is in fact a major biological system in the medical field, underlying a lot of morbidity that goes way, way beyond drug abuse. (2005)

Repetition is the key to the brain-reward system, the existence of which, as Kuhar said, "reinforces certain actions [that] turn out to be things that are good for your survival—food, water, salt, sex." Kuhar explained: "Those things are turned on by the reward system. If we didn't have reward systems, we'd have been gone a long time ago. The reward system is the secret to life" (2005). Thus did a scientific enterprise once trained on marginalized, stigmatized "deviants" become a key to the very "secrets of life" (Keller 1992). More than a route to garner public support, the construction of the brain-reward system as the supposed secret to life has enabled scientists to justify their views on drug policy. As Kuhar put it, given the number of chemical compounds, "it isn't surprising that some few are going to activate that reward system, maybe by mistake, just by chance." He continued:

> Those things are the drugs that turn out to be abuse drugs. They activate that reward system, the reinforcing system. Understanding that there is this naturally occurring system in the brain, the view of drug addiction has changed tremendously. It's now physiologically based. This is a physiologically based brain disorder, like Parkinson's disease, [and] we can develop medications now to treat these things. Treatment is a lot more effective and cheaper than incarceration. (2005)

The political perspective on the futility of incarceration is a convergent perspective among scientists who study drug dependence.

Genetically based explanations can lead to claims of persistent and even irreversible alteration, as in the following excerpt from my interview with Kuhar.

> One of the other major discoveries goes like this. When you take a drug, the drug binds to receptors. The receptors are activated and then things happen inside the cell . . . because this receptor's being activated. [T]herefore the brain on drugs is a different brain. It's chemically different. It's chemically changed. That's a great realization because a reasonable strategy for treatment is restore the old balance, and you've got somebody unaddicted. I think that may be true. In other studies, there were other striking findings, and people didn't believe it at first. It was found that these changes in the brain last a long time. We're talking about months and months, maybe years. That's why drug addiction is a chronic relapsing disease, because the changes that are caused are very long-lasting. (2005)

One reason for pausing to reflect before jumping on the neuroscientific bandwagon is that the approach leaves much to be desired when it comes to evolving treatment methods to cope better with relapse and recovery. Not everyone agrees that persistence of changes in the brain accounts for behavioral change. Eric Nestler and David Landsman explain:

> The cardinal feature of addiction is its chronicity. Individuals can experience intense craving for drugs and remain at increased risk for relapse even years after abstinence, so addiction must involve very stable changes in the brain. But it has been difficult to identify such changes at the molecular, cellular, or circuit levels. The molecular and cellular adaptations related to tolerance, sensitization, and dependence do not persist long enough to account for the more stable behavioral changes associated with addiction. (2001)

The hope is that neuroscience will lead to understandings of how "cellular and molecular mechanisms . . . mediate the transition between occasional, controlled drug use and the loss of behavioral control over drug seeking and drug taking that characterizes chronic addiction" (Koob and Bloom 1998, 467). The idea that chronicity might be a feature not of the brain on drugs but of social worlds in which people learn to use drugs in chronic ways remains difficult for neuroscientists to grasp, because so few are in close touch with chronic drug users. The apparent triumph of neurogenetic approaches ought to be at least as troubling as earlier approaches. Happily, there are a few exemplary research groups that display a sense of historical continuity with the addiction research enterprise and a concern for close social proximity with research subjects.

BRINGING LIFE INTO THE LAB: THE SEARCH FOR THE "PSYCHE" IN THE NEUROIMAGING LABORATORY

Abraham Wikler's scientific heir apparent, Charles P. O'Brien,[15] learned to "superimpose research on good treatment" when he was drafted during Vietnam. He directed the Philadelphia Naval Hospital psychiatric unit between 1969 and 1971, during his medical residency. O'Brien recalled: "One of the major reasons for my patients being unfit for duty was because of drug abuse, which provoked other kinds of psychiatric problems. . . . I got interested because it was so clinically important, and there was so little science" (2005). O'Brien was then recruited to start a treatment program at the Philadelphia Veterans Administration Medical Center. Thus, during President Nixon's 1972 presidential reelection campaign, O'Brien found himself running one of the first VA programs dealing with heroin-addicted veterans returning from Vietnam.

Describing his treatment program as "science-based" from its inception, O'Brien became interested in Wikler's animal conditioning model. In 1977, he validated Wikler's model by demonstrating that craving and withdrawal were conditioned responses in human beings. He began using addiction as a model for memory: "This is how we came to the idea that addiction is a chronic disease—because it's a memory. It's not a brain lesion, it's a very much overlearned memory, like learning how to ride a bicycle or play the piano" (O'Brien 2005). When asked why Wikler, who had access to human subjects for much of his career, had not made the jump to thinking of addiction as a form of overlearned memory, O'Brien said:

> He was very helpful to me because I wrote to him very early on and told him what I wanted to do. He wrote back and thought it was a great idea, but he only actually studied rats. He talked to people, but he only did experiments on rats. I was the first one to do experiments on human beings on this. Wikler had been influenced by Pavlov, who did the first work in conditioning of drug effects. . . . What I did, essentially, was design in Philadelphia something like they have in Russia. By coincidence, I got invited to Russia [in 1974] along with a VA delegation, and I visited some of Pavlov's students, [but] by that time he was dead. (2005)

Like Pavlov's lab in Russia, Wikler's lab at Lexington took on new life in Philadelphia.

Near the end of his career, Wikler reflected on his long search for the "psyche" in drug dependence. He described how he had evolved his research plan from his first brush with Pavlov, who, having shown that decorticated dogs could not be conditioned, had concluded that the cerebral cortex was essential to development of conditioned reflexes. "Groping for an operational definition of the 'psyche,'" Wikler inferred that if an organism could "learn, i.e. could acquire conditioned reflexes, it had a 'psyche'; if not, then, no 'pysche'" (Wikler 1974, 2). He transformed the problem into a puzzle to be solved via laboratory logic: by what practical techniques could the learning patterns of the "psyche" be made evident in a demonstrable way? By the 1970s, Wikler felt the clues were clearer than they had been when he had embarked on his quest more than three decades previously. Summoning the ghost of psychoanalyst Sandor Rado, Wikler closed his 1974 Nathan B. Eddy Memorial Award lecture before the College on Problems of Drug Dependence thusly: "Regardless of whether or not there is any validity in Rado's dictum, '. . . not the toxic agent but the impulse to use it makes an addict out of a given individual,' the evidence is abundant that both the 'toxic agent' and the schedules of reinforcement under which it is self-administered are crucial in the development of the disease *sui generis* that is called drug dependence" (10).[16] His hybrid integration of behaviorist and psychoanalytic lexicons was linked to new research, such as O'Brien's demonstration that "classically conditioned tearing, yawning, lacrimation, systolic blood pressure elevation, respiratory irregularities and skin temperature decreases can be developed in subjects maintained on methadone in response to conditioned stimuli such as an odor or a tone coupled with saline injection, after the odor or tone had been paired repeatedly with injections of naloxone, the unconditioned stimulus" (Wikler 1974, 10). Finally, Wikler spoke of a suggestive polygraph study in which postaddict subjects appeared to respond differently to opioid-related images than they did to neutral slides. Lamentably, the polygraph had broken during the study.

Polygraphs (so-called lie detectors) were initially employed by O'Brien's group to study learned responses to opiate cues by measuring arousal reactions. The idea fit into cognitive-behavioral therapy designed to teach people to extinguish arousal responses. Hired in 1981 to work with behavioral and polygraphic assessment of response to drug cues, Anna Rose Childress moved cue studies into the neuroimaging laboratory, adopting SPECT (single photon emission computed tomography) neuroligand imaging in 1991; PET scanning in 1996; and nonradioactive functional, or "fast," magnetic resonance imaging (fMRI), which can be used for longitudinal studies because the process does not use ionized radiation and therefore can be repeated in single subjects.[17] Imaging technologies were adopted for the study of drug addiction because they allow noninvasive mapping of the neuroanatomical and neurochemical substrates of desire, or "appetitive drug motivation."[18] The Philadelphia laboratory moved from studying opiates to studying cocaine. They produced data sets on drug craving, showing the activation of particular regions of the brain in response to videos depicting drug paraphernalia and visual images associated with local drug subcultures.

Neuroimaging technologies are useful for understanding relapse after long periods of not using drugs. Successive generations of imaging technologies have supplanted the polygraph's crude physiological measurements and today attempt to corroborate the physical changes that memory makes in the brain. O'Brien observed:

> Clearly my patients have a memory that won't go away. When I show them cues that are associated with addiction, they develop craving; they have blood pres-

> sure, pulse, and respiration changes. [W]e've been able to demonstrate that they have brain changes, which they can't control. So when they are in the brain imaging chamber, and we show them a video of people using drugs, there's a reflex that goes on. We see brain activation. It's not something that you can command off by just saying no. (2005)

Brain imaging experiments narrow in on the powerful urge to return to drug use. By bringing into the lab images of the everyday objects, sights, and sounds that cue research subjects that opiates may be coming, researchers are trying to visualize "emotional memories" that serve as triggers for relapse. In Moyers's "The Hijacked Brain," Childress referred to these "feeling memories" as powerful and long-lived memories that concern things that enhance survival. The purpose of her PET scan studies, Childress explained on camera, was mapping where such emotional memories are stored so as to develop signatures of craving in the brain. To accomplish this, she and her patients produce true-life videos to capture associations that trigger people to remember their feeling states when high. These associations are social cues—the persons, places, and things—said to trigger relapse in the lexicon of popular recovery discourse.

Neuroimaging studies did not completely displace behavioral study. In fact, Vocci describes fMRI as "married to behavioral tasks that people do in the magnet" (2005). Again, the social location and material conditions of the research site matter. The University of Pennsylvania Center for Studies of Addiction is connected to a treatment research institute and a treatment center that enable interactions between researchers and patients actively struggling to end their addictions—or, in the lexicon of those who study them, to inhibit their responses to social and environmental cues. Childress refers to the patients she works with as "collaborators" and relies on them to coach her research team on how to better induce craving "in the magnet" in order to study why craving persists "outside the magnet." The process of bringing life into the lab replicates to some extent the social and material conditions available to the ARC when it was at Lexington. The original 1948 study that formed the basis for Wikler's conditioning theory involved the experimental readdiction of a single human subject who shared his free associations, manifest dream content, and interpretations in psychoanalytic interviews two or three times a week for several months (Wikler 1948b, 1952d). Although this study could not be replicated today, cue-triggered responses from subjects undergoing neuroimaging similarly integrate behavioral and neuropharmacological approaches. Likewise, an fMRI cocaine study performed at Massachusetts General Hospital in Boston asked subjects who were regular, untreated cocaine users to report their subjective states following a placebo injection and an injection of cocaine (Brieter et al. 1997). By correlating imaging data with subjects' rating of their state of "craving," "rush," "high," and "low" throughout an imaging sequence, researchers identified brain regions they believe are implicated in the subjective sensations experienced by cocaine users. Vocci explained:

> [Neuroimaging studies have shown that] individuals' responses, what they felt, and what their brains were doing were not necessarily concordant, but the ones that got the highest response in their brain were the ones that relapsed. . . . [This] suggests that there are brain systems that are impacted by drugs of abuse to the point where, although the person looks just the same as somebody else who's gone through a treatment program and they're not using drugs at that time, their probability of relapsing is very high. The guy next to them who doesn't have that response is low. We've always wondered, why does one guy make it and the other one doesn't? From these technologies, it's starting to look like you might be able to pick these folks out during or after treatment, and say, this one's got a brain signature that's suggestive of relapse, and this one doesn't. (2005)

The hope that science will someday indicate which treatments might be effective for whom obviously has the downside of marking those on whom treatment would be a lost cause. For employers, parole boards, child protective services, and other authorities, this could easily become grounds for new forms of discrimination. At the same time, such a process, if fairly implemented, could be useful for channeling public health resources. However, there are as yet no practical implications resulting from this domain.

The outcome of neuroanatomical mapping is a "brain signature," which supposedly shows what is happening in the brain at a particular moment in time. Such images do not yield knowledge of the underlying neurochemistry necessary to develop medications. In fact, when O'Brien and colleagues tried to use cue-reactivity paradigms to screen medications supposed to block or blunt cue-induced cravings, their results were "underwhelming" (as explained on their Web site, cited in n. 18). They then strategically retreated from the goal, returning to basic research focused simply on understanding addictive states. What, then, does a brain signature do? Photoneurorealism provides a convincingly objectified map of subjective variation and is thus thought to hold the key to the long-pursued questions of addiction research: Why do only some people become addicts? Why do only some people relapse? Neuroimaging is today's version of the old attempt to render subjective effects objective and to hold at bay questions of social and economic context. What will we do once we know the answers, and what will that knowledge be used to accomplish?

Rapid technological development of imaging technologies propelled a rush to embrace metabolic and physiological models of drug dependency. Sociological, anthropological, and psychological models have been displaced. Whatever addiction may be, the expert communities who deal with it in our time no longer consider it a social problem. Recently, social and cultural factors have paradoxically reentered through the backdoor of genetics. There are possibly fundamental barriers in the way of interpreting addiction as a primarily cellular process, rendering emotional motivations and behavioral expressions as purely molecular matters. First, there is little knowledge of how molecular events translate into cellular interactions and, so the story goes, into complex social behaviors. Second, there is little knowledge about the effects of long-term exposure, a critical component of a chronic relapsing disorder supposed to fundamentally alter brain structure and function. The CRBD construct itself drives research in a particular direction. Third, the potential contribution of genetics to vulnerability is admittedly poorly understood, although neuroscientific optimists pursue vulnerability genes and hope eventually to explain the role of genetic risk factors and protective mechanisms (National Academy of Sciences Committee to Identify Strategies 1997, 47). One need not argue against neuroscientific or genetic research in order to notice that the explanations so far offered share that most salient feature of all drug addiction research over the past century—they are limited, partial, and incapable of addressing the role of social context or integrating all levels of analysis.

In addiction research, a most public science, conceptual models provide answers to ongoing questions about what kinds of knowledge are most useful to govern drug use and drug users. By the end of the twentieth century, that answer was that social behavior can be understood through molecular means elaborating the neurobiochemical and genetic pathways that reward users and reinforce their behavior. What haunts this technoscientific construction of addicts as a fundamentally altered species structurally and functionally different from the rest of us? Leshner himself answered this question in a special, 1997 edition of *Science* magazine on addiction: "Addiction is not *just* a brain disease" (46). Its social meanings mark the presence of continued concerns with deviance or aberrant behavior that remain part of the cultural repository of ideas and images that underlie our assumptions about governance. Current NIDA director Nora Volkow refers to drug addiction as "disrupted volition"

(2006) or "behavior gone awry" (Volkow and Li 2004). Volkow and Ting-Kai Li observe:

> Drug addiction manifests as a compulsive drive to take a drug despite serious adverse consequences. This aberrant behaviour has traditionally been viewed as bad "choices" made voluntarily by the addict. However, recent studies have shown that repeated drug use leads to long-lasting changes in the brain that undermine voluntary control. This, combined with new knowledge of how environmental, genetic and developmental factors contribute to addiction, should bring about changes in our approach to the prevention and treatment of addiction. (2005, 1430)

The wording of the preceding quotation reveals that continued activity of the old moral lexicon since the nineteenth century has constructed addiction as a "disease of the will" subject to voluntary control. The work of Volkow, Li, and other neuroimagers testifies to the convergence between behavioral and neuroscientific approaches in the study of what constitutes volition itself and what processes lead to "disrupted volition" (Volkow 2006). With that amnesiac gesture toward its own repressed past, the addiction research enterprise comes full circle into the present.

Redefining addiction as a chronic relapsing brain disease in the waning decades of the twentieth century provides a striking example of amnesia with which to close this chapter. Back in 1966, Warren P. Jurgensen, the deputy medical officer in charge of the Lexington Hospital, told the American Correctional Association that addiction was a "chronic, often relapsing affliction, which may require treatment intermittently for a period of years." Like many at Lexington, he defined addiction as an "illness with relapses often to be expected," adding: "It is believed that periods of abstinence can be lengthened, and in some cases extended indefinitely. Indeed, this is characteristic of the medical treatment of many chronic illnesses."[19] Although this problem definition did not stick in the 1960s, it preceded by decades the adoption of the strangely similar definition used to court neuroscientists to the field in the 1990s. Subject to cycles of learning, forgetting, and relearning, the social worlds of addiction research continue to face the intractability of the drug problem in the United States. How they will do so in the future owes something to the ways they have done so in the past.

Conclusion

ARC researcher Abraham Wikler maintained:

> We must be able to give up our time-hallowed but useless quest for "ultimate realities" in exchange for limited, but useful patches of knowledge. But even a patch-work quilt may be beautiful as well as warm. (1952c, 98)

All knowledge is partial, limited, produced from multiple standpoints. Taking more perspectives into account yields more useful knowledge—this is one of the lessons of situated knowledges. Without the "junkie monkeys" of Michigan or the postaddicts of Lexington, researchers would have discovered addiction differently. Scientific concepts and claims emerge as retrospective products of the social process of discovery—they are socially constituted products that cannot be said to pre-exist their discovery in any simple way. Barbara Herrnstein Smith has characterized the process of "discovery" thusly:

> [T]his image of scientific agency and alignment of intentions, actions, and outcomes is clearly the product of retrospective selection and schematization. If one looks at the record of the events leading to the discovery, one sees not a straight line but a "meandering path" that includes false assumptions, vague hunches, unsuccessful experiments, lucky accidents, and, at every point, the contribution of useful ideas, methods, and technical adjustments by many different people. (2005, 54)

"Addiction" evolved from the meandering interplay of multiple methods, subfields, experimental subjects, and objects of knowledge. Like the Wasserman test about which Ludwik Fleck wrote in *Genesis and Development of a Scientific Fact,* the concept of "addiction" has been produced and reproduced through a "harmony of illusions" (1979, 28). The task of a sociology of knowledge or "comparative epistemology" is to follow the trail of hazy protoideas as they move from one thought style to another on their way to being "preserved as enduring, rigid structures" (Fleck 1979, 28).

Understanding the tenacious grip exerted by the conceptual frameworks through which "addiction" has been discovered and rediscovered has been one goal of this book. Fleck argued that "evidence conforms to conceptions just as often as conceptions conform to evidence" (1979, 28). If we are amnesiac about the degree to which "addiction" is a social construct in this age of evidence-based medicine, that forgetfulness marks the success of the "creative fictions" to which we subscribe (Fleck 1979, 32). The harmony of illusions does not undermine the lived realities of addiction so much as cast them as historical products subject to change. The ongoing work of the scientific communities concerned with addiction lies in fashioning laboratory logics that better recognize lived realities and cultural differences in ways that can be reconciled with both individual variation and social patterning. Outside the walls of Lexington or the cages of the monkey colony, drug dependence looks and feels different from how it looks and feels in the closed worlds of addiction researchers. Although researchers were and are aware that different forms of addiction are discovered and enacted in the laboratory as opposed to those witnessed outside institutions, their science could not stretch to encompass perspectives that might have given them other insights.

What if knowledge about psychoactive drugs had been produced via logics, practices, and perspectives beyond those related in this book? The science of substance abuse would look different if the research enterprise worked from social contexts in which people use drugs or if it considered how experiences of drug effects vary between social groups and cultural geographies. Drug policy would look different if it was not based on controlling supply, convincing people to abstain from drugs to which they have easy access, and punishing those who do not meet that standard. Policing, prohibition, and abstinence are powerless in the face of drug markets that proliferate availability, decrease price, and increase purity. What if knowledge was produced in order to be more useful to those who use psychoactive drugs?

When the relative of a close friend died from a heroin overdose, my friend peppered me with questions in the struggle to make sense of his death: How long did he suffer? What did he really die from? Was there anything that anyone could have done? Did his most recent detox have anything to do with his death? Was there something different about his brain, mind, or body? What do we know about what went wrong for him? How do we know it? Who knows it? As I answered as best I could, my mind reeled back to the night that two comatose prisoner patients at Lexington were brought back to life by administration of a narcotic antagonist that can prevent overdose deaths. I found myself asking my own questions: Where was the political will to step in to prevent overdose deaths, slow down transmission of HIV, or reduce other adverse health consequences associated with drug use? How can policy makers be persuaded to craft and implement harm-reducing public health policies? What role can science play in constituting addiction in ways that could redirect the trajectory of U.S. drug policy?

Discovering Addiction was written to jog conversations about drug policy and science beyond venues currently dominated by the criminal justice enterprise, the Drug Enforcement Administration, the FDA, and the pharmaceutical industry. The social privilege of science is such that substance abuse researchers and treatment professionals potentially could offer an untapped force for changing global drug policy regimes. But there are numerous obstacles to alliances between scientific communities, treatment providers, multiple publics, policy makers, and activist communities. These obstacles first need to be addressed before there is much chance of enrolling scientific communities in taking a leadership role to change regulatory regimes, the conduct of clinical trials, the treatment of persons living with addictions, or the outcomes of problematic opiate use.

Science speaks with plural voices concerning mind-shaping and mood-altering drugs, but few people even hear these voices. Ordinary citizens could use better understandings of the scientific claims made about the strengths and weaknesses, promises and failures, and possibilities and shortcomings of the drugs they consume. Disagreement within science and between science and its publics can engender wider conversations about the governance of drugs and the ethical conduct of research. The question is not whether human experimentation is going to take place but how it should be organized and who should participate in it. After a brief theoretical discussion of ethical agency, this conclusion takes up historical lessons for the socially responsible conduct of clinical trials, for making research more relevant to the treatment of those living with drug dependence, and for remaking the trajectory of U.S. drug policy.

ENACTING A SITUATED ETHICS: THE AMBIVALENT SCENE OF AGENCY

Criminalization has been the main response to addiction among persons of color, and poor and working-class people, as well as the mentally ill, a significant proportion of whom now fall under the control of the criminal justice system. The census of the federal narcotics farms at Lexington and Fort Worth declined in direct proportion to the rise of the current treatment infrastructure, scaled up in the 1970s. Despite different administrators, modalities, providers, and addicted persons, drug treatment remains class-stratified, especially in the criminal justice system, where so many now spend "deinstitutionalized" lives. Medicalization remains the province of the insured middle and upper classes. Many of the scientists whose everyday laboratory lives were reenacted in this book lament these structural circumstances but have nonetheless played a part in extending into everyday life Michel Foucault's "carceral continuum" (1979, 303). Insiders pursued research of their choosing, but from an outsider's perspective, addiction science has fitted seamlessly into the disciplinary regimes of drug control. Hence drug policy reformers—along with users, treatment providers, activists, and advocates—rarely see scientists as allies in struggles for social justice.

This is partly because professional research enterprises connected to therapeutic practices typically adopt practices that place them on Foucault's carceral continuum, which "provides a communication between the power of discipline and the power of the law, and extends without interruption from the smallest coercions to the longest penal detention" (1979, 303). Clinicians and scientists became integral to the regime of "examinatory justice" through which disciplinary power was extended over drug consumption (Foucault 1979, 304–5). Professional judgment is integral to the administrative processes through which the carceral continuum works. Foucault maintained that under such conditions, it is "useless to believe in the good or bad consciences of judges, or even of their unconscious," because "it is the economy of power that they exercise, and not that of their scruples or their humanism, that makes them pass 'therapeutic' sentences and recommend 'rehabilitating' periods of prison" (1979, 304). Although scientists involved in drug addiction research are not directly judging drug users, they are certainly making the data on which policy regimes sort out what should happen to addicted persons.

This book has shown that Foucault's thoroughgoing skepticism toward the conscience and scruples of judges does not quite fit this case. Be they scientists or social workers, doctors or teachers, Public Health Service officers, or prison officials, those who carry out the institutional routines of examinatory justice in democratic societies have some room to follow the dictates of conscience or compassion. Situated ethics are not entirely colonized by institutional constraints, for extralocal rules and norms also govern professional conduct. For considering the lessons of twentieth-century addiction research, rethinking the relationship between ethical agency and social structure is essential. Judith Butler explained in *The Psychic Life of Power: Theories in Subjection* (1997):

> [W]hat is enacted by the subject is enabled but not finally constrained by the prior working of power. Agency exceeds the power by which it is enabled. One might say that the purposes of power are not always the purposes of agency. To the extent that the latter diverge from the former, agency is the assumption of a purpose *unintended* by power, one that could not have been derived logically or historically, that operates in a relationship of contingency and reversal to the power that makes it possible, to which it nevertheless belongs. (15)

Ethical subjectivity cannot be reduced to social role, for subjects find themselves in the predicament, described by Butler, of "how to take an oppositional relationship to power that is, admittedly, implicated in the very power one opposes" (17). Taking up the possibilities present in the ambivalent scene of agency means departing from what you are supposed to do within the prevailing social norms and indigenous moralities that structure the spaces you inhabit—whether you are a prisoner, patient, inmate, addict or postaddict, researcher, clinician, policy maker, treatment provider, or administrator.

Ethics often focuses on the individual actions of autonomous moral agents making singular decisions on the basis of personal integrity. Bringing to life the long-dead laboratories discussed in this book has shown that ethical action is based less on individual scruples or attitudes than on the collective processes that coordinated research, often at a distance. Ethical subjectivity is not atomistic but socially situated and directed from particular social standpoints. By reenacting the ethical dilemmas in which scientists who worked within these material and institutional structures were caught, this account of situated ethics captured the changing social and institutional structures through which addiction has been discovered since the 1920s. Three additional changes have significantly impacted the social relevance of substance abuse research: the changing conduct of clinical trials, therapeutic innovation, and the emergence of harm reduction drug policy.

BROKERING SOCIALLY RESPONSIBLE CLINICAL TRIALS

Bringing to life the laboratory logics that animated twentieth-century substance abuse research allowed me to trace the intellectual and ethical history of the addiction research enterprise. If all knowledge is situated knowledge, how does scientific work taking place inside the walls of a prison-hospital differ from studies conducted in noncaptive populations? Considering this question forced me to confront the limits of analysis, the partiality of all perspectives, and the construction and maintenance of science as social privilege. Bringing more voices to the table will not allay legitimate public fears about the most problematic of scientific practices, such as those at issue in experimentation on unwitting subjects or subjects from whom valid informed consent simply cannot be obtained. However, closing the social distance between the scientific world and the multiple counterpublics who have stakes in scientific arenas would go some way toward building better ways to produce more socially relevant science. Fear about past abuse encourages ongoing vigilance toward the unresolved ethical dilemmas enacted in this book. Believing this to be a healthy state of skepticism, I have here set out not to resolve the practical and ethical dilemmas encountered in my historical research but to bring up unresolved questions about the role of science in social life, the role of human and animal experimentation in science and politics, and the role played by "good" and "bad" drugs in the lives of a significant fraction of the global population.

Technological innovations have reduced the need for human and animal subjects early in the drug development process. But most people believe that large-scale human experimentation remains necessary. In an age when "treatment-naive" subjects have become few and far between, many potential participants are disqualified for having used too many licit or illicit drugs. Despite greater attention to screening, privacy, and informed consent, clinical testing is now conducted with less controlled conditions, human contact, and attention to the experimental situation than was present at the ARC when it was in Lexington. Testing occurs in a commercialized domain with no checks and balances designed to distinguish public interests from commercial interests. The social inequities of clinical trials are produced by a basic, underlying problem: that high levels of risk and scrutiny are trained on the poor, while the relatively rich participate at much lower levels. Yet social and economic class is rarely acknowledged as an important marker within scientific studies, which typically lack a historical, sociological, or even epidemiological approach.

Class and race issues have again come to the forefront due to the revival of the prison research controversy decades after federal prison research was suspended. In 2006, a National Academy of Sciences (NAS) report from the Institute of Medicine (IOM), titled *Ethical Considerations for Research Involving Prisoners,* recommended stepping up federal oversight and allowing federal prisoners to resume participating in the later phases of clinical trials required for the FDA drug approval process (IOM 2006). Ironically, prisoners involved in research lacked protective federal regulations during the massive expansion of the carceral system. The demise of federal prison research ended federal public sector research but allowed private sector and state-level projects to continue in U.S. prisons. Such projects occur outside the federal purview and beyond the reach of institutional review boards. The IOM, advisory to the NAS, suggested remedying this lack of oversight by updating the ethical framework and bringing research in federal penitentiaries under federal oversight.[1]

That a mainstream scientific advisory body was willing to reopen the debate suggests that the stakes have changed since the 1970s. The IOM was asked to do so by the federal Department of Health and Human Services due to claims that the protections put into place at the end of the 1970s were no longer compatible with the current penal system. Since the early 1980s, the United States has witnessed the privatization and expansion of the prison system. Similarly, the scale of human experimentation itself has expanded radically (if unevenly) in terms of race, class, and ethnicity. Although only one in twenty North Americans has participated in a clinical trial, many more people's lives outside the United States have been touched since the new human subjects regime was put into place. Some subjects, such as AIDs activists, have become much more familiar with the limits of informed consent for ensuring fairness and more apt to question the need for placebo-controlled, double-blind studies. Given that federal prisoners no longer participate in risky Phase 1 and 2 studies, it is worth asking who does participate in them. In other words, the race and class politics of prisoner participation today differ from what they were in the 1970s, because pharmaceutical globalization has changed the political playing field.

Nonetheless, press coverage and public response to the 2006 IOM report reverted to the strident and polarized postures of the 1970s. Subjects of the dermatology experiments conducted by the University of Pennsylvania at the Holmesburg Prison in Philadelphia (Hornblum 1998) publicly protested, insisting they were never going back to being research subjects, a stance that made it seem as if all prison research had been completely shut down for the past thirty years. This was far from the case, yet Holmesburg survivors depicted the IOM as calling for barbaric research to resume in the abusive and exploitive form that had characterized it at Holmesburg. Nothing could be further from the case. The panel simply advised extending human subjects protections to all prisoners, finding "no ethically defensible reason to exclude certain prisoners from most, if not all, human subjects protections afforded by federal regulation" (IOM 2006, 3). Mindful of what the panel called the dark history of prisoner research, the IOM report outlined a new "ethic of collaborative responsibility," in which prisoners themselves would "collaborate" with researchers, administrators, and advocates at every step of the research process. The intemperate response to *Ethical Considerations for Research Involving Prisoners* indicates the confused state of thinking about prison research. Some responded as if the IOM was suggesting a return to the very past abuses it sought to avoid. I am led to wonder whether the underlying assumptions of many stakeholders may now preclude reasonable discussion of the form that biomedical research should take in prisons.

Derived from the principle of justice set out in *The Belmont Report* (National Commission for the Protection of Human Subjects 1978), the IOM panel viewed an "ethic of collaboration" as a way to "cope with the reality that each institution has its own unique conditions" and as a means to facilitate an open research environment (2006, 11). The collaborative working relationship would be brought about by the creation of a new social role, the Prison Research Subject Advocate (PRSA), who would guard against exploitation by monitoring each research project. Like the new social role of the "informed outsider," who was to mediate between current patient-subjects, future subjects, and researchers (Barber et al. 1979, 196), the PRSA role is imagined as a way to overcome the structural unfairness inherent in prison research. Such participatory mechanisms as the PRSA role have become more common since the women's health, civil rights, and HIV/AIDs movements successfully pressured NIH for more say in how science is done (Epstein 1996). Such participation remains optional due to perceptions that it delays research or makes it impossibly conflictual. Even the best participatory bodies do not yet incorporate all elements necessary to achieve socially responsible drug trials. Despite a chorus of critical voices calling for the democratization of science, there have been only modest attempts to do so, and the critical force of these voices has been contained.

In this respect, the 2006 IOM report advocated human subjects protection that is better than what generally prevails in most pharmaceutical research conducted outside prison environments. While I applaud making prisoner advocacy central to the research process, I fear that collaboration cannot be the sole solution to a structural situation in which social inequalities are inherent. Participation can do little to restrain commercial entities from exploiting research subjects, nor can it buffer researchers from commercial pressures as did the NRC committee described in this book. It is not yet clear to me where such buffering capacity might reside inasmuch as the NAS no longer supports specific standing committees. The NAS discontinued sponsorship of CPDD in 1976, just about the same time as the human testing facilities at Lexington were closed (May and Jacobson 1989, 198). This forced CPDD to become a large membership association to survive, and the venerable professional association no longer coordinates the focused research effort it maintained through 1975, although it still runs a small testing program. No other body has emerged to play the role of "honest broker" that CPDD once did through the NAS and the NRC. Yet some entity along the lines of the old NRC committee, which restrained commercial interests in ways that prevented direct conflicts of interest and direct exploitation within the addiction research enterprise, remains necessary to ensure socially responsible clinical trials.

The IOM panel recognized some of the most problematic aspects of prison research: "Justice requires more than the protection of prisoners from harm caused by the research itself. Ethical research carries with it the responsibility to grapple with the fact that potential harm is ubiquitous in everyday prison life" (NAP 2006, 12). Prisons inevitably inflict harm on those punished—that is their purpose, albeit one from which many dissent (see the final section of this conclusion for an alternative policy trajectory more in line with clinical and scientific understandings of drug addiction). The inescapable vulnerability of prison populations is compounded when they contain "people with diseases (addiction, hepatitis, HIV, hypertension, diabetes) that may or may not be treated during imprisonment" (NAP 2006, 12). However, the IOM panel fell short of suggesting that access to health care during incarceration be widened or improved, a goal of the current prison reform movement. Instead, it suggested severely limiting biomedical research in prison, while disallowing riskier Phase 1 and 2 studies altogether, on grounds that safety and efficacy are unknown until these earlier phases are complete. Phase 1 and 2 studies cannot assure that benefits to individual prisoners are commensurate with the risks of participation.

Significantly, the panel said nothing about Phase 3 studies, which are typically expensive and hard for pharmaceutical companies or clinical research organizations to recruit or enroll subjects in and to complete. Using prisoners to accomplish Phase 3 studies would be seen as attractive by pharmaceutical companies for precisely the same reason that they are hard to complete on the outside: a captive audience is more likely to remain enrolled all the way through to the completion of a large clinical trial. However, the conditions under which the panel suggested federal prison research could resume were similar to those that had arisen in the 1970s: half the subjects had to be non-prisoners, and there had to be a "strongly favorable benefit-risk ratio for the prisoner" (NAP 2006, 10). The panel argued that all human subjects research should be brought under uniform regulations—no matter who the sponsor was or which federal agency had jurisdiction. Lastly, the panel recommended a national database to "bring clarity to the currently murky landscape of research involving prisoners" (NAP 2006, 7). The unsettled nature of the controversy has returned to haunt the present, but to my mind, the debate need not assume its former contours.

One positive development is that the relevant scientific communities and advocacy communities have both become more sophisticated about the stakes involved in biomedical and behavioral research. One of the most vehement opponents from the 1970s, National Prison Project litigator Alvin Bronstein, stated in a *New York Times* article: "[W]ith the help of external review boards that would include a prisoner advocate, I do believe that the potential benefits of biomedical research [in prisons] outweigh the potential risks" (quoted in Urbina 2006). The demise of research in federal prisons that Bronstein helped bring about in the 1970s did not end exploitive experimentation. Indeed, it can be said to have opened a new era of clinical entrepreneurialism in the form of privatized clinical trials.

Phasing out prison research introduced problematic practices that make even the most questionable practices of the Lexington era look relatively benign. Today's clinical trials industry routinely depends on economically disenfranchised people as research subjects (Fisher 2005; Petryna 2006; Shah 2006). Where trials are the only way people can secure access to health care for themselves or family members, there is a coercive element involved. This also applies to physician researchers who conduct trials to keep their practices afloat amid time constraints imposed by managed care and the changing financial structure of medical care delivery. That the context in which clinical trials are conducted often produces injustice, venality, and carelessness is documented in the emerging literature on the clinical trials industry. Mechanisms to counteract these problems are unlikely to come from the pharmaceutical industry or from the FDA, the existing regulatory body that is so often perceived as "captive" to the industry.

More generally, public institutions have proven incapable of truly governing the pharmaceutical industry by restraining its tendencies to commodify health and health care, expand market share by promoting lifestyle drugs and look-alikes, and exploit intellectual property monopolies. One of the major constraints to genuine monitoring and public oversight has been the industry's successful engineering of an antiregulatory consensus under the mantle of "commercial free speech" and "free markets" (Ronald 2006). If public interests are to prevail, a new regulatory consensus will have to be reached, and the most likely source of that will be a combination of scientific and advocacy-oriented communities. Although participatory mechanisms would be a good start, new and revised institutions are also needed not only to ensure socially responsible clinical trials and postmarketing surveillance but to broker deals to bring "public interest drugs" to market. Although nongovernmental organizations could play "honest broker" roles, they are unlikely to have the authority or resources that it will take to mediate the social conflicts involved in marrying private interests to public goals. Government-funded scientists are caught between a privatized, deregulated industry and a public that constructs them as agents of social control. Despite the dependency of the pharmaceutical industry on the public purse (Goozner 2004), there are political and economic obstacles to inducing private industry to serve public purposes.

The possibility of honest brokering by government is not far-fetched, as is shown by the example of buprenorphine, the sort of drug in which the CDAN/CPDD invested. The FDA finally approved buprenorphine in 2003 for treating drug addiction through office-based medical maintenance therapy. Its promise had first become evident during initial testing at the ARC in Lexington (Jasinski 2003). Lack of coordination between public and private interests delayed development far longer than the notoriously slow FDA approval process. To bring "bupe" to market, NIDA worked to stimulate private interest and gain "orphan drug" status for the drug on behalf of Reckitt and Coleman, the company ultimately responsible for marketing the drug in the United States (Jasinski 2003; Johnson 2005; O'Keefe 2005; Vocci 2005). Buprenorphine was handled as a bellwether drug, and a new nonprofit entity was developed to carry out an extensive (and expensive) postmarketing surveillance program designed to detect and respond to abuse quickly (Cicero 2006). This is one example of the general point that emerged from the history of addiction research: the relatively sensible practices of addiction researchers ought to prompt a full-scale revisiting of the public priorities involved in clinical trials—before the next "wonder drug" becomes the next public health crisis.

BRIDGING TWO CULTURES: THE GAPS BETWEEN CLINIC AND LABORATORY

What might induce substance abuse researchers to pursue more socially relevant research questions more of the time? Getting this to happen will require improved relationships between researchers, subjects, and treatment providers. Poor relations between the addiction research enterprise and the therapeutic side of Lexington seeded an ongoing struggle between those who treat and those who study. By the end of the twentieth century, this conflict had flowered into a full-blown "two cultures problem." Treatment providers complain that basic research is disengaged from everyday practice. Their calls for a research culture that is more attuned and accountable to addicted persons have yet to result in increased involvement of clients, consumers, or providers in setting research priorities, generating hypotheses, designing studies, or interpreting data. Clinicians adopt whatever methods become available, whereas researchers constantly question these methods in order to build and refine the knowledge base. Research findings introduce uncertainties that treatment providers perceive as threatening. They then dismiss research as irrelevant to practice, in a cycle of blame that pits theory against practice. Who has the political will and cultural capital to democratize research and treatment, much less mediate relations between clinic and laboratory settings? What would it take to de-escalate the two cultures problem?

One policy maker seeking to infuse "evidence-based thinking" through a statewide treatment system expressed frustration that research simply affirms "what treatment providers and people in the self-help groups have known for years, [that] people, places and things are toxic." The policy maker continued:

> They might not have known it's because there's an amygdala section of the brain that's triggering relapse and cues. They knew this intuitively by watching thousands and thousands of addicts and alcoholics. [I]t's very nice that NIDA can now confirm with brain scans what they already know. . . . I've looked right at them and said, "What's your recommendation for what a clinician should do with this knowledge? In an individual session, when do I share with them about their amygdala? Do I do it when they're first coming in the door? Not really abstinent? Do I do it three weeks in? When and how do I use this information about the neurobiological nature of their disease?" They can't tell me that. They look at me and say, "That would be a great study."

As I learned through ethnographic research with practitioners and policy makers, such sentiments are not uncommon. The two cultures problem in the field of the addictions was exacerbated by a federal reorganization in the 1990s that detached service delivery from research.[2]

Entrenched bureaucratic and cultural divisions among the criminal justice system, the mental health system, and the substance abuse research and treatment infrastructure make jails and prisons unlikely scenes for the democratization of research or treatment innovation. Writing this book did not convince me that prisons are therapeutic, rehabilitative, or educative. Lexington stands as an exemplary failure of the ideals of "moral therapy" and the project of normalization. Locking people up is a stupid way to deter them from using drugs, for incarceration does more to amplify and proliferate the harms associated with drug problems. Although I applaud efforts to expand drug treatment in prisons, it is always an exercise of power that can tip over into domination, surveillance, and social control. Research—wherever conducted—can also be a form of domination, especially where researchers have direct financial ties or commercial interests in outcomes. Despite safeguards, new reports arise concerning conflicts of interest, poorly designed studies, and badly executed research stemming from failure to address power relations and differing levels of knowledge and responses to risk. Must research reenact the scene of disenfranchisement and extract "interest" from the poor, the sick, or the vulnerable?

The degree to which a given research project is exploitive depends on how it is conceptualized and carried out, what its goals and objectives are, with whom it is conducted, and what forms of ethical subjectivity are brought to it. When research is conceived as the top-down production of treatment technologies to be transferred or adopted without variation to other settings, there will continue to be a disjunct with treatment providers. Failing to acknowledge the validity of local or indigenous knowledge, technology transfer programs ride roughshod over cultural particularities and prevent full partnerships from forming between the research and treatment communities. What would it mean for treatment providers to scrutinize the basic assumptions on which research paradigms are based? If providers could participate more in the political process of priority setting so central to resource allocation, that might create a greater degree of responsiveness between researchers, clinicians, and subjects.

What would it mean for those most affected by addiction research and treatment to have collaborated in selecting research questions? If, as discussed already, there was an ethic of collaboration involving imprisoned persons, should there not also be one involving treatment practitioners? The priorities of the research agenda are now set without such participatory design, a fact brought out in the 1997 report *Bridging the Gap between Research and Practice,* cosponsored by NIDA, the federal agency most identified with the research culture, and the Center for Substance Abuse Treatment (CSAT), the federal agency most identified with the treatment culture. The report documented "cultural and attitudinal differences" between clinicians and researchers that were amplified by frustrations in both cultures. Chief among the complaints of clinicians were the "apparent failure of research to provide practical and relevant answers to important clinical and programmatic questions" and the pursuit of a "methodological rigor [that] breeds narrowly defined research that often ignores the complexities of real-world environments" (Substance Abuse and Mental Health Services Administration 2001). Both federal agencies sought to relate differently to their constituencies by building decentralized infrastructures that addressed ongoing tensions between the two cultures: the nationwide regional structure of the Addiction Technology Transfer Center Network; the NIDA Clinical Trials Network, initiated in 2000; and CSAT's Practice Research Network (PRN).

CSAT's effort directly took on the two cultures problem.[3] The Practice Research Network was supposed to demonstrate the "blending" of cultures, easing movement between them by giving providers a stake in making science. Instead, a turf war resulted, in which NIDA took a proprietary approach to what counts as science and "research." The institute declared the treatment agency's use of the term *research* invalid. A federally mandated name change forced the New York State Practice Research Collaborative to become the Practice Improvement Collaborative (PIC). An anonymous participant to a February 27, 2002, PIC meeting complained, "NIDA claims that word [i.e., *research*], [whereas] we're funded by an organization that doesn't have ownership of that word." The regional PRN groups in New York state refused to stop using the high-status word, because they were aware that it was a path to scientific credibility, cultural capital, and social status. Providers felt palpably shut out by the focus on high-end, laboratory-based research modeled on clinical trials.

Soon after this skirmish, however, NIDA began an ongoing series of "blending" conferences and "bridging" initiatives where those who straddle the two cultures meet. Going beyond bridging and blending to truly connect science-as-usual to everyday practice will take a serious rethinking of the federal research infrastructure. Practitioners and researchers navigate different social norms, expectations, and structures, with differing beliefs and commitments. Having explored the tensions that drew the two cultures apart, I want, in closing, to consider harm reduction as a possible rapprochement that might narrow the social distance between them.

CONSCRIPTING THE CLINICAL GAZE: SHIFTING PUBLIC HEALTH TOWARD HARM REDUCTION

U.S. drug policy is based on two misguided assumptions. The first is that the distinction between "medical" and "nonmedical" use still holds (for a full-scale examination of the collapse, see DeGrandpre 2006). The second is the prohibitionist ideal that abstinence will someday prevail. "A drug-free nation" is a view in which the absence of drugs is idealized in ways that foreclose the space for talking about other approaches to public health and social good. Both scientific and therapeutic projects have been harnessed to these assumptions. The clinical gaze of addiction researchers and treatment providers has been conscripted to serve the projects of criminalization, resistance to medicalization, and prohibition, despite the personal scruples and humane intentions of many inhabitants of the social worlds of substance abuse research and treatment.

The conscription of the clinical gaze has dangerous effects, one of which has been to prevent biomedical researchers and medical personnel from advocating policies aimed at reducing the social harms and negative health consequences of drug use. Even if researchers believe in harm reduction, they must disclaim the label as a "dirty word" in policy circles (Shaw and Campbell forthcoming). Ultimately, a harm reduction approach toward legal pharmaceuticals and illegal drugs offers a pragmatic route beyond the impasse. Drugs can be dangerous if used in dangerous ways, but drugs can be relatively safe if used in situations structured to minimize harm. Where will the political will to restructure U.S. drug policy and public health around a politics of harm reduction come from, if not from the expert communities who deal with drug dependence?

Mundane and tragic, the continuum of problematic drug effects ranges from none to death. Ironically, we live in a world where the risks and benefits of pharmaceutical drugs are promoted and listed as if they are the sole ingredients of good decision making about which drugs to consume and which to stay away from. Yet the risks and benefits of illegal substances are shrouded in sanctioned ignorance. Those who use illegal drugs and (as is becoming most common) those who use legal drugs in illegal ways lack the knowledge to do so safely. The assumption is that withholding such knowledge is good because condoning drug use is bad. Thus when "neurobiology goes awry," many people do not know how to respond, because useful knowledge has been kept from them.

The interviews and archival research that I conducted for this book led me to believe that substance abuse researchers have a crucial role to play in shifting drug policy toward public health and harm reduction. Scientific communities contribute data for drug control decisions, and my microlevel perspective enabled a close look at the production of (to again quote Wikler's comment with which I started this conclusion) "limited, but useful patches of knowledge." Some readers might wish my analysis had hovered above, in search of "ultimate realities" and moral judgments, but this would have been a different book had those been my goals. Instead, the close and constructive engagement I had with the scientific communities involved opened my eyes to what could be a way out of a tragic predicament: drawing scientists and clinicians into the drug policy reform movement by convincing drug policy reformers and prison advocates to start taking them seriously as allies. Effectively contesting the morally judgmental argument that harm reductionists advocate "coddling the sick" or "condoning drug use" requires the cultural authority of science. Researchers should be courted by the drug policy reform movement—rather than being scorned for studying monkeys or rats or prisoners. I state it this way not to equate all research subjects but to indicate how much disdain has been directed toward scientists and research participants themselves by those who construct all experimental subjects as "guinea pigs." If more scientists could be convinced to stop endorsing the impossible dream that prohibition will lead to a drug-free nation, they might help policy makers craft a way beyond the unimaginative polarity of criminalization and medicalization.

Harm reduction offers a metaphor for care and an ethical sensibility "attuned to the play of power" (Schram 2006, 162). An alternative to the idea that abstinence is the only way to live, harm reduction follows from addiction researchers' recognition that addiction is better thought of as a chronic relapsing condition than as something to which individuals can simply say no. Harm reduction focuses on the actual harms that occur as people lead lives filled with pain, boredom, and structural violence. Substance abuse research does not really question why so many people are drawn to self-medicate or what social structures produce "addiction" as a route toward self-definition, for this would mean incorporating the social rather than disqualifying or controlling for it. Short of engaging the ambitious project of asking why so many people turn to drugs when and how they do, modest steps toward reducing harm and expanding access to health care and drug treatment offer the most workable drug policy.

Bringing to life the laboratory logics and indigenous moralities of the addiction research enterprise has changed my perspective on the social relevance of the sciences of craving, appetite, and addiction; on the definition of ethical conduct; and on the clinical usefulness of the outcomes of basic research. Getting close to the multiple social worlds of drug addiction unsettled my assumptions about what science ought to be and do. Given the pains and pleasures, rewards and punishments integral to research and writing, I hope *Discovering Addiction* provokes readers to question assumptions about drug addicts, drug policy, and the social role of science. I hope that it provides addiction researchers a fuller sense of their history as a community constituted in diversity. Finally, I hope policy reformers, advocates, activists, and policy makers find value and inspiration in realizing that harm reduction and critical public health approaches have a longer and richer history than many imagine.

Notes

INTRODUCTION

1. Called by names ranging from "addiction" to "drug dependence" to "substance abuse," the concept has generated a rich critical literature: see, for example, Davies 1992; DeGrandpre 2006; Forbes 1994; Fraser and Gordon 1994; Keane 2002; Lenson 1999. No synonym has gained as much traction as "addiction," a term returning to today's scientific parlance (O'Brien, Volkow, and Li 2006).

2. There is a flourishing literature on drug policy history: see Courtwright 1982/2001; Musto 1973/1999; Tracy and Acker 2004. Howard I. Kushner (2006) argues for looking more closely at the history of science.

3. Walsh also published an article (1973a) specifically on the institution that housed the ARC and on its transfer from the National Institute of Mental Health to the Bureau of Prisons.

4. Some social worlds cohere more than others. Behavioral pharmacologists comprise a well-defined group, but neuroimagers are relative newcomers whose networks are dispersed across social worlds. Social worlds are "universes of mutual discourse" (Mead 1938/1972, 518 [quoted in Clarke 1998, 289 n. 21]) that form the basic building blocks of the social organization of knowledge. Social worlds or arenas form coherent units of analysis despite contentious politics and heterogeneities within them (Clarke 2005, 48).

5. The field of science and technology studies has analyzed sciences as varied as biochemistry, crystallography, genetics, geology, physics, primatology, and the reproductive sciences (Clarke 1998; Frickel 2004; Fujimura 1996; Gilbert and Mulkay 1984/2003; Haraway 1976, 1989, 1997; Kohler 1991 and 2002; Latour and Woolgar 1986; Traweek 1988). Yet only Acker (1995, 1997, 2002) has written about the search for a nonaddicting analgesic. I am indebted to her landmark chronicle of the formative generation of addiction researchers up through World War II.

6. Having previously written a book on gender and drug policy, I am acutely aware of the appalling lack of women and persons of color who study addiction. Thomas Babor notes, "One thing that is clear from the selection process that brought these people into the field is that it favoured the recruitment of men rather than women," raising the question of the "possible influence of gender bias in the disciplines from which addiction has built its workforce" (quoted in Edwards 2002, 384).

7. These conflicts often involve accusations of secrecy, betrayal, and ethical lapse (Crease 2003; Hayden 2003). The Tuskegee Study of Untreated Syphilis in the Negro Male still stands as an exemplar of the moral failing of science the world over (Jones 1981/1992; Reverby 2000). Failure to disclose covert military and intelligence drug exper-

iments has heightened distrust of government, particularly in communities of color (U.S. Congress 1973, 1975, 1977a, 1977b). A countervailing example is provided by the U.S. Department of Energy Advisory Committee on Human Radiation Experiments.

CHAPTER 1

1. Michel Foucault's insight into the place of the "dangerous" delinquent in the "carceral continuum" rightly noted continuities between prison and "work begun elsewhere, which the whole of society pursues on each individual through innumerable mechanisms of discipline." Nothing, he wrote, distinguished the forms of authority directed toward sentencing, supervising, transforming, correcting, and improving individuals other than the "singularly 'dangerous' character of the delinquents, the gravity of their departures from normal behavior" (1979, 303). For Foucault, the power to punish was indistinguishable from the power to educate or even to "cure."

2. Harry M. Marks describes "medical individualism" as a cultural barrier to clinical research in the United States (1997, 51). Several factors exacerbated conflict between the clinic and laboratory in ways that made clinicians relatively uninterested in treating drug addiction. Once blamed for addicting patients, physicians began to avoid or underprescribe opiates even to patients in need of them (Jaffe 1985). So-called self-administration studies are discussed further in chapter 4 in the present book.

3. Himmelsbach 1972, 3. Many thanks to Jon M. Harkness for sharing copies of Himmelsbach 1972 and of his own interview with Himmelsbach, completed with Gail Javitt on November 2, 1994, under the auspices of the U.S. Department of Energy Advisory Committee on Human Radiation Experiments.

4. See Terry 1999 on a similar undertaking to define markers of lesbianism in the 1920s.

5. The federal Hygienic Laboratory was established in 1887 to pursue broader research programs than could municipal, state, or private laboratories (H. Marks 1997, 48). Although it had regulatory responsibility to test serums, vaccines, and industrial compounds, it lacked access to patients and did not have the capacity to do clinical research.

6. Although Robert Koch visualized the tubercle bacillus in 1882, U.S. clinicians integrated germ theory into practice slowly, because they still subscribed to miasmatic thought or feared that the new bacteriology would displace the medical arts. However, germ theory was popularly and commercially embraced. The personification of germs was central to the developing public health bureaucracy of the Progressive Era (Brandt 1985; Kraut 1994).

7. Carter et al. quoted in Terry and Pellens 1928/1970, 613. On hormone research in this period, see Oudshoorn 1994, 2003.

8. Terry and Pellens 1928/1970, 542. Paul Sollier's assistants at the Sanatorium of Boulogne conducted hematological studies to trace leukocyte reactions, which they interpreted as signaling a "true crisis" of the body along the lines of an infectious disease, rather than a mere "psychical breaking up of a habit." (Terry and Pellens 1928/1970, 541).

9. Some of the early psychoanalytic material is reprinted in Yalisove 1997.

10. The pharmacotoxic orgasm offered an objectless "executive process by which the

discharge of the entire psycho-sexual excitation is accomplished, like the function of onanism in children" (Rado 1926, 403).

11. Rado's Columbia lectures, delivered from 1945 to 1955, were published in 1969.

12. Addiction researchers trace their lineage not to psychoanalysis but to behaviorism, crediting Olds with discovering the "brain reward system," the neurological substrate for motivation and learning foundational to "brain mapping" and neurobehavioral drug-screening approaches. See Olds and Milner 1954; Olds 1955, 1956, 1958. Yet Olds was rarely cited in addiction studies until after a late 1960s review of work on drug effects on "brain-stimulation reward" (Kornetsky 2003a, 2003b).

13. On how such gendered conceptions play out in institutional settings, see Lunbeck 1994. On the longer history of such attribution patterns, see Tuana 1989, 1993.

CHAPTER 2

1. For Becker, the term *drug* is not a pharmacological category but a reflection of "how a society has decided to treat a substance" (2001).

2. At the May 28–29, 1970, symposium that marked Seevers's retirement, Nathan B. Eddy credited Seevers with realizing that monkeys could be used as a primary research tool, an idea that became the basis of a "world-recognized regimen for screening agents for morphine-like physical dependence capacity" (quoted in Domino 2004, 5). Eddy's own foundational work at Michigan and, later, at the National Institutes of Health was the main basis for Seevers's realization that monkeys could be used in this way.

3. By then, the bench program had synthesized 125 morphine derivatives and 350 other compounds and tested many in animals, according to Swain (1991, 18).

4. Reid Hunt to Charles W. Edmunds, April 30, 1936, Charles W. Edmunds Papers, box 1, Bentley Historical Library, Ann Arbor, Michigan. Edmunds lectured against patent medicine advertising and served as an expert witness in a case brought by the forerunner of the Food and Drug Administration, the U.S. Department of Agriculture's Bureau of Chemistry, against manufacturers of "Buffalo lythia waters," who claimed they relieved arthritis and rheumatism. He chaired the national standards committee on the desirability of biological assays for the United States Pharmacopeia and was active with the NRC committee until his sudden death in 1941.

5. Seevers later had Gerry A. Deneau translate Claude Bernard's article "Experimental Studies on Opium and Its Alkaloids" from the French. Bernard subcutaneously injected the active principles of opium into dogs, cats, rabbits, guinea pigs, rats, pigeons, sparrows, and frogs. He mentioned that two Paris physicians had conducted similar trials in man. After explaining the difficulty of comparison due to species differences, Bernard wrote: "The animal experiments facilitate the physiological analysis which will clarify and explain the pharmacological effects in man. We will see, in effect, that everything which we establish in man will be confirmed in animals, and vice versa, except for the particulars which differences in species explain; but basically the nature of the physiological actions is the same. It should not be otherwise, because without that there would never be physiological science nor medical science" (1864, 406). The unpublished translation was in Seevers's files at the University of Michigan. For access to this and otherwise unavailable material pertaining to Seevers, I thank James Woods.

6. Seevers later refuted his dual-action hypothesis (Domino 2004, 24–27).

7. The lecture was published in 1939 in the *Sigma Xi Quarterly*. Elsewhere, I explore antidrug reformers' use of "orientalizing" and "primitivizing" registers (Campbell 2000, 60–71). Seevers's use of the scientific register was designed to counter the caricatures of popular imagery for the purpose of grounding what he called a sane approach to drugs and drug policy.

8. While at Wisconsin, Seevers became an authority on monkey handling, as indicated by a letter of November 28, 1934, to him from K. K. Chen of the Lilly Research Laboratories in Indianapolis, Indiana. "Contemplating doing some work with monkeys," Chen sought advice on where to get them and how to feed them. Prompt and extensive, Seevers's reply included diagrams; detailed advice on housing, feeding, and handling; and a warning: "Utmost vigilance must be maintained at all times since they are always alert to escape or bite with any relaxation of the captor or at the unexpected time" (Maurice Seevers to K. K. Chen, December 3, 1934).

9. Many thanks to postdoctoral fellow Graham Florry for rescuing the monkey movies and screening them during my visit on March 19, 2005. Dated 1936, the film I saw and hereafter quote from was no. 5818.2, titled *Opiate Addiction in the Monkey*. It resembled *A Cinematic Study of Macaca mulatta*, a Seevers June 1936 publication listed in the *Journal of Pharmacology and Experimental Therapeutics*. The film depicted group-housed monkeys outside, quarreling and resisting capture, with a caption speculating about what the monkey wants—"only dilaudid, desire handling or injection?"

10. On Harlow, see Haraway 1989, 231–43; Blum 2002.

11. This undated film script from the Department of Pharmacology at the University of Wisconsin listed numbered scene shots organized by drug, time, and animal subjects—named "Cody," "Meyer," "Dillinger," "Morphy," "Jocko," and "Boss."

12. A positive stimulus had to take place within two or three minutes, the length of the monkey's "mental set" (a term used instead of the anthropomorphic term *memory*).

13. Victor Laties has posted an invaluable set of materials on Spragg at http://www.apa.org/divisions/div28/archive/History/pan/briefspragg.html.

14. Maurice Seevers to William Charles White, chair of CDAN, March 21, 1940.

15. This was a novel request from a researcher outside Lexington. On October 8, 1940, Seevers acknowledged receipt of five hundred grams of morphine sulfate to Lyndon Small at NIH. Small supplied the laboratories at Lexington and Michigan with morphine and other compounds, sometimes purifying as many as ten pounds at a time for research purposes (Lyndon Small to Maurice Seevers, October 31, 1941).

16. William Charles White to Maurice Seevers, April 9, 1940.

17. Clifton Himmelsbach to Maurice Seevers, January 16, 1941. The subject of the correspondence was Seevers's attempt to convene a subgroup of "morphinists" (who studied morphine) at an annual meeting of the Federation of American Societies for Experimental Biology.

18. Wailoo (1997) argues that social contexts make disease identity coherent by assigning meaning to physiological symptoms. Because the anemias have shed their moral character, his case offers a contrast to the persistence of the moral discourse of addiction.

19. Minutes from the first postwar CDAN meeting on October 2, 1947, National Research Council, Washington, DC, appendix and p. 9. Proceedings and minutes can be

consulted at the National Academy of Sciences Archives in Washington, DC, or at the National Library of Medicine in Bethesda, MD. I am grateful to Jim Woods and Louis Harris for allowing me access to their personal collections.

20. Kelsey trained under E. M. K. Geiling, who showed that a drug released by Massengill under the name Elixir Sulfanilamide caused over one hundred deaths in 1937. The event led to the 1938 Food, Drug, and Cosmetic Act that established the FDA (Stephens and Brynner 2001, 44–45).

21. Supply problems necessitate the reuse of animals. Later animal rights and antivivisectionist movements also troubled the supply of research primates (Blum 1994). The original problems Seevers faced in establishing the colony were related to the large numbers of animals used to produce and test polio vaccine and antimalarial drugs (Deneau 1970, 213). Popular protests eventually led India to cut off the traffic in monkeys in 1955, and it resumed only after the United States promised to use Indian monkeys solely for biomedical research that benefited "all humanity," rather than in military or space research (Haraway 1989, 121). The embargo prompted the NRC to start a secure domestic breeding colony on the island of Cayo Santiago near Puerto Rico. In 1978, India again banned export of rhesus monkeys, of which it was the only supplier. On animal models, see Rader 2004; Rowan 1984.

22. Seevers spoke to the Proprietary Association in the proceedings of the Annual Research and Scientific Development Conference held at the Biltmore Hotel in New York City on December 8, 1960 (Seevers 1960, 4–12). Dedicated to steady growth and dissemination of scientific knowledge among pharmaceutical manufacturers, the society was reactivating its Therapeutic Research Foundation in response to the Kefauver hearings that led to the 1962 amendments to the Food, Drug, and Cosmetic Act of 1938. Seevers's paper on test planning utilized Henry K. Beecher's CDAN-sponsored studies (see chap. 4 of the present book). Seevers joked that aspirin would not have survived the animal and human screens typically used to determine safety and efficacy (1960, 10).

23. Thanks are due Jeremy Nordmoe, archivist at the Eskind Biomedical Library at Vanderbilt University in Nashville, Tennessee, which holds the archives of the American College of Neuropsychopharmacology. He remembered that this film predating 1965 was among the collected papers of Keith and Eva Killam. CDAN was listed as the film's sponsor, and it was in 1965 that CDAN adopted the name change that made it the Committee on Problems of Drug Dependence.

24. Eddy related the following anecdote at Seevers's retirement: "The only time Dr. Seevers and I ever exchanged sharp words had to do with a deadline. We were members of a World Health Organization study group on drug dependence. I happened to be chairman and Dr. Seevers was asked to head a subcommittee to write a description of the concept of dependence. We gave them a free day and I waited a little longer for their statement. Then I chided Dr. Seevers for the delay; we had only a week and we had to approve the statement for our report. In his usual forceful language, Dr. Seevers said that maybe we would get the statement and maybe we wouldn't; it had to be right" (quoted in Domino 2004, 5).

25. The negative connotations of the term *dependency* in Anglophone cultures were not fully recognized by this coalition. See Fraser and Gordon 1994; Schram 2006, 136–52. As these sources make clear, the term was advanced to destigmatize

pauperism but was recycled as a "postindustrial pathology" associated with bad habits and addiction.

CHAPTER 3

1. *Porter Act,* Public Law 203, 71st Cong., 1st sess. (May 13, 1930).

2. Research did not occur at Forth Worth until 1965, when the small Social Research Unit opened in collaboration with the Institute for Behavioral Research headed by Saul B. Sells of Texas Christian University. See U.S. Department of Health, Education, and Welfare, 1967.

3. For a sense of how this multidisciplinary research team functioned until World War II, see Himmelsbach 1972, 1994; Martin and Isbell 1978, 13–24.

4. Clinical observation led William R. Martin, ARC director from 1963 to 1977, to classify multiple opiate receptors (kappa, sigma, and mu) and correctly predict their location in the brain before they were visualized (Acker 1997).

5. The U.S. District Court ruled in 1936 that Lexington could not hold voluntary patients against their will (*Ex parte Lloyd,* 13 F. Supp. 1005 [D.C. Ky. 1936]). At first, only male opiate addicts were admitted, but President Roosevelt opened Lexington to "neuropsychiatric" patients in 1942, and many came from veterans hospitals. See *Operations Manual,* part A, chapter 1: History, NIMH Clinical Research Center, Lexington, Kentucky, 1971, found in Record Group 511 ADAMHA Alcohol, Drug Abuse, and Mental Health, Administrative Office, Clinical Research Center, Lexington, KY, Lexington General Operations, box 8, folder "Lexington History and Operations," NARA Southeast, Morrow, GA.

6. Soon after the women were moved into the main building, patience wore thin due to the "living and working of both men and women in the same building" (Annual Report of the General Services Section 1957, 1). Social control at the Lexington Hospital was eroding by the late 1950s, when there began to be more "adverse behavior reports," bribery, and attempts to introduce contraband, all of which administrators viewed as disruptive to withdrawal, treatment, and research. Half the voluntary patients stayed for less than thirty days, which was considered "destructive to efficient use of staff and morale since very little treatment is accomplished" (Record Group 511 ADAMHA Alcohol, Drug Abuse, and Mental Health, Administrative Office, Clinical Research Center, Lexington, KY, Administrative Records 1957–1974, Statistical Data Annual Statistical Summary 1957–1964, box 1, NARA Southeast, Morrow, GA).

7. The bureaucratic history is confusing due to Lexington's hybrid status and the separation of the research unit from the larger institution. The PHS was transferred out of the Treasury Department on July 1, 1938, to the Federal Security Agency, which became the Department of Health, Education, and Welfare in 1953. The Division of Mental Hygiene was abolished when NIMH was established in 1948. After that, Lexington and Fort Worth fell under the jurisdiction of the Division of Hospitals, and the ARC became an NIMH research unit in 1949. Not until 1967 was the hospital operation transferred to NIMH and renamed the Clinical Research Center. In 1968, the Health Services and Mental Health Administration was established, along with the Division of Narcotic Addiction and Drug Abuse (DNADA), under the auspices of which fell both the ARC and the NIMH Clinical Research Center.

8. Sanford Bates to Walter Treadway, May 28, 1935, Record Group 129, Bureau of Prisons, National Archives II, box 746 NC-43, correspondence file 4-13-0, 1930–1937, College Park, MD.

9. Bates to Treadway, May 28, 1935. This prophecy held only until the mid-1970s, when the facility reverted to a federal prison.

10. Sanford Bates, director of the BOP, to Lawrence Kolb, May 28, 1935, NARA Record Group 129, file 4-13-0, box 746 NC-43.

11. James V. Bennett, commissioner of prison industries, to Lawrence Kolb, November 4, 1936, NARA 4-13-3-29, box 47.

12. Lawrence Kolb, "Drug Addiction among Women," n.d. Record Group 511 ADAMHA Alcohol, Drug Abuse, and Mental Health, Administrative Office, Clinical Research Center, Lexington, KY, Public Relations, box 1, NARA Southeast, Morrow, GA.

13. Lexington staff were reluctant to engage policy debates without definitive data, although they testified on behalf of more humane treatment on June 2, 3, and 8, 1955 (U.S. Congress 1955).

14. Sanford Bates to Eleanor T. Glueck, Institute of Criminal Law, Kendall House, Cambridge, MA, December 17, 1930, NARA 4-13-0.

15. WHO 1950 was submitted by Nathan B. Eddy, National Institutes of Health, and was based on Isbell's data produced at the ARC, illustrating how tightly interwoven CDAN was with the WHO expert committee.

16. *Annotated Bibliography of Papers from the Addiction Research Center, 1935–1975* (DHEW no. [ADM] 77-435, 1978) includes addenda covering the years 1976 and 1977.

17. Bates to Treadway, May 28, 1935.

18. Bates to Treadway, May 28, 1935.

19. Chestang 1970. Many thanks to Professor Gwendolyn Hall for allowing me to use the materials she gathered in the spring of 1970.

20. The research staff held different political beliefs than clinical and support staff. These were often implicit, because they marked researchers as "outsiders." For instance, Wikler's eldest daughter Marjorie Senechal, who lived on the Lexington grounds from the age of one to the age of fourteen, has noted that though her parents, Eastern European Jews from New York's Lower East Side, forbade their children to voice the family's left-liberal political views, "the glaring absence of Monopoly among the board games on our porch would have tipped off the politically aware" (Senechal 2003, 189).

21. Sociologist Howard S. Becker taped the book-length oral history of Marilyn Bishop, which was edited by Helen McGill Hughes, wife of Everett C. Hughes, and published as *The Fantastic Lodge: The Autobiography of a Girl Drug Addict* (1961). Bishop's pseudonym was "Janet Clark."

22. Record Group 511 ADAMHA Alcohol, Drug Abuse, and Mental Health, Administrative Office, Clinical Research Center, Lexington, KY, box 6, folder "Forms," NARA Southeast, Morrow, GA.

23. Correspondence addressed to attorney general, Washington, DC, 18 October 1942, NA Record Group 129, box 25, by Perry and Gladys Youts.

24. Availability of drugs other than those used in ARC studies depended on fluctuating levels of security. Senechal recollects finding drugs and paraphernalia on the grounds as a child (2003, 192). The pharmacist who mixed preparations for the ARC in the 1970s noted changes over time (Johnson 2005). An inmate, Eddie Flowers, inter-

viewed in 2004 by J. P. Olsen and Luke Walden in the course of making their film *The Narcotics Farm,* recounted entering the research program specifically to get drugs.

25. Dropout rates as high as one-third were recorded in studies of narcotic antagonists, which most people do not experience as pleasant. Participants could and did opt out, according to National Commission 1976a.

26. The earliest instruments, the Morphine Abstinence Syndrome Intensity (MASI) scale developed by Himmelsbach and Kolb's K-classification system, categorized addicts in terms of psychological profile, behavior, and physiological state. In the mid-1950s, Harris Hill, Charles Haertzen, and Richard Belleville developed the Addiction Research Center Inventory (ARCI), which is still in use (Martin and Isbell 1978, 161).

27. The second interview was conducted as part of the Oral History Project of the U.S. Department of Energy's Advisory Committee on Human Radiation Experiments (Himmelsbach 1994). Himmelsbach did not return to addiction research after he left Lexington in 1944.

28. The concepts "normal" and "abnormal" shift in relation to time and place: "It must be admitted that the normal man knows that he is so only in a world where every man is not normal. . . . The normal man is he who lives with the assurance of being able to arrest within himself what in another man would run its course. In order for the normal man to believe himself so, and call himself so, he needs not the foretaste of disease but its projected shadow" (Canguilhem 1991, 286).

29. The meeting was held on April 29, 1961, as part of a three-year PHS project that culminated in a report issued by the Law-Medicine Research Institute titled "A Study of the Legal, Ethical, and Administrative Aspects of Clinical Research Involving Human Subjects," issued on March 31, 1963. Thanks to Jon M. Harkness for sharing the meeting transcripts, which identify speakers by initials. The transcripts are housed at the Mugar Memorial Library at Boston University.

30. Wikler wrote about the neuropathology of Horner's syndrome, cases of which he encountered between 1938 and 1940 at the PHS Marine Hospital in St. Louis, Missouri.

31. Soon after Lexington opened in 1935, Robert H. Felix became persuaded that the electroencephalograph would be useful for studying the effects of addiction on the brain. He went to Providence, Rhode Island, for training, where he met biophysicist Howard L. Andrews and convinced him to move to Lexington. There, Andrews installed the first electroencephalograph west of the Alleghenies (Kay and Andrews in Martin and Isbell 1978, 140–54). Andrews did not leave Lexington until 1942, when he departed "with a distinct sense of disappointment and personal failure" because the technology had not enabled him to draw conclusions of basic significance (Martin and Isbell 1978, 153). Wikler took over Andrews's lab in 1943 and expanded the facility with a government surplus ink-writing EEG machine that was used to study sleep patterns, metabolic and tissue tolerance to alcohol and barbiturates, and the effects of mescaline and psilocybin.

32. From 1942 to 1943, Wikler went to the University of Chicago, the Illinois Neuropsychiatric Institute, the Northwestern University Institute of Neurology, the Yale University Laboratory of Physiology, and the Rockefeller Institute for Medical Research at the New York State Psychiatric Institute and New York Hospital.

33. Wikler's first publication of national scope was coauthored with Jules H. Masserman, with whom Wikler studied at the University of Chicago (1943). They conditioned responses using conflict in an operant conditioning situation to produce "experimental neuroses" and recorded the experiments on film. Masserman had a psychoanalytic orientation and an "avowed anthropomorphism" (Iversen and Iversen 1981, 35).

34. He cited Lawrence Kubie and Roy R. Grinker, Sr., both experimental psychiatrists, although Grinker had been psychoanalyzed by Freud himself. Grinker studied anxiety as an objective, observable behavior (1979, 45, 50).

35. The idea resembles Rado's "pharmacothymic orgasm," which he claimed was equivalent to the pregenital alimentary orgasm of a baby at the breast. Robert D. Chessick (1960) later attempted to confirm the existence of this phenomenon.

36. The Social Science Section found high relapse rates in a "fairly low percentage" and argued, "[G]enerally discouraging conclusions which have been drawn from other studies may, therefore, be based largely on the fact that these studies have chosen to use the most negative of the possible measurements" (O'Donnell 1964).

CHAPTER 4

1. Sigmund Freud quoted in Greenacre 1953.

2. Psychopharmacology's usefulness was contested; for instance, Felix was reluctant to establish the NIMH Psychopharmacology Service Center. Yet historians claim, "[I]ntroduction of chlorpromazine and reserpine in the mid-1950s held out the promise of healing the long-standing division between biological and psychodynamic psychiatrists and promoting the reintegration of the specialty with medicine generally" (Grob 1991, 154). The Psychopharmacology Service Center's Early Clinical Drug Evaluation Unit conducted clinical trials until the 1970s, standardizing data collection, protocols, and rating scales. David Healy claimed, "This was almost a new form of science, one that acknowledged that techniques drive progress as much as, if not more than, anything else—a form of science that was looked down upon by university-based scientists, for whom experiments were conducted to test already existing theories" (2002, 282). See Healy 1996, 239–63; Cole 1970.

3. We have been "becoming neurochemical selves" for a long time (Rose 2003).

4. Benedict (1960) quoted heavily from Huxley's "Drugs That Shape Men's Minds" (1958), while stressing the "deadly amorality" of government mind control research, which he correctly insisted was neither science fiction nor prophecy.

5. The first edition of Nelson Algren's *The Man with the Golden Arm* (1951) won the National Book Award in 1949. It became a major motion picture—directed by Otto Preminger and starring Frank Sinatra—that was notorious for getting around the Hollywood censorship codes. Addiction researcher Conan Kornetsky (2003b) remarked on its accurate portrayal of heroin.

6. The figure of the monkey encodes a stunning array of social phobias, polarities, and political agendas about the "enemy within," controlled by external forces as is *The Manchurian Candidate*'s Raymond Shaw, who embodies qualities opposite to those of the democratic citizens of the free world. Drug issues provide "chemical curtains" for racist sentiments.

7. Internalist accounts refute serendipity. See Dews 1985, 3.

8. Donald Klein, interview by Jackie Orr, March 29, 1996, quoted in Orr 2006, 171. Thanks to Jackie Orr for sharing her interview with Klein, who worked at Lexington as a psychiatrist and assistant surgeon from 1954 to 1956.

9. Evelyn Fox Keller reminds us that claims to universality are political, not scientific (1992, 180–81). The putative universality of ethnopharmacology still surfaces in debates over how to regulate psychoactive substances in the face of global inequality.

10. The movie *The Snakepit* was made at the Rockland State Hospital prior to Kline's arrival (Healy 2002, 104).

11. This passage is from a guidebook to the "new territory" (Barchas et al. 1977, 528).

12. In *Useful Bodies: Humans in the Service of Medical Science in the Twentieth Century* (2003), Jordan Goodman, Anthony McElligott, and Lara Marks argue that focusing on informed consent "skews the study of human experimentation toward an ethical analysis rather than a practice" (4). More significant, they say, is how the "modern state increasingly used its prerogative to lay claim to the individual body for its own needs, whether social, economic, or military" (2).

13. Pharmacologist Harry Gold of Cornell is credited with developing the double-blind test "virtually alone" (Shapiro and Shapiro 1997; cf. Kaptchuck 1998, which argues for a much longer history).

14. Beecher's Anesthesiology Laboratory at Massachusetts General Hospital was the world's first facility for the clinical study of anesthetic agents (Harkness 1999).

15. See Ellison C. Peirce, Jr., "Anesthesia Safety and Mortality Studies in the 1950's through 1970's," at http://www.apsf.org/about/rovenstine/part3.mspx.

16. Beecher studied drug effects on performance of physical and mental tasks. According to Tousignant 2006, the U.S. Army Medical Research and Development Board funded Beecher's first large-scale clinical trial of methadone, and he conducted military-supported field trials of methadone in Korea.

17. The expansion of experimentation by clinicians was not legally recognized as a legitimate part of the physician's activities in the late 1950s. Beecher regarded it as essential and believed its necessity should be legally recognized.

18. Information on Louis Lasagna (deceased) is taken from Lasagna 1994 and Healy 2002. There is little information on Jane Denton. See Anthony Petrosino's entry on Charles Frederick (Fred) Mosteller in the James Lind Library (http://www.jameslindlibrary.org). See also Beecher et al. 1953; Lasagna et al. 1954.

19. The Cornell group published dozens of papers from 1940 to the mid-1950s, when Hardy turned to other interests (see Hardy, Wolff, and Goodell 1940, 1952; Schumaker et al. 1940). The dolorimeter enjoyed a brief heyday in the early days of Lexington, falling out of favor by the early 1950s (Tousignant 2006).

20. Rothman argues that due to the construction of the Nazis as fundamentally different, U.S. clinical researchers did not perceive implications for their own work (1994, 62–63).

21. Bridgman's concept of "operationalism" was famously attacked by Herbert Marcuse in *One-Dimensional Man* (1964).

22. Wikler participated in a phenomenology reading group convened by Erwin Strauss, who edited *Phenomenology: Pure and Applied* (1964), to which Wikler contributed.

23. Wikler wrote: "In achieving an impressive degree of mastery over the world about us, the growth of the natural sciences has been characterized by an ever-increasing supplementation of 'private operations' (sensing, feeling, inducing, deducing) with 'public' ones (control and manipulation over measurable variables). As one result, even our 'private' ways of perceiving the world have changed from those of our prescientific ancestors, so that at sunset, we no longer 'see' the sun sinking into the sea, but 'see' it disappearing beneath the horizon" (Wikler 1965, 85).

24. Beecher here cites two letters received from Wikler, penned August 7 and September 6, 1956.

25. The thalidomide controversy broke during Senator Estes Kefauver's hearings on price-fixing and profit margins in the pharmaceutical industry (Stephens and Brynner 2001).

26. The committee explored Puerto Rico, a common pharmaceutical testing ground, but never followed up (Committee on Drug Addiction and Narcotics 1954b). On the use of Puerto Rico as a "laboratory," see Briggs 2002).

27. Under the auspices of the National Institute on Drug Abuse, Charles Gorodetzky added a voice-over in the 1970s.

CHAPTER 5

1. Sydney A. Halpern has defined an "indigenous morality" as a set of statements and practices that pervades the scientific problem groups and social networks that comprise a clinical research. She has defined "scientific problem groups" as networks of "researchers who address common questions, share materials and techniques, review one another's scientific papers, and debate the meaning of empirical findings" (2004, 9–10). The concept is useful for studying the social organization of science (Mulkay, Gilbert, and Woolgar 1975).

2. Harry M. Marks criticized sociologists of science for focusing on the laboratory and ignoring the clinic (1997, 8). Movement was bidirectional at the ARC, where researchers took cues from clinicians and corrected the evidence base on which they acted. Although oriented toward basic research, ARC findings were useful to clinicians.

3. Frank Jewett, president of the National Academy of Sciences, responded thusly to a 1943 proposal to introduce venereal disease into a prison population in hopes of finding an effective chemoprophylaxis: "[P]rison populations are not free populations and . . . so-called volunteers are not true volunteers in the ordinary sense. Their volunteering is or can be alleged to have been brought about by reasons which are entirely absent in a free population" (quoted in H. Marks 1997, 104).

4. Flowers testified in the Kennedy hearings (U.S. Congress 1973) beside Harris Isbell and Lexington inmate John Henderson Childs, who worked for Isbell. Flowers has been interviewed several times by filmmakers J. P. Olsen and Luke Walden, and I remain indebted to their willingness to share the fruits of their labor. John Marks also interviewed Flowers for his book *The Search for the Manchurian Candidate* (1979), which I discuss in chapter 6 of the present book.

5. For instance, Wikler wrote: "[C]linical and electroencephalographic effects of these drugs are determined not only by the chemical properties of these agents but also by other factors which are not clearly defined. However, the 'personality' of the individ-

ual, his past experiences with drugs and the meaning to him of the experimental situation appear to modify drug effects" (1954, 174).

6. Industry had to look elsewhere to build its clinical research infrastructure. It often looked to poor populations within the United States and Puerto Rico (Briggs 2002; Fisher 2005; Petryna 2006; Shah 2006).

7. At Lexington, methadone was used to ease withdrawal, not as a form of maintenance. Not until the 1960s did Vincent Dole and Marie Nyswander, architects of methadone maintenance, develop the clinical logic of the "methadone blockade" at Rockefeller University. Dole was a highly respected scientist trying to solve the "opium problem" evident on the streets of New York City, but Nyswander's credibility in the scientific community was low. During her 1945 residency at Lexington, she was perceived as "threatening" or "naive" in the tiny professional enclave at the ARC (Senechal 2004). One especially telling anecdote presaging his views on the "methadone mess" was recounted late in life by Harris Isbell in an interview with Marjorie Senechal, Abraham and Ada Wikler's daughter, who lived on the Narco campus until age twelve. Isbell recalled preventing Nyswander from distributing morphine shots as Christmas presents to Lexington inmates (Senechal 2003, 193). Outsiders to the "research establishment," Dole and Nyswander were criticized for prematurely announcing methadone's efficacy as a maintenance agent and for being "not pharmacological" enough (Courtwright, Joseph, and Des Jarlais 1989, 337). They in turn disparaged prior addiction research, as evidenced by Dole's remark that there "was no research talent in the field, just some pharmacologists working with animals who didn't have a concept of human epidemiology" (quoted in Courtwright, Joseph, and Des Jarlais 1989, 332).

8. At the January 1953 CDAN meeting, Isbell urged Beecher to include nalorphine as a control and to run clinical trials of a nalorphine-morphine combination to establish nalorphine's analgesic efficacy in cases of postoperative pain. According to May and Jacobson, this suggestion had come up in the late 1940s (1989, 190).

9. The series ran from November 26 to December 1 and catalyzed conferences sponsored by the New York City Office of the Mayor, the New York City Welfare Council, the New York Academy of Medicine, and the Josiah Macy, Jr., Foundation (Campbell 2000, 98–102).

10. Lobotomy was atypical at Lexington because it did not have discernible therapeutic effects. Kolb Hall housed a couple hundred veterans or retired members of the Coast Guard who were neuropsychiatric patients (the population for whom lobotomies were commonly recommended at the time).

11. My account is drawn from an informal interview with Edward F. Domino in March 2006, as well as from Domino 1995 and my formal interview with him in 2006.

12. The drug was also tested at Lexington (Isbell and Fraser 1953).

13. As mentioned earlier, the ARC evaluated the abuse potential of many branded compounds central to the medical market of the 1950s, such as Seconal and other barbiturates, Dromoran, or Miltown (meprobamate, the first popular minor tranquilizer). See Isbell 1951a, 1951b; Hill and Belleville 1953; Isbell and Fraser 1953. Isbell 1951a reported on a study in which ten barbiturate-addicted patients were maintained on large doses of secobarbital (Seconal) for lengthy periods (Addiction Research Center 1978, 53). Severe impairment was found, leading to warnings that consumers could not anticipate emergencies and should not operate machinery on the drug.

14. Cancer research at the Jewish Chronic Disease Hospital in Brooklyn, hepatitis research at Willowbrook School on Staten Island, and the Tuskegee Study of Untreated Syphilis in the Negro Male stand as examples of unethical human subjects research. The Tuskegee scandal catalyzed the National Commission for the Protection of Human Subjects of Biomedical Research (Reverby 2000). Soon after the scandal broke in the summer of 1972, another human subjects scandal regarding military and Central Intelligence Agency (CIA) testing of psychoactive drugs as "incapacitating agents" implicated the ARC, which studied LSD-25 and other hallucinogens. Most research on LSD occurred at the Edgewood Arsenal; Fort Detrick, Maryland; Fort Bragg, North Carolina; Fort McClellan, Alabama; Fort Benning, Georgia; and Dugway Proving Ground, Utah (Moreno 2001, 256). By contrast, the ARC studied these drugs through their usual protocols and techniques and in comparison to the opiates with which they usually worked (Wikler 1954).

15. Unlike opiate research, LSD research was not centrally coordinated. Instead, the army and the CIA competitively funneled money through private foundations for clandestine LSD studies, in which prisoners served as unwitting subjects of convenience. See Lee and Schlain 1985; Campbell 1995; Goliszek 2003; Hewitt 2002; J. Marks 1979; Moreno 2001.

16. Kennedy's Interdepartmental Committee on Narcotics recommended that the federal narcotics hospitals shift "from their present emphasis on treatment of Federal narcotic prisoners and probationers as well as volunteers, to full-time research-oriented programs, examining all aspects of narcotic and drug abuse" (memorandum from the secretary of the Department of Health, Education, and Welfare to the surgeon general, n.d., Record Group 511 ADAMHA Alcohol, Drug Abuse, and Mental Health, Administrative Office, Clinical Research Center, Lexington, KY, Study of Narcotic Problems—Forms—Civil Commitment Reports, box 6, folder "Policy 1963–1966," NARA Southeast, Morrow, GA). Although President Johnson reportedly viewed the committee's report skeptically, on July 15, 1964, he directed all units into maximum activity (Office of the White House Press Secretary, Statement by the President, July 15, 1964 Record Group 511 ADAMHA Alcohol, Drug Abuse, and Mental Health, Administrative Office, Clinical Research Center, Lexington, KY, Study of Narcotic Problems—Forms—Civil Commitment Reports, box 6, folder "Policy 1963–1966," NARA Southeast, Morrow, GA). His directive spurred a study of the PHS neuropsychiatric and narcotic hospitals as part of the attempt to devolve responsibility for treatment to states and municipalities, while continuing the federal research mandate. Ironically, since voluntary patients had never participated in ARC studies, the president's commission recommended that they be accepted "only to advance research aims" (briefing memorandum to the secretary of the Department of Health, Education, and Welfare from Rufus E. Miles, Jr., assistant secretary for administration, "Design for a Study on the Future of the Neuropsychiatric and Narcotic Hospitals of the Public Health Service,"1964, Record Group 511 ADAMHA Alcohol, Drug Abuse, and Mental Health, Administrative Office, Clinical Research Center, Lexington, KY, Study of Narcotic Problems—Forms—Civil Commitment Reports, box 6, folder "Policy 1963–1966," NARA Southeast, Morrow, GA, 3).

17. Likening responses to drug addiction to past responses to insanity or witchcraft, the *Robinson* opinion advocated modern medical treatment. Addicts, Justice Douglas wrote for the majority, were under the sway of compulsions they could not manage

without professional help. An addict was defined as "a person who habitually takes or otherwise uses to the extent of having lost the power of self-control any opium, morphine, cocaine, or other narcotic drug" (*Robinson v. California* 370 U.S. 660 [1962]).

18. Most NARA patients were considered "too antagonistic or disruptive to participate in the institution treatment program" (Maddux in Martin and Isbell 1978, 239).

19. Sidney Cohen, acting director of DNADA, formed a panel to transition Lexington to a "model treatment facility" and named Harold Conrad chief of the CRC.

20. Bertram S. Brown to the Secretary of the Department of Health, Record Group 511 ADAMHA Alcohol, Drug Abuse, and Mental Health, Administrative Office, Clinical Research Center, Lexington, KY, box 5, NARA Southeast, Morrow, GA.

21. Record Group 511 ADAMHA Alcohol, Drug Abuse, and Mental Health, Administration Office, Clinical Research Center, Lexington, KY, box 4, NARA Southeast, Morrow, GA.

22. Paul Q. Peterson, acting deputy surgeon general, "Program Review of the Clinical Research Center, Lexington, Kentucky," August 7, 1970, Record Group 511 ADAMHA Alcohol, Drug Abuse, and Mental Health, Administrative Office, Clinical Research Center, Lexington, KY, Administrative Records 1957–74, box 4, NARA Southeast, Morrow, GA.

23. At the request of Jerome H. Jaffe, director of the White House Special Action Office for Drug Abuse Prevention and an alumnus of Lexington, William Bunney, director of DNADA, dispatched William Pollin and Richard Belleville (once at the ARC) to Lexington the week of October 16, 1972. Earlier that year, the CRC shifted priorities from treatment to research at DNADA's behest. Their report reflected the dissatisfaction of the CRC researchers with their lower prestige relative to the ARC. On November 30, 1972, Bunney responded to Jaffe's request for recommendations. He noted that the ARC was necessary to carry out the Department of Health, Education, and Welfare's responsibility for assessing the abuse potential of new compounds, warning "there is no other federal laboratory which can carry out the present or expanded responsibilities" (Record Group 511 ADAMHA Alcohol, Drug Abuse, and Mental Health, Administrative Office, Clinical Research Center, Lexington, KY, Lexington General Operations, box 8, NARA Southeast, Morrow, GA). Believing that the ARC might have to take on tasks carried out in Ann Arbor, Bunney advocated merging the ARC and the CRC. Nowhere did he mention the possibility of discontinuing the ARC's human research program.

CHAPTER 6

1. See Joseph Sturgell, "Description of Hospital Treatment Program," appendix B, in Committee on Drug Addiction and Narcotics 1955, 1033–36.

2. Atlanta Record Group 511 ADAMHA Alcohol, Drug Abuse, and Mental Health, Administrative Office, Clinical Research Center, Lexington, KY Study of Narcotic Problems—Forms, box 5, NARA Southeast, Morow, GA.

3. Early sociology of bioethics documented social norms among biomedical researchers. Barber et al. (1979) analyzed the first national survey of the institutional review boards mandated in 1966 at every institution that conducted research on human

subjects with PHS funding. Originally published in 1973, the book revealed a "permissive" minority of biomedical researchers that held low-status positions in the social hierarchy of science and who would approve studies that most considered ethically questionable. Barber et al. wrote: "The research community is itself pathogenic, at least to a degree, and perhaps we will never adequately regulate the use of humans in research until we better understand the pathology" (1979, x). Emphasizing the pattern through which "'good guys' [were turned] into 'bad guys,'" the sociologists contrasted their approach to the individualistic terms of Beecher and others who did not situate ethical actions within social context (Barber et al. 1979, xiii).

4. See U.S. Congress 1969, 5689; Mitford 1973a; Rugaber 1969.

5. I support the National Prison Project, which has been crucial for expanding prisoners' rights and changing prison conditions in the United States.

6. U.S. Congress 1973.

7. Commission members were Joseph V. Brady, professor of behavioral biology, Johns Hopkins University; Robert E. Cooke, vice chancellor for health sciences, University of Wisconsin; Dorothy I. Height, president of the National Council of Negro Women; Albert R. Jonson, associate professor of bioethics, University of California at San Francisco; Patricia King, associate professor of law, Georgetown University; Karen Lebacqz, consultant in bioethics, California State Department of Health; David W. Louisell, professor of law, University of California at Berkeley; Donald W. Seldin, professor and chair of the Department of Internal Medicine, University of Texas at Dallas; Elliott Stellar, provost and professor of physiological psychology, University of Pennsylvania; and Robert H. Turtle, attorney. Only Brady was familiar with the ARC.

8. U.S. Congress 1975.

9. MKULTRA was the code name for a CIA contract research program on the controlled alteration of human behavior. It ran from 1953 to 1963 and used research materials obtained through "standing arrangements with specialists in universities, pharmaceutical houses, hospitals, state and federal institutions, and private research organizations." Testing was carried out in many sites other than the "Lexington Rehabilitation Center," as it was called in the Church committee hearings.

10. *The Belmont Report* built on ten reports issued by the committee between 1974 and 1978. Its principles—respect for persons, beneficence, and justice—remain in effect (Callahan 2003). See http://www.nihtraining.com/ohsrsite/guidelines/belmont.html.

11. Biographical information on Carlson was taken from Keve 1991.

12. Correspondence dated March 1, 1976, from Norman A. Carlson, director of the BOP, to the Honorable Robert W. Kastenmeier indicated that use of prisoners with a history of narcotic abuse in tests of the addictive properties of new drugs would be phased out at the ARC in Lexington, Kentucky. Carlson's letter was mentioned several times in *Research Involving Prisoners: Report and Recommendations,* by the National Commission for the Protection of Human Subjects (1976b).

13. NIDA was established in September 1972 and given statutory authority in 1973. The ARC was not absorbed into it until 1974. Until 1992, when it became part of the NIH, NIDA was administered by the Alcohol, Drug Abuse, and Mental Health Administration (ADAMHA) under the auspices of the U.S. Department of Health, Education, and Welfare (DHEW).

14. Lexington went through a particularly deplorable incarnation not long after the ARC's departure. My thanks to Scott Christianson for pointing out the notorious "experimental" basement unit where women political prisoners were subjected to sensory deprivation and behavior modification designed to break their will. The "Lexington Unit" closed in 1988 in a major victory for prison activists.

15. James V. Lowry, "Opening Remarks," in Committee on Drug Addiction and Narcotics 1955, 1031–32.

16. Norm Carlson sat on the advisory board of the CEC.

17. The ARC had no direct fiscal relationship with the pharmaceutical industry. CPDD and the FDA have small testing programs that are widely regarded by the scientific community as inadequate to prevent such public health crises as those involving Oraflex (Ronald 2006) or OxyContin, both painkillers of the class that the ARC would have once investigated.

18. The industry reconsidered drug research in prisons in August 1973 at a conference held in Airlie, Virginia (Harkness 2003, 253–55). Pharmaceutical Manufacturers' Association president C. Joseph Stetler announced the conference at the Kennedy hearings (U.S. Congress 1973) as he indicated how deeply dependent the industry was on prisoners.

19. *Otis Clay, Plaintiff-Appellant v. Doctor William R. Martin et al. and The United States Surgeon General et al. and The United States Defendants-Appellees,* 509 F.2d 109–14 (2d Cir. 1975). A government motion to dismiss Clay's 1975 appeal was granted in June 1977. On September 8, 1978, the U.S. government filed a motion for summary judgment, which is considered a harsh remedy that is granted only where material issues of fact no longer remain to be tried. The Court partly granted this motion after determining that Clay's heart attack was not caused by drugs administered at the ARC. However, the Court viewed as unsettled the issue of whether Clay's consent was voluntary and informed, and thus it allowed an investigation to determine whether the naltrexone experiment was conducted in a "negligent and reckless" manner. Three days after these matters were tried on March 12, 1979, the Court dismissed Clay's complaint in its entirety with prejudice.

20. "Prisoner Claims Inhuman Treatment in Medical Experimentation," *Citation* 31.12 (October 1, 1975), 138; *Clay v. Martin,* 509 F.2d 109.

21. I am grateful to Jon M. Harkness for sharing a copy of this letter, obtained through Freedom of Information Act request no. 91-3171, with me. Unless otherwise noted, all letters quoted in this chapter came from this source.

22. The last three conditions first appeared in Morris and Mills 1974 (quoted in Harkness 2003, 319 n. 114).

23. Political and bureaucratic pressures converged on Carlson: his task force on medical research wanted to phase out ARC participation, and the ACA called for abandoning all such projects in a position statement issued by its board of directors on February 20, 1976. Thus the ACA terminated use of federal prisoners as research subjects before the National Commission for the Protection of Human Subjects decided what its approach would be.

24. In his March 2, 1976, letter to the deputy attorney general, Carlson described receiving "an irate call" from DuPont indicating "we had reneged on an earlier com-

mitment concerning phasing out of the project." Carlson wrote, "I firmly believe, however, that we should get out of the project as soon as possible." His March 1, 1976, letter to Kastenmeier explained that all other research on federal prisoners had already been phased out over the preceding five years. Carlson received inquiries—including one (dated January 4, 1974) from Senator Sam J. Ervin, Jr., chair of the powerful Committee on the Judiciary—about the scope of prison research and the nature of BOP policy.

25. The authorship of this report, which is dated December 19, 1972, is unclear. With the help of archivist Jeremy Nordmoe, it was located among the collected papers of Heinz Lehmann, in a folder titled "Lexington Talk," in the archives of the American College of Neuropsychopharmacology, Eskind Biomedical Research Library, Vanderbilt University, Nashville, Tennessee.

26. William R. Martin to Joseph V. Brady, September 3, 1975, Georgetown University, Kennedy Institute of Ethics, Papers of the National Commission for the Protection of Human Subjects, meeting 11, box 3. My thanks to Jon Harkness for sharing copies of these letters with me.

27. William R. Martin to Joseph V. Brady, December 5, 1975, Georgetown University, Kennedy Institute of Ethics, Papers of the National Commission for the Protection of Human Subjects, meeting 14, box 4.

28. E. Leong Way to Kenneth John Ryan, March 24, 1976, Georgetown University, Kennedy Institute of Ethics, Papers of the National Commission for the Protection of Human Subjects, meeting 17, box 7.

29. Leo Hollister to Philip Handler, President, National Academy of Sciences, April 9, 1976, National Academy of Sciences Archives, Record Group 78-016-1. "ALS: D.Med: CPDD: Chairman's letters (3) on Human Experimentation Transmitted by President, NAS, 1976," box 1.

30. Keith F. Killam, President, American College of Neuropsychopharmacology, to Kenneth John Ryan, March 26, 1976, Georgetown University, Kennedy Institute of Ethics, Papers of the National Commission for the Protection of Human Subjects, meeting 17, box 7.

31. Phase 1 testing at Jackson halted after twelve years; nearly thirty thousand participants were involved, only sixty-four of whom experienced a "medically significant event," mainly adverse drug reactions from which all recovered completely (Harkness 2003, 203–10).

32. *Henry Fante et al. v. Department of Health and Human Services et al.*, U.S. District Court, Eastern District of Michigan, Southern Division, Civil Action no. 80-72778. Records from this case, which I obtained through Jon Harkness, are housed at the Great Lakes Regional Archives in Chicago, accession no. 21-88-0016, location no. 331792-332283, box 269. FDA officials announced the indefinite stay, which remained in effect at the time this book went to press. See *Federal Register* 46 (July 7, 1981): 35085.

33. NARA was used as the vehicle for the criminalization of LSD (Hewitt 2002). See Isbell et al. 1956 for an example of what the Lexington group published about LSD in peer-reviewed scientific journals and the medical press. This research was not covert. See also the entry on Harris Isbell's Lilly Research Prize lecture, given on March 15, 1956, in Indianapolis and titled "Studies on the Diethylamide of Lysergic Acid: Development of Tolerance and Effects of Tranquilizing Drugs on the Reaction" (Annotated Bibliog-

raphy of Papers from the Addiction Research Center, 1935–75, DHEW no. [ADM] 77-435, 1978, 70).

34. The few relevant pages of this report were found in the files of Heinz Lehmann, a member of the National Advisory Council subcommittee, among his collected papers in the archives of the American College of Neuropsychopharmacology, Eskind Biomedical Research Library, Vanderbilt University, Nashville, Tennessee.

35. Materials considered by the task force included the NIDA ARC's annual report for the period July 1, 1974, to June 30, 1975, and Wikler 1972. A similar review of the clinical, pharmacological, physiological, and biochemical investigations was submitted in the same time frame by Martin.

36. The only prison industry for which ARC participants were eligible was the printing trades, and they could not earn meritorious compensation for both participating in studies and working in the print shop. A "Schedule for Meritorious Compensation" appeared as attachment 3 in the report of the National Commission for the Protection of Human Subjects (1976a). Compensation was set at five dollars per study day and could not exceed six study days per month for single-dose studies or forty dollars per month for chronic studies. "Routine jobs" were capped at twelve dollars per month. At the end of their stay at the ARC, patients received a fifty-dollar bonus for each year of participation but could not receive more than one hundred dollars. This schedule responded to former criticisms—made in the pre-NARA days—that the ARC environment was "seductive."

37. Information in this paragraph appears on the Web site of the Advisory Committee on Human Radiation Experiments, at http://www.hss.energy.gov/healthsafety/ohre/roadmap/achre/chap9_4.html. In 1971, DHEW produced an institutional guide to its policy on protection of human subjects, in an attempt to regularize federal policy on the use of human subjects.

38. This laboratory was involved in the visualization of opiate receptors, which catapulted neuropharmacology into public visibility in 1973. See Goldstein 1997.

39. Despite his pioneering animal models, Wikler never believed they could "furnish a complete inventory of the variables that determine human adaptation," although they served as "limited models of 'learning' that may apply to man as well" (1957, 225–26).

40. Petersen compiled a list of all extramural projects, which was published in July 1975 as the first two volumes of the NIDA Research Monograph series. *Findings of Drug Abuse Research, 1967–1974* illustrates both rapid expansion and lack of coordination in the addiction research enterprise, summarizing over thirty-five hundred studies supported by over ten federal agencies and conducted by 650 researchers. Neither volume acknowledged the existence of an intramural program.

41. Although the intramural program became a poor second cousin, working in it had its advantages for those whose approaches were not underwritten by the more publicly visible extramural program of this highly politicized field. Two examples of such approaches suffice: Tsung Ping Su's career-long research on kappa receptors, which did not appear to play a role in opiate addiction but may hold the key to understanding the action of amphetamines (Su 2003); and genetic research undertaken in George Uhl's laboratory shortly after NIMH's retraction of claims about the genetics of schizophrenia (Uhl 2003).

42. Bernard Barber, "Prepared Statement," in U.S. Cong. 1973.

43. Six experiments involving mixed viruses and mycoplasmas were done on humans in a Ramsey, Texas, prison unit between September 19, 1970, and June 2, 1974; two more were done in 1976; and recombinant DNA experiments took place from 1974 through 1979, when little was known about its effects (Tabenanika 2002). Similarly, infectious disease research at the Maryland House of Detention in Jessup, Maryland, indicated lack of respect for human life and dignity (Gilchrist 1974). Yet in August 1979, *Bailey et al. v. Lally,* the ACLU test case at Jessup, was concluded in favor of the University of Maryland researchers who were the defendants. The ruling held that prisoners could volunteer even in generally poor prison conditions. The scientists had already withdrawn from the prison in January 1976, before the trial got under way and long before the ruling on their behalf. Finally, the Jackson program, although ethical, involved direct contact between commercial interests, researchers, and subjects, with few layers of oversight. It shut down in 1989; the stigma of prison research rendered its continuance impractical.

CHAPTER 7

1. Those who follow scientists at work speak of "epistemic cultures" (Knorr-Cetina 2001) or "epistemic communities," defined by Haas as professional networks whose members share "recognized expertise and competence in a particular domain and an authoritative claim to policy-relevant knowledge within that domain or issue-area" (1992, 3). Although members of an epistemic community hail from a variety of disciplines, they share a consistent set of normative principles and beliefs that provide the rationale for their activities, a set of causal beliefs derived from how they go about analyzing problems central to their domain, and a basis for linking their findings to policy. They also share ideas about how to validate knowledge in their expert domain. Finally, they see themselves as engaged in a common research and policy enterprise to enhance human welfare. The social worlds (or arena analysis) approach points to the translation of shared beliefs and commitments into practice (Clarke 1998, 2000, 2005).

2. Behavioral pharmacologists I interviewed include Robert Balster, George Bigelow, Thomas Crowley, Roland Griffiths, Chris-Ellyn Johanson, Charles R. (Bob) Schuster, and James (Jim) Woods. The present chapter is based on their interviews and publications, visits to their laboratories, and a literature review that included all extant internal histories of behavioral pharmacology. The generosity of these scientists was tangible, and I hope that this account does justice to the complexity of their views, practices, and politics.

3. This statement, made in the course of my 2005 interview with Becker, captures the spirit of the behavioral pharmacology enterprise, despite Becker himself being a critic of behaviorism (as was his mentor, Herbert Blumer). See Plummer 2003.

4. Publications of interest include Dews 1955, 1958; Morse 1955; Ferster and Skinner 1957.

5. CPZ is a major tranquilizer marketed in the United States by Smith Kline and French Laboratories under the trade name Thorazine. See Brady's foreword to Thompson and Schuster 1968; Dews 1985, 3–5.

6. CPZ was synthesized in the attempt to find an antihistamine to better manage stress. Invented in the 1920s by David Macht, the "rope-climbing test" was the pharmaceutical industry's first screening technique using animals. CPZ rendered rats "indifferent" to food rewards; they refused to climb a rope even to escape aversive shock. The drug was included in medical kits to manage "battlefield stress" in Korea (Healy 2002, 82).

7. The formalization of behavioral pharmacology included the First International Conference of Neuropsychopharmacology, held in Rome in 1958, and the formation of the Behavioral Pharmacology Society in 1957.

8. Thompson and Schuster cite a decrease in LD-50 (lethal dose for half of the subjects) when animals are on amphetamines and subjected to stress or crowding (Weiss, Laties, and Blanton 1961).

9. For a similar attempt to map such a convergent interdisciplinary domain configured around mutagenesis, see Frickel 2004.

10. Actively working on a "two-factor learning theory" of relapse, Abraham Wikler cited presentations on animal self-administration by Weeks, Schuster, and Thompson at the 1963 CDAN meeting in Ann Arbor, Michigan. Wikler's first factor was "temporal contiguity" between onset of abstinence and specific environments; his second was a version of hustling called the "reinforcement of instrumental activity" or "morphine acquisitory behavior" (Wikler 1965, 89). Wikler saw the new behaviorist vocabulary as a route to operationalize "mentalistic" concepts or such cultural activities as hustling.

11. Red Rodney was known as a "musician's musician." He was a long-term heroin addict who made several trips to Lexington.

12. On associations between heroin and jazz, see Davis 2003; Jonnes 1996.

13. This meeting was held in 1963, prior to when the NRC committee changed its name to the Committee on Problems of Drug Dependence in 1965.

14. A lifelong cigar smoker, Seevers knew something about the strength of desire and underwent a notable conversion in the late 1960s when he was appointed to chair the American Medical Association's Committee on Tobacco and Health. He prohibited smoking in the department, ended sale of tobacco products in the University of Michigan hospital, and encouraged Schuster and Lucchesi to study the effects of intravenous nicotine on human subjects (healthy adult volunteers of both genders). The study attracted the interest of Jerome H. Jaffe, serving as the basis for Schuster's subsequent move to Chicago.

15. Tomoji Yanagita, the Japanese scientist responsible for the technical innovation of the backpack apparatus necessary for behavioral study of monkeys, concurred with this statement in an interview that Schuster conducted with him.

16. Douglas Candland contrasted the physical sciences, where the goal is to eliminate variance because it confounds predictive accuracy, to the behavioral sciences, where the goal is to accept and measure variance as a descriptive technique. "Measures of variance," he argued, "can be just as reliable as formulas that strive to eliminate or reduce variance" (1993, 357), yet popular conceptions of the physical sciences as reliable or rigorous remain deeply interred in the distinction between the "hard" and the "soft."

17. Analysis of specific sites, or receptors, in the brain where drugs exert rewarding and reinforcing effects did not become technically feasible until after behavioral tech-

niques and procedures were developed and validated (Cozzens 1989; Pert 1997; Snyder 1989).

CHAPTER 8

1. By joint resolution in 1989, the Decade of the Brain (1990–2000) was designated by the U.S. Senate and House of Representatives and a presidential proclamation by George Bush, Sr., in July 1990 (Jones and Mendell 1999).

2. Evelyn Fox Keller describes sociotechnical "borrowings" between physics and molecular biology that are not unlike how substance abuse research has incorporated neuroscience and genetics: "I want to argue that physics and physicists provided a resource of far greater import for the success of molecular biology than any particular skills; namely, they provided social authority. That authority was, of course, acquired in the first place through the formidable displays of technological and instrumental power issuing from physics itself, but this initially technical authority soon became available for deployment far beyond the domain of their technical triumphs; it became, in short, an authority that could be called upon for the essentially social process of reframing the character and goals of biological science. This borrowing proceeded in a variety of ways—first, through the borrowing of an agenda that was seen as looking like the agenda of physics; second, by borrowing the language and attitude of physicists; and finally, by borrowing the very names of physicists" (1992, 98).

3. I thank Kathryn Keller for bringing to my attention the special issue of *Science* with Bloom's article.

4. The field of science and technology studies offers a vast literature on eugenics and genetic determinism (e.g., Duster 2003; Gould 1981; Kevles 1985; Rafter 1997; Roberts 1997; Stepan 1982).

5. The extent to which it is accurate or legitimate to refer to cycles of drug use as "epidemics" is debatable. The importation of epidemiological discourse into the drug field was furthered by Hughes and Jaffe 1971 and Hughes et al. 1972. Courtwright (1982/2001) is an example of a drug policy historian who makes great use of epidemiological mapping.

6. The 1990 OTA report claimed, "That drug abuse is a chronic relapsing condition and that drug abusers are a heterogeneous population with other social and behavioral problems pose obstacles to effective treatment" (1). The OTA report repeated the phrase "chronic relapsing disorder" without citing its origins or examining its meaning, while castigating thirty years of federally funded addiction research for failing to produce "studies that attempt to conform more closely to research principles" (10). Suggesting that the lack of rigor and unsophisticated, anecdotal, and uncontrolled studies were endemic to the field, the OTA advised new studies designed to "dissect" treatment programs so as to determine which components were effective for which "client groups." The report advanced targeted study and individually tailored treatment as the solution: "Ultimately, research on drug abuse treatment should lead to what has been a common practice in medicine, namely a case management approach with an individual tailored plan to maximize the likelihood of treatment effectiveness" (10). The OTA report cited NIDA favorably for embarking on randomized, controlled trials. Although this damn-

ing assessment was hardly recognizable by those within the field, it galvanized the turn toward neuroscience.

7. Campbell 2000 provides a detailed critique of biological determinism in drug policy discourse. For instance, the CRBD could be used to cast punishment as ineffective, inhumane, or nonscientific. By contrast, it could be used to justify congregate care or orphanages for the children of addicts or to write off continued allocation of public resources toward treatment and research.

8. These claims are made within specific structural and social contexts that have professionalized the frontline treatment workforce (Payne, Schreiber, and Riley 2004). Although anecdotal accounts circulate about resistance to science and evidence-based thinking among addiction treatment professionals, my ethnographic observations have led me to believe that there has been a sea change. Many treatment providers regularly appeal to such scientific constructs as the CRBD, tout neuroscience as the path to enlightenment, and cite science as a "tool" for dealing with difficult people and complex problems.

9. This can be best glimpsed through a comparison to the form that neuroscience has taken elsewhere (Xie 1999).

10. Ehrlich's earliest reference occurred within a 1913 speech before the general session of the Seventeenth International Congress of Medicine in London; subsequent references can be found in the first volume of his collected papers (1956).

11. On previous preoccupations with unveiling the "deep femininity" lodged in the brain, see Ludamilla Jordanova 1989, 56–58. In "Nature Unveiling Herself before Science," Jordanova discusses the "physiognomic mentality" that encouraged the move from "visual signifiers to other, invisible, inner signifieds" (1989, 92). She writes: "The process of looking is central to the acquisition of valid knowledge of nature. From classical times, science and medicine have been explicitly concerned with the correct interpretation of visual signs, and skill in those fields was pre-eminently seen as a form of visual acuteness" (1989, 91). Carolyn Merchant refers to the figure of *Nature Revealing Herself to Science,* a statue by French sculptor Louis-Ernest Barrias that Merchant says "suggests the sexuality of nature in revealing her secrets to science" (1980, 190).

12. The quotation echoes Francis Bacon's "Enough if, on our approaching her with due respect, she condescends to show herself" (quoted in Keller 1992, 57). Merchant (1980) and Keller (1985, 1992) have shown that courtship metaphors are gentle versions of the scientific assault on feminized nature.

13. Lecturing at Stanford University in the late 1960s, Vincent Dole motivated molecular pharmacologist Avram Goldstein to take up opiate biochemistry. Dole and Nyswander hypothesized that addiction was a metabolic disease in which genetics played some role (1967, 19–24). Goldstein (1976) postulated existence of an endogenous reward system.

14. The clinically effective dosage is believed to be the dose that occupies a certain fraction of receptors for that class of drugs.

15. Information on Charles P. O'Brien comes from O'Brien 1998 and 2005.

16. My thanks to Graham Florry for sending me this paper along with similar retrospective accounts by Harris Isbell and Maurice H. Seevers.

17. Information on fMRI is taken from Savoy 2001. I would like to thank Rachel Dowty, Colin Beech, and Sal Restivo for illuminating conversations on fMRI.

18. Information can be found at http://www.uphs.upenn.edu/trc/conditioning/studies.html. I also relied on a segment of the Bill Moyers special "The Hijacked Brain," which involved Childress explaining her research, as well as on Childress 2006.

19. Record Group 511 ADAMHA Alcohol, Drug Abuse, and Mental Health, Administrative Office, Clinical Research Center, Lexington, KY, Public Relations, 1939–1973, folder 2, 2. Jurgensen presented this paper on August 30, 1966, in Baltimore, Maryland. He was departing Lexington to head the narcotics farm in Fort Worth, Texas.

CONCLUSION

1. Chartered in 1970 as a component of the National Academy of Sciences, the IOM is a nonprofit science advisory board and honorific membership organization that provides science-based advice to government agencies by relying on unpaid, volunteer experts.

2. NIDA was subsumed into NIH in 1992, leaving the public service aspects of treatment and prevention in the Department of Health and Human Services division of the Substance Abuse and Mental Health Services Administration (SAMHSA). SAMHSA created the Center for Substance Abuse Treatment (CSAT) to expand access and enhance quality of treatment services and established the Center for Substance Abuse Prevention for the purpose of technology transfer of prevention materials to treatment providers.

3. The concept behind the Practice Research Network is a social innovation used in many fields, including social work, psychiatry, and medicine. I conducted an institutional ethnography within a statewide PRN initiative that was part of CSAT's 1999–2003 Practice Research Collaborative grant program. Primary investigators were John Coppolla, executive director of the Alcoholism and Substance Abuse Providers Association, and Frank McCorry of the New York State Office of Alcoholism and Substance Abuse Services. My position as a participant-observer from fall 2001 through fall 2005 offered a fascinating vantage on how the social machinery of credibility of substance abuse research operates in the field of clinical practice. I thank everyone involved for their generosity in allowing me both to observe and participate.

Selected Bibliography

Acker, Caroline. "Addiction and the Laboratory: The Work of the National Research Council's Committee on Drug Addiction, 1928–1939." *Isis* 86 (1995): 167–93.

Acker, Caroline. "Planning and Serendipity in the Search for a Nonaddicting Opiate Analgesic." In *The Inside Story of Medicines,* ed. Gregory J. Higby and Elaine C. Stroud (Madison, WI: American Institute for the History of Pharmacy, 1997): 139–59.

Acker, Caroline. *Creating the American Junkie: Addiction Research in the Classic Era of Narcotics Control.* Baltimore: Johns Hopkins University Press, 2002.

Adams, Aileen, and Geoffrey Cowan. "The Human Guinea Pig: How We Test New Drugs." *World,* December 5, 1971, 20.

Addiction Research Center. *Annotated Bibliography of Papers from the Addiction Research Center, 1935–1975.* ADM 77-435. Rockville, MD: U.S. Department of Health, Education, and Welfare, 1978.

Advisory Committee on Human Radiation Experiments. *Final Report.* Washington, DC: U.S. Government Printing Office, 1995.

Algren, Nelson. *The Man with the Golden Arm.* New York: Pocket Books, 1951.

Anderson, O. D., and R. Parmenter. "A Long-term Study of Experimental Neurosis in the Sheep and Dog." *Psychosomatic Medicine,* Monograph Suppl. 2 (1941).

Andrews, Howard L., and Clifton K. Himmelsbach. "Relation of the Intensity of the Morphine Abstinence Syndrome to Dosage." *Journal of Pharmacology and Experimental Therapeutics* 81.3 (1944): 288.

Anonymous. Interview by Gwendolyn Hall. Oral History of Methadone Collection. Bentley Historical Library. University of Michigan, Ann Arbor, 1970.

Anslinger, Harry J., and William F. Tompkins. *The Traffic in Narcotics.* New York: Funk and Wagnalls, 1953.

Ariens, E. J., ed. *Molecular Pharmacology: The Mode of Action of Biologically Active Compounds.* New York: Academic Press, 1964.

Bakalar, David. "In Medicine, Acceptable Risk Is in the Eye of the Beholder." *New York Times,* June 20, 2006.

Bakan, David. "Behaviorism and American Urbanization." *Journal of the History of the Behavioral Sciences* 11.1 (1966): 5–28.

Ball, John. "Addiction Scientists from the USA." In *Addiction: Evolution of a Specialist Field,* ed. Griffith Edwards, 29–38. Malden, MA: Blackwell Science, 2002.

Balster, Robert L. Interview by the author. San Juan, PR, June 2004.

Balster, Robert L. and George E. Bigelow. "Guidelines and Methodological Reviews Concerning Drug Abuse Liability Assessment." *Drug and Alcohol Dependence* 90 (2003): S13–S40.

Barber, Bernard, John Lally, Julia Loughlin Makarushka, and Daniel Sullivan. *Research on Human Subjects: Problems of Social Control in Medical Experimentation.* New Brunswick, NJ: Transaction, 1979.

Barchas, Jack D., Philip A. Berger, Roland D. Ciaranello, and Glen R. Elliott, eds. *Psychopharmacology: From Theory to Practice.* New York: Oxford University Press, 1977.

Bass, Allan D. "Growth." In *The American Society for Pharmacology and Experimental Therapeutics: The First Sixty Years,* ed. K. K. Chen, 155–74. Washington, DC: Judd and Detweiler, 1969.

Becker, Howard S. *The Outsiders: Studies in the Sociology of Deviance.* New York: Free Press, 1963.

Becker, Howard S. "Les drogues: Que sont-elles?" [Drugs: What Are They?]. In *Qu'est-ce qu'une drogue?* ed. Howard S. Becker, 11–20. Anglet: Atlantica, 2001.

Becker, Howard S. Interview by the author. Telephone, January 2005.

Beecher, Henry K. *Experimentation in Man.* Springfield, IL: Charles C. Thomas, 1959a.

Beecher, Henry K. *Measurement of Subjective Responses: Quantitative Effects of Drugs.* New York: Oxford University Press, 1959b.

Beecher, Henry K. "Ethics and Clinical Research." *New England Journal of Medicine* 74 (1966): 1354–60.

Beecher, Henry K., *Research and the Individual.* Boston: Little, Brown, 1970.

Beecher, Henry K., Arthur S. Keats, Frederick Mosteller, and Louis Lasagna. "The Effectiveness of Oral Analgesics (Morphine, Codeine, Acetylsalicylic Acid) and the Problem of Placebo 'Reactors' and 'Non-reactors.'" *Journal of Pharmacology and Experimental Therapeutics* 109 (1953): 393–400.

Beecher, Henry K., and D. P. Todd. "Study of the Deaths Associated with Anesthesia and Surgery." *Annals of Surgery* 140 (1954): 2–34.

Benedict, John. "Mind Control: The Ultimate Tyranny." *American Mercury* 90.435 (1960): 12–27.

Bernard, Claude. Experimental Studies on Opium and Its Alkaloids. *C. r. Acad. Sci.* 59 (1864): 406–15.

Berridge, Virginia. "Digitizing and Democratizing Historical Research." *Addiction* 101 (2006): 1533–35.

Bigelow, George. "Human Drug Abuse Liability Assessment: Opioids and Analgesics." *British Journal of Addiction* 86 (1991): 1615–28.

Bigelow, George. Interview by the author. Orlando, FL, June 2005.

Bigelow, George, and Roland Griffiths. "An Experimental Approach to Treating Chronic Alcoholism: A Case Study and One-Year Follow-up." *Behaviour Research and Therapy* 11 (1973): 321–25.

Blank, Robert H. *Brain Policy: How the New Neuroscience Will Change Our Lives and Our Politics.* Washington, DC: Georgetown University Press, 1999.

Bloom, Floyd E. "The Science of Substance Abuse." *Science* 278 (October 3, 1997): 15.

Blum, Deborah. *The Monkey Wars.* Oxford: Oxford University Press, 1994.

Blum, Deborah. *Love at Goon Park: Harry Harlow and the Science of Affection.* Cambridge, MA: Perseus, 2002.

Boyd, Graham. "The Drug War Is the New Jim Crow." *NACLA Report on the Americas* 35.1 (July–August 2001): 18–22.

Brady, Joseph V. *History of Behavioral Pharmacology.* Kalamazoo, MI: Association for Behavior Analysis, 2004.

Brandt, Allan M. *No Magic Bullet: A Social History of Venereal Disease in the United States since 1880.* New York: Oxford University Press, 1985.

Braslow, Joel. *Mental Ills and Bodily Cures: Psychiatric Treatment in the First Half of the Twentieth Century.* Berkeley: University of California Press, 1997.

Bridgman, Percy W. *The Logic of Modern Physics.* New York: Macmillan, 1928.

Brieter, Hans C., Randy L. Gollub, R. M. Weisskoff, David N. Kennedy, Nicos Makris, J. D. Berke, J. M. Goodman, H. L. Kantor, David R. Gastfriend, J. P. Riordan, R. T. Mathew, Bruce R. Rosen, and Steven E. Hyman. "Acute Effects of Cocaine on Human Brain Activity and Emotion." *Neuron* 19.9 (1997): 591–611.

Briggs, Laura. *Reproducing Empire: Race, Sex, Science, and U.S. Imperialism in Puerto Rico.* Berkeley: University of California Press, 2002.

Bunk, Steve. "NIDA Boss Touts Addiction Studies." *Scientist* 12.3 (February 1998): 1.

Butler, Judith. *The Psychic Life of Power: Theories in Subjection.* Stanford, CA: Stanford University Press, 1997.

Caldwell, Anne E. *Origins of Psychopharmacology: From CPZ to LSD.* Springfield, IL: Charles C. Thomas, 1970.

Callahan, Daniel. *What Price Better Health? Hazards of the Research Imperative.* Berkeley: University of California Press, 2003.

Campbell, Nancy D. "Cold War Compulsions: U.S. Drug Science, Policy, and Culture." PhD diss., University of California, Santa Cruz, 1995.

Campbell, Nancy D. *Using Women: Gender, Drug Policy, and Social Justice.* New York: Routledge, 2000.

Candland, Douglas K. *Feral Children and Clever Animals.* Oxford: Oxford University Press, 1993.

Canguilhem, Georges. *The Normal and the Pathological.* Trans. Carolyn R. Fawcett. New York: Zone Books, 1991.

Castel, Robert, Francoise Castel, and Anne Lovell. *The Psychiatric Society.* Trans. Arthur Goldhammer. New York: Columbia University Press, 1982.

Chein, Isidor. In *Narcotic Drug Addiction Problems,* ed. Robert B. Livingston, 146–58. Bethesda, MD: U.S. Department of Health, Education, and Welfare and National Institute of Mental Health, 1958.

Chen, K. K., ed. *The American Society for Pharmacology and Experimental Therapeutics: The First Sixty Years.* Washington, DC: Judd and Detweiler, 1969.

Chessick, Robert D. "The 'Pharmacogenic Orgasm' in the Drug Addict." *Archives of General Psychiatry* 3 (1960): 117–28.

Chestang, Earl. Interview by Gwendolyn Hall. 1970. Oral History of Methadone Collection, Bentley Historical Library, University of Michigan, Ann Arbor.

Childress, Anna Rose. Interview by the author. Phoenix, AZ, June 2006.

Cicero, Theodore. Interview by the author. Phoenix, AZ, June 2006.

Claridge, Gordon. *Drugs and Human Behavior.* New York: Praeger, 1970.

Clark, William G., and Joseph del Guidice. *Principles of Psychopharmacology.* 2nd ed. New York: Academic Press, 1978.

Clarke, Adele E. *Disciplining Reproduction: Modernity, American Life Sciences, and the Problem of Sex.* Berkeley: University of California Press, 1998.

Clarke, Adele E. "Maverick Reproductive Scientists and the Production of Contraceptives, 1915–2000+." In *Bodies of Technology,* ed. Anna Saetman, Nellie Oudshoorn, and M. Kirejczyk, 37–89. Columbus: Ohio State University Press, 2000.

Clarke, Adele E. *Situational Analysis: Grounded Theory after the Postmodern Turn.* Thousand Oaks, CA: Sage, 2005.

Clarke, Adele E., and Theresa Montini. "The Many Faces of RU-486: Tales of Situated Knowledges and Technological Contestations." *Science, Technology, and Human Values* 18.1 (Winter 1993): 42–78.

Cohn, Victor. "Prisoner Test Ban Opposed." *Washington Post,* March 14, 1976.

Cole, Jonathan O. "The ECDEU Program: A View from Both Sides of the Table." *Psychopharmacology Bulletin* 6 (1970): 74–81.

Committee on Drug Addiction and Narcotics. "Minutes of the Sixth Meeting." Washington, DC, March 1950.

Committee on Drug Addiction and Narcotics. "Minutes of the Eleventh Meeting." Lexington, KY, January 1953.

Committee on Drug Addiction and Narcotics. "Minutes of the Thirteenth Meeting." Rathway, NJ, Nutley, NJ, and New York, January 1954a.

Committee on Drug Addiction and Narcotics. "Minutes of the Fourteenth Meeting." Rensselaer, NY, October 1954b.

Committee on Drug Addiction and Narcotics. "Minutes of the Fifteenth Meeting." Lexington, KY, January 1955.

Committee on Public Health Relations. *Drug Addiction among Adolescents.* New York: New York Academy of Medicine and Josiah Macy, Jr. Foundation, 1952.

Conhurst, William F. "A 'New Deal' for the Drug Addict." *Baltimore Sun,* July 14, 1935.

Cook, Len. Interview by Steve Fowler. Division 28 Oral History Project, American Psychological Association, Washington, DC. 1991.

Cooke, Robert A., Arnold S. Tannenbaum, and Bradford Gray. *A Survey of Institutional Review Boards and Research Involving Human Subjects.* Ann Arbor, MI: Survey Research Center, 1977.

Courtwright, David C. *Dark Paradise: A History of Opiate Addiction in America.* Cambridge, MA: Harvard University Press, 1982/2001.

Courtwright, David C., Herman Joseph, and Don Des Jarlais. *Addicts Who Survived: An Oral History of Narcotic Use in America, 1923–1965.* Knoxville: University of Tennessee Press, 1989.

Cozzens, Susan E. *Social Control and Multiple Discovery in Science: The Opiate Receptor Case.* Albany: State University of New York Press, 1989.

Crease, Robert P. "Fallout: Issues in the Study, Treatment, and Reparations of Exposed Marshall Islanders." In *Science and Other Cultures,* ed. Robert Figueroa and Sandra Harding, 106–25. New York: Routledge, 2003.

Crowley, Thomas. Interview by the author. Orlando, FL, June 2005.

Davies, John Booth. *The Myth of Addiction: An Application of the Psychological Theory of Attribution to Illicit Drug Use.* Philadelphia, PA: Harwood Academic Publishers, 1992.

Davis, Richard. "Thoughts on Jazz Musicians and Dope Addiction." In *Of Human Bondage: Historical Perspectives on Addiction,* ed. Douglas L. Patey, 135–42. Smith College Studies in History 52. Northampton, MA: Smith College, 2003.

DeGrandpre, Richard. *The Cult of Pharmacology: How America Became the World's Most Troubled Drug Culture.* Durham, NC: Duke University Press, 2006.

De Jongh, D. K. "Some Introductory Remarks on the Conception of Receptors." In *Molecular Pharmacology: The Mode of Action of Biologically Active Compounds,* ed. E. J. Ariens, 1: xi–xviii. New York: Academic Press, 1964.

Deneau, Gerry A. "The Monkey Colony in Studies of Tolerance and Dependence." *University of Michigan Medical Center Journal* 36.4 (October–December 1970): 212–15.

Denton, Jane E., and Henry K. Beecher. "New Analgesics." "Methods in the Clinical Evaluation of New Analgesics, Part 1." *Journal of the American Medical Association* 141 (1949a): 1051–57.

Denton, Jane E., and Henry K. Beecher. "New Analgesics." "A Clinical Appraisal of the Narcotic Power of Methadone and Its Isomers, Part 2." *Journal of the American Medical Association* 141 (1949b): 1146–48.

Denton, Jane E., and Henry K. Beecher. "New Analgesics." "A Comparison of the Side Effects of Morphine, Methadone, and Methadone's Isomers in Man, Part 3." *Journal of the American Medical Association* 141 (1949c): 1148–53.

Department of Health, Education, and Welfare. "Report of the President's Biomedical Research Panel." (05) 76–500. Washington, DC: U.S. Department of Health, Education, and Welfare, 1976.

De Ropp, Robert S. *Drugs and the Mind.* New York: Grove, 1957.

Dewey, William. Interview by the author. Orlando, FL, June 2005.

Dews, Peter B. "Studies on Behavior." Part 1, "Differential Sensitivity to Pentobarbital of Pecking Performance in Pigeons Depending on the Schedule of Reward." *Journal of Pharmacology and Experimental Therapeutics* 115.4 (1955): 393–401.

Dews, Peter B. "Stimulant Actions of Methamphetamine." *Journal of Pharmacology and Experimental Therapeutics* 122.1 (1958): 137–47.

Dews, Peter B. Introduction to *Behavioral Pharmacology: The Current Status,* ed. Lewis S. Seiden and Robert L. Balster. New York: Alan R. Liss, 1985.

Dews, Peter B., and Travis Thompson, eds. *Advances in Behavioral Pharmacology.* Vol. 1. New York: Academic Press, 1977.

Dillon, George. *Contending Rhetorics: Writing in the Academic Disciplines.* Bloomington: Indiana University Press, 1991.

Dole, Vincent. "Biochemistry of Addiction." *Annual Review of Biochemistry* 39 (1970): 821–40.

Dole, Vincent, and Marie Nyswander. "Heroin Addiction: A Metabolic Disease." *Archives of Internal Medicine* 120 (1967): 19–24.

Domino, Edward F. Interview by Chris Gillan. 1995. Archives of the American College of Neuropsychopharmacology, Vanderbilt University, Nashville, TN.

Domino, Edward F. *Sixty-one Years of University of Michigan Pharmacology.* Ann Arbor, MI: NPP Books, 2004.

DuMez, A. G. "Increased Tolerance and Withdrawal Phenomena in Chronic Morphinism." *Journal of the American Medical Association* 72 (1919): 1069.

DuMez, A. G., and Lawrence Kolb. "Absence of Transferable Immunizing Substances in the Blood of Morphine and Heroin Addicts." *Public Health Reports* 40 (1925): 548–59.

DuMez, A. G., and Lawrence Kolb. "Experimental Addiction of Animals to Opiates." *Public Health Reports* 46 (1931): 698.

Dumit, Joseph. *Picturing Personhood: Brain Scans and Biomedical Identity.* Princeton, NJ: Princeton University Press, 2003.

DuPont, Robert L. *The Selfish Brain: Learning from Addiction.* Washington, DC: American Psychiatric Press, 1997.

DuPont, Robert. "The Addiction Research Center: The Second Forty Years." In *Drug Addiction and the U.S. Public Health Service,* ed. William R. Martin and Harris Isbell, 260–66. Rockville, MD: U.S. Department of Health, Education, and Welfare, 1978.

Duster, Troy. *Backdoor to Eugenics.* 2nd ed. New York: Routledge, 2003.

Dynes, J. B., and J. L. Poppen. "Lobotomy for Intractable Pain." *Journal of the American Medical Association* 140 (May 7, 1959): 15–19.

Eddy, Nathan B. *The National Research Council Involvement in the Opiate Problem, 1928–1971.* Washington, DC: National Academies Press, 1973.

Eddy, Nathan B., H. Halbach, Harris Isbell, and Maurice Seevers. "Drug Dependence: Its Significance and Characteristics." *Bulletin of the World Health Organization* 32 (1965): 721–33.

Edwards, Griffith, ed. *Addictions: Personal Influences and Scientific Movements.* New Brunswick, NJ: Transaction, 1991.

Edwards, Griffith, ed. *Addiction: Evolution of a Specialist Field.* Malden, MA: Blackwell Science, 2002.

Efron, Daniel H., Bo Holmstedt, and Nathan S. Kline, eds. *Ethnopharmacological Search for Psychoactive Drugs.* Bethesda, MD: U.S. Department of Health, Education, and Welfare, 1967.

Ehrlich, Paul. *The Collected Papers of Paul Ehrlich.* Ed. F. Himmelwait. London: Pergamon Press, 1956.

Epstein, Steven. *Impure Science.* Berkeley: University of California Press, 1996.

Felix, Robert H. "Comments on the Psychopathology of Drug Addiction." *Mental Hygiene* 23 (1939): 567–82.

Felix, Robert H. "An Appraisal of the Personality Types of the Addict." *American Journal of Psychiatry* 100 (1944): 462–67.

Felix, Robert H. Interview by Milton J. E. Senn. March 8, 1979. Child Guidance Series, Senn Oral History Collection, National Library of Medicine, Bethesda, MD.

Ferster, Charles, and B. F. Skinner. *Schedules of Reinforcement.* New York: Appleton-Century-Crofts, 1957.

Figueroa, Robert, and Sandra Harding, eds. *Science and Other Cultures.* New York: Routledge, 2003.

Fisher, Jill. "Pharmaceutical Paternalism and the Privatization of Clinical Trials." PhD diss., Rensselaer Polytechnic Institute, 2005.

Fleck, Ludwik. *Genesis and Development of a Scientific Fact.* Ed. Thaddeus J. Trenn and

Robert K. Merton. Trans. Fred Bradley and Thaddeus J. Trenn. Chicago: University of Chicago Press, 1979.

Flowers, Eddie. Interview by J. P. Olsen and Luke Walden. Alexandria, VA, 2004.

Forbes, David. *False Fixes: The Cultural Politics of Drugs, Alcohol, and Addictive Relations.* Albany: State University of New York Press, 1994.

Fort, Joel P. "Heroin Addiction among Young Men." *Psychiatry* 17.3 (1954): 251–60.

Fort, Joel P. "Public Health Pioneer, Criminologist, Reformer, Ethicist and Humanitarian." Interview by Caroline C. Crawford, Berkeley, CA, 1991, 1992, and 1993. Regional Oral History Office, The Bancroft Library, University of California, Berkeley, 1997.

Foucault, Michel. *The Birth of the Clinic: An Archaeology of Medical Perception.* Trans. A. M. Sheridan Smith. New York: Vintage Books, 1975.

Foucault, Michel. *Discipline and Punish: The Birth of the Prison.* Trans. Alan Sheridan. New York: Vintage Books, 1979.

Fox, Renee C. *Experiment Perilous: Physicians and Patients Facing the Unknown.* Glencoe, IL: Free Press, 1959/1998.

Fraser, H. Franklin, and J. A. Grinder, Jr. "Treatment of Drug Addiction." *American Journal of Medicine* 14 (1953): 571–77.

Fraser, H. Franklin, Abraham Wikler, Anna J. Eisenman, and Harris Isbell. "Use of N-allylnormorphine in Treatment of Methadone Poisoning in Man: Report of Two Cases." *Journal of the American Medical Association* 148 (1952): 1205–7.

Fraser, Nancy, and Linda Gordon. "A Genealogy of 'Dependency': Tracing a Keyword of the U.S. Welfare State." *Signs* 19.2 (1994): 309–36.

Freud, Sigmund. *Beyond the Pleasure Principle.* Trans. James Strachey. New York: W. W. Norton, 1961.

Freud, Sigmund. *Three Essays on the Theory of Sexuality.* Trans. James Strachey. New York: Basic Books, 1975.

Frickel, Scott. *Chemical Consequences: Environmental Mutagens, Scientist Activism, and the Rise of Genetic Toxicology.* New Brunswick, NJ: Rutgers University Press, 2004.

Fujimura, Joan H. *Crafting Science: A Sociohistory of the Quest for the Genetics of Cancer.* Cambridge, MA: Harvard University Press, 1996.

Gerard, Ralph W. "Drugs for the Soul: The Rise of Psychopharmacology." *Science* 125 (August 2, 1957): 201–3.

Gilbert, Nigel. "The Transformation of Research Findings into Scientific Knowledge." *Social Studies of Science* 6 (1976): 281–306.

Gilbert, Nigel, and Michael Mulkay. *Opening Pandora's Box: A Sociologists' Analysis of Scientists' Discourse.* Cambridge: Cambridge University Press, 1984/2003.

Gilchrist, Irving. *Medical Experimentation on Prisoners Must Stop: Documents Generated during the Course of a Struggle.* College Park, MD: Urban Information Interpreters, 1974.

Glick, Stanley D., and Joseph Goldfarb, eds. *Behavioral Pharmacology.* St. Louis, MO: C. V. Mosby, 1976.

Goffman, Erving. *Stigma: Notes on the Management of Spoiled Identity.* Englewood Cliffs, NJ: Prentice Hall, 1963.

Goffman, Erving. *Asylums: Essays on the Social Situation of Mental Patients and Other Inmates.* New York: Anchor Books, 1981.

Goldberg, Steven R. "The Behavioral Analysis of Drug Addiction." In *Behavioral Pharmacology,* ed. Stanley D. Glick and Joseph Goldfarb, 283–316. St. Louis, MO: C. V. Mosby, 1976.

Goldstein, Avram. "Opioid Peptides (Endorphins) in Pituitary and Brain." *Science* 193 (December 3, 1976): 1081–86.

Goldstein, Avram. "A Rewarding Research Pathway." *Annual Review of Pharmacology and Toxicology* 37 (1997): 1–28.

Goliszek, Andrew. *In the Name of Science: A History of Secret Programs, Medical Research, and Human Experimentation.* New York: St. Martin's Press, 2003.

Goodman, Jordan, Anthony McElligott, and Lara Marks, eds. *Useful Bodies: Humans in the Service of Medical Science in the Twentieth Century.* Baltimore: Johns Hopkins University Press, 2003.

Goozner, Merrill. *The $800 Million Pill: The Truth behind the Cost of New Drugs.* Berkeley: University of California Press, 2004.

Gorodetzky, Charles. Interview by the author. Kansas City, MO, July 2003.

Gould, Stephen Jay. *Mismeasure of Man.* New York: W. W. Norton, 1981.

Greenacre, Phyllis. "Psychoanalysis and the Cycles of Life." *Bulletin of the New York Academy of Medicine* 29.10 (1953): 796.

Greenshaw, Andrew J., and Colin T. Dourish, eds. *Experimental Psychopharmacology.* Clifton, NJ: Humana, 1987.

Griffiths, Roland. Interview by the author. Orlando, FL, June 2005.

Grinker, Roy S., Sr. *Fifty Years of Psychiatry: A Living History.* Springfield, IL: Charles C. Thomas, 1979.

Grob, Gerald N. *From Asylum to Community: Mental Health Policy in Modern America.* Princeton, NJ: Princeton University Press, 1991.

Haas, Peter. "Epistemic Communities and International Policy Coordination." *International Organizations* 46.1 (Winter 1992): 1–35.

Hall, Gwendolyn. Interview of anonymous patient. 1970. Oral History of Methadone Collection. Bentley Historical Library, University of Michigan, Ann Arbor.

Halpern, Sydney A. *Lesser Harms: The Morality of Risk in Medical Research.* Chicago: University of Chicago Press, 2004.

Hamilton, F. E., and G. J. Haynes. "Prefrontal Lobotomy in the Management of Intractable Pain." *Archives of Surgery* 58 (June 1949): 731.

Haraway, Donna J. *Crystals, Fabrics, and Fields: Metaphors of Organicism in Twentieth-Century Developmental Biology.* New Haven, CT: Yale University Press, 1976.

Haraway, Donna J. "Situated Knowledges: The Science Question in Feminism as a Site of Discourse on the Privilege of Partial Perspective." *Feminist Studies* 14.3 (1988): 575–600.

Haraway, Donna J. *Primate Visions: Gender, Race, and Nature in the World of Modern Science.* New York: Routledge, 1989.

Haraway, Donna J. *Modest Witness@SecondMillenium.FemaleMan_Meets_OncoMouse.* New York: Routledge, 1997.

Harden, Virginia A. *Inventing the NIH: Federal Biomedical Research Policy, 1887–1937.* Baltimore: Johns Hopkins University Press, 1986.

Harding, Sandra. *Whose Science? Whose Knowledge? Thinking from Women's Lives.* Ithaca, NY: Cornell University Press, 1991.

Hardy, H., George Wolff, and Helen Goodell. "Studies on Pain: A New Method for Measuring Pain Threshold: Observation on Spatial Summation of Pain." *Journal of Clinical Investigation* 19 (1940): 649–57.

Hardy, H., George Wolff, and Helen Goodell. *Pain Sensations and Reactions.* Baltimore: Williams and Wilkins, 1952.

Harkness, Jon M. "Henry Knowles Beecher." In *American National Biography,* ed. John A. Garraty and Mark C. Carnes, 465–67. Oxford: Oxford University Press, 1999.

Harkness, Jon M. "Research behind Bars: A History of Nontherapeutic Experimentation on American Prisoners." PhD diss., University of Wisconsin–Madison, 1996.

Harrington, Anne, ed. *The Placebo Effect: An Interdisciplinary Exploration.* Cambridge, MA: Harvard University Press, 1997.

Hayden, Corinne. *When Nature Goes Public: The Making and Unmaking of Bioprospecting in Mexico.* Princeton, NJ: Princeton University Press, 2003.

Healy, David. *The Psychopharmacologists.* Vol. 1. New York: Altman (Chapman and Hall), 1996.

Healy, David. *The Psychopharmacologists.* Vol. 2. London: Hodder Arnold, 1998.

Healy, David. *The Psychopharmacologists.* Vol. 3. London: Arnold, 2000.

Healy, David. *The Creation of Psychopharmacology.* Cambridge, MA: Harvard University Press, 2002.

Hertzman, Marc, and Douglas E. Feltner, eds. *The Handbook of Psychopharmacology Trials: An Overview of Scientific, Political, and Ethical Concerns.* New York: New York University Press, 1997.

Hewitt, Kim. "Psychedelics and Psychosis: LSD and Changing Ideas of Mental Illness, 1943–1966." PhD diss., University of Texas at Austin, 2002.

Hill, H. E., and Richard E. Belleville. "Effects of Chronic Barbiturate Intoxication on Motivation and Muscular Coordination." *Archives of Neurology and Psychiatry* 70 (1953): 180–88.

Himmelsbach, Clifton K. "Malaria in Narcotic Addicts at the United States Penitentiary Annex, Fort Leavenworth, Kansas." *Public Health Reports* 48 (1933): 1465.

Himmelsbach, Clifton K. "The Morphine Abstinence Syndrome, Its Nature and Treatment." *Annals of Internal Medicine* 15 (1941): 829–30.

Himmelsbach, Clifton K. Interview by Wyndham D. Miles. May 4, 1972. Oral History Interviews, Accession 613, History of Medicine Division, National Library of Medicine.

Himmelsbach, Clifton K. Interview by Jon M. Harkness and Gail Javitt, Advisory Committee for Human Radiation Experiments. Washington, DC, November 2, 1994.

Hornblum, Allan M. *Acres of Skin: Human Experiments at Holmesburg Prison.* New York: Routledge, 1998.

Hughes, Helen M. *The Fantastic Lodge: The Autobiography of a Girl Drug Addict.* Boston: Houghton Mifflin, 1961.

Hughes, Patrick H., Noel W. Barker, Gail A. Crawford, and Jerome H. Jaffe. "The Natural History of a Heroin Epidemic." *American Journal of Public Health* 62.7 (1972): 995–1001.

Hughes, Patrick H., and Jerome H. Jaffe. "The Heroin Copping Area: A Location for Epidemiological Study and Intervention." *Archives of General Psychiatry* 24 (1971): 394–400.

Hursh, Steven R. "Behavioral Economics of Drug Self-Administration and Drug Abuse Policy." *Journal of the Experimental Analysis of Behavior* 56.2 (1991): 377–93.

Huxley, Aldous. *The Doors of Perception.* New York: Harper and Brothers, 1954.

Huxley, Aldous. *Heaven and Hell.* New York: Harper and Brothers, 1955.

Huxley, Aldous. "Drugs That Shape Men's Minds." *Saturday Evening Post,* October 18, 1958, 28, 108–13.

Huxley, Aldous. *Moksha.* Ed. Michael Horowitz and Cynthia Palmer. Los Angeles: J. P. Tarcher, 1977.

Institute of Medicine. *Pathways of Addiction.* Washington, DC: National Academies Press, 1996.

Institute of Medicine (IDM). *Ethical Considerations for Research Involving Prisoners.* Washington, DC: National Academies Press, 2006.

Isbell, Harris. *Acute and Chronic Barbiturate Intoxication.* Veterans Administration Technical Bulletin 10–76. Washington, DC: U.S. Department of Veterans Affairs, 1951a.

Isbell, Harris. "The Treatment of Barbiturate Addiction." *Postgraduate Medicine* 9 (1951b): 256–58.

Isbell, Harris. "Nalline, a Specific Narcotic Antagonist: Clinical and Pharmacological Observations." *Merck Report* 62 (1953): 23–26.

Isbell, Harris. "Rapid Diagnosis of Addiction to Morphine." *Journal of the American Medical Association* 154 (1954): 414.

Isbell, Harris. "Clinical Research on Addiction in the United States." In *Narcotic Drug Addiction Problems: Proceedings of the Symposium on the History of Drug Addiction Problems,* ed. Robert B. Livingston, 114–30. Bethesda, MD: National Institutes of Health and U.S. Department of Health, Education, and Welfare, 1958.

Isbell, Harris. "Neurophysiological and Neuropsychiatric Aspects of Opioid Dependence." In *Drug Addiction and the U.S. Public Health Service,* ed. William R. Martin and Harris Isbell, 63–88. Rockville, MD: U.S. Department of Health, Education, and Welfare, 1975.

Isbell, Harris. "The Search for a Non-addicting Analgesic: Has It Been Worth It?" *Clinical Pharmacology and Therapeutics* 22.4 (October 1977): 377–84.

Isbell, Harris. Interview by Marjorie Senechal. Lexington, KY, 1986.

Isbell, Harris, Richard E. Belleville, H. Franklin Fraser, Abraham Wikler, and C. R. Logan. "Studies on Lysergic Acid Diethylamide (LSD-25)." Part 1, "Effects in Former Morphine Addicts and Development of Tolerance during Chronic Intoxication." *Archives of Neurology and Psychiatry* 76 (1956): 468–78.

Isbell, Harris, Anna J. Eisenman, Abraham Wikler, and Karl Frank. "The Effects of Single Dose of 6-Dimethlyamino-4-4-Diphenyl-3-Heptanone (Amidone, Methadon, or '10820') on Human Subjects." *Journal of Pharmacology and Experimental Therapeutics* 92.1 (1948): 83–89.

Isbell, Harris, and H. Franklin Fraser. "Actions and Addiction Liability of Dromoran Derivatives in Man." *Journal of Pharmacology and Experimental Therapeutics* 107.4 (1953): 524–30.

Isbell, Harris, H. Franklin Fraser, Abraham Wikler, Richard Belleville, and Anna J. Eisenman. "An Experimental Study of the Etiology of Rum Fits and *Delirium Tremens.*" *Quarterly Journal of Studies on Alcohol* 16.1 (March 1955): 1–33.

Isbell, Harris, Abraham Wikler, Nathan B. Eddy, John L. Wilson, and Clifford F. Moran. "Tolerance and Addiction Liability of 6-Dimethylamino-4-4-Diphenylheptanone-3 (Methadon)." *Journal of the American Medical Association* 135 (1947): 888–94.

Isbell, Harris, Abraham Wikler, Anna J. Eisenman, Mary Daingerfield, and Karl Frank. "Liability of Addiction to 6-Dimethlyamino-4-4-Diphenyl-3-Heptanone (Methadon, 'Amidone' or '10820') in Man: Experimental Addiction to Methadone." *Archives of Internal Medicine* 82 (1948): 362–92.

Iversen, Susan D., and Leslie L. Iversen. *Behavioral Pharmacology.* 2nd ed. Oxford: Oxford University Press, 1981.

Jaffe, Jerome H. "Drug Addiction and Drug Abuse." In *The Pharmacological Basis of Therapeutics,* 3rd ed., ed. Louis Goodman and Alfred Gilman, 285–311 (New York: Macmillan, 1965).

Jaffe, Jerome H. "Impact of Scheduling on the Practice of Medicine and Biomedical Research." *Drug and Alcohol Dependence* 14 (1985): 403–18.

Jaffe, Jerome H. Interview in *Addiction: Evolution of a Specialist Field,* ed. Griffith Edwards, 284–304. Malden, MA: Blackwell Science, 2002.

Jaffe, Jerome H. Interview by the author. Baltimore, MD, January 2007.

Jasinski, Donald. Interview by the author. Baltimore, MD, June 2003.

Johanson, Chris-Ellyn. Interview by the author. San Juan, PR, June 2004.

Johnson, Rolley E. Interview by the author. Orlando, FL, 2005.

Jones, Edward D., and Lorne M. Mendell. "Assessing the Decade of the Brain." *Science* 284 (April 30, 1999): 739.

Jones, James. *Bad Blood: The Tuskegee Syphilis Experiment.* New York: Free Press, 1981/1992.

Jonnes, Jill. *Hep Cats, Narcs, and Pipe Dreams: A History of America's Romance with Illegal Drugs.* New York: Scribner, 1996.

Jordanova, Ludamilla. *Sexual Visions: Images of Gender in Science and Medicine between the Eighteenth and Twentieth Centuries.* New York: Harvester Wheatsheaf, 1989.

Joseph, Herman. "Medical Methadone Maintenance: The Further Concealment of a Stigmatized Condition." PhD diss., City University of New York, 1995.

Joseph, Herman. Interview by the author. Troy, NY, August 2005.

Kaptchuck, Theodore J. "Powerful Placebo: The Dark Side of the Randomized Controlled Trial." *Lancet* 351 (1998): 1722–25.

Kay, David C., and Howard L. Andrews. "Electroencephalographic and Sleep Studies of Psychoactive Drugs." In *Drug Addiction and the U.S. Public Health Service,* ed. William R. Martin and Harris Isbell, 140–54. Rockville, MD: Department of Health, Education, and Welfare, 1978.

Keane, Helen. *What's Wrong with Addiction?* New York: New York University Press, 2002.

Keller, Evelyn Fox. *Reflections on Gender and Science.* New Haven, CT: Yale University Press, 1985.

Keller, Evelyn Fox. *Secrets of Life, Secrets of Death.* New York: Routledge, 1992.

Keve, Paul W. *Prisons and the American Conscience: A History of U.S. Federal Corrections.* Carbondale and Edwardsville: University of Illinois Press, 1991.

Kevles, Daniel J. *In the Name of Eugenics: Genetics and the Uses of Human Heredity.* New York: Alfred A. Knopf, 1985.

Kleber, Herb. Interview by the author. San Juan, PR, 2004.

Kleinman, Daniel Lee. *Politics on the Endless Frontier: Postwar Research Policy in the United States.* Durham, NC: Duke University Press, 1995.

Kline, Nathan S. "Clinical Applications of Reserpine." In *Psychopharmacology,* ed. Nathan S. Kline, 81–108. (Washington, DC: American Association for the Advancement of Science and the American Psychiatric Association, 1956).

Knorr-Cetina, Karin. *Epistemic Cultures: How the Sciences Make Knowledge.* Cambridge, MA: Harvard University Press, 2001.

Kohler, Robert E. *Lords of the Fly: Drosophila Genetics and the Experimental Life.* Chicago: University of Chicago Press, 1991.

Kohler, Robert E. *Landscapes and Labscapes: Exploring the Lab-Field Border in Biology.* Chicago: University of Chicago Press, 2002.

Kolb, Lawrence, Sr. "Drug Addiction in Its Relation to Crime." *Mental Hygiene* 9 (1925a): 74–89.

Kolb, Lawrence, Sr. "Pleasure and Deterioration from Narcotic Addiction." *Mental Hygiene* 9 (1925b): 699–724.

Kolb, Lawrence, Sr. "Types and Characteristics of Drug Addicts." *Mental Hygiene* 9 (1925c): 300–313.

Kolb, Lawrence, Sr., and Clifton K. Himmelsbach. "Clinical Studies of Drug Addiction." Part 3, "A Critical Review of the Withdrawal Treatments with Method of Evaluating Abstinence Syndromes." *American Journal of Psychiatry* 94 (1938): 759–97.

Kolb, Lawrence, Sr., and William F. Ossenfort. "The Treatment of Addicts at the Lexington Hospital." *Southern Medical Journal* 31 (1938): 914–20.

Koob, George F., and Floyd E. Bloom. "Neuroscience of Addiction." *Neuron* 21.9 (September 1998): 467–76.

Kornetsky, Conan. Interview. *Addiction* 98 (2003a): 875–82.

Kornetsky, Conan. Interview by the author. Boston, MA, June 2003b.

Krasgenor, Norman A., D. B. Gray, and Travis Thompson, eds. *Advances in Behavioral Pharmacology.* Vol. 5, *Developmental Behavioral Pharmacology.* Hillsdale, NJ: Lawrence Erlbaum Associates, 1986.

Kraut, Alan M . *Silent Travelers: Germs, Genes, and the "Immigrant Menace."* New York: Basic Books, 1994.

Kreeger, Karen Young. "Drug Institute Tackles Neurology of Addiction." *Scientist,* 9.16 (August 21, 1995): 12.

Kuhar, Michael. Interview by the author. Orlando, FL, June 2005.

Kushner, Howard I. "Taking Biology Seriously: The Next Task for Historians of Addiction?" *Bulletin of the History of Medicine* 80.1 (Spring 2006): 115–43.

La Barre, Weston. "Anthropological Perspectives on Hallucination and Hallucinogens." In *Hallucinations: Behavior, Experience, and Theory,* ed. Ronald K. Siegel and Louis J. West, 9–52. London: John Wiley and Sons, 1975.

Ladimer, Irving. "Law and Medicine: Ethical and Legal Aspects of Medical Research on Human Beings." *Journal of Public Law* 3.1 (Spring 1954): 466–511.

Lasagna, Louis. Interview by Jon M. Harkness and Suzanne White-Junod. Rochester, NY, 1994.

Lasagna, Louis. "Towards a Rapprochement between Clinical Pharmacology and Behavioral Pharmacology." In *Behavioral Pharmacology of Human Drug Dependence,* ed. Travis Thompson and Chris-Ellyn Johanson, 21–26. NIDA Research Monograph 37. Rockville, MD: National Institute on Drug Abuse, 1981.

Lasagna, Louis, Frederick Mosteller, John Von Felsinger, and Henry K. Beecher. "A Study of the Placebo Response." *American Journal of Medicine* 16 (1954): 770–79.

Lasagna, Louis, John M. Von Felsinger, and Henry K. Beecher. "Drug-Induced Mood Changes in Man." Part 1, "Observations in Healthy Subjects, Chronically Ill Patients, and Postaddicts." *Journal of the American Medical Association* 157 (1955): 1006–20.

Laties, Victor G. "Lessons from the History of Behavioral Pharmacology." In *Advances in Behavioral Pharmacology,* vol. 5, *Developmental Behavioral Pharmacology,* ed. Norman A. Krasgenor, D. B. Gray, and Travis Thompson, 21–39. Hillsdale, NJ: Lawrence Erlbaum Associates, 1986.

Laties, Victor G. "Behavioral Analysis and the Growth of Behavioral Pharmacology." *Behavior Analyst* 26 (2003): 235–52.

Latour, Bruno. *Science in Action: How to Follow Scientists and Engineers through Society.* Cambridge, MA: Harvard University Press, 1987.

Latour, Bruno, and Steve Woolgar. *Laboratory Life: The Construction of Scientific Facts.* Princeton, NJ: Princeton University Press, 1979.

Law-Medicine Research Institute (LMRI). "A Study of the Legal, Ethical, and Administrative Aspects of Clinical Research Involving Human Subjects." Final Report of Administrative Practices in Clinical Research. Boston: Law-Medicine Research Institute, 1963.

Leake, Chauncey D. *An Historical Account of Pharmacology to the Twentieth Century.* Springfield, IL: Charles C. Thomas, 1975.

Le Carre, John. *The Constant Gardener.* New York: Pocket Star Books, 2001.

Lederer, Susan E. *Subjected to Science: Human Experimentation in America before the Second World War.* Baltimore: Johns Hopkins University Press, 1995.

Lee, Martin A., and Bruce Schlain. *Acid Dreams: The Complete Social History of LSD; The CIA, The Sixties, and Beyond.* New York: Grove Weidenfeld, 1985.

Lenoir, Timothy. *Instituting Science: The Cultural Production of Scientific Disciplines.* Palo Alto, CA: Stanford University Press, 1997.

Lenson, David. *On Drugs.* Minneapolis: University of Minnesota Press, 1999.

Leshner, Alan I. "Addiction Is a Brain Disease, and It Matters." *Science* 278 (October 3, 1997): 45–47.

Levine, Robert J. "Drug Testing in Prisons." In *Troubling Problems in Medical Ethics: The Third Volume in a Series on Ethics, Humanism, and Medicine,* ed. Marc D. Basson, Rachel E. Lipson, and Doreen L. Ganos, 73–78. New York: Alan R. Liss, 1981.

Levine, Robert J. *Ethics and Regulation of Clinical Research.* Baltimore: Urban and Schwarzenberg, 1986.

Lindemann, Eric, and L. D. Clarke. "Modifications of Ego Structure and Personality Reactions under the Influence of the Effects of Drugs." *American Journal of Psychiatry* 108 (1952): 561–67.

Lindesmith, Alfred. "Can Chimpanzees Become Morphine Addicts?" *Journal of Comparative and Physiological Psychology* 39 (April 1946): 109–17.

Lindesmith, Alfred. *Opiate Addiction.* Bloomington, IN: Principia, 1947.

Livingston, Robert B., ed. *Narcotic Drug Addiction Problems: Proceedings of the Symposium on the History of Drug Addiction Problems.* Bethesda, MD: National Institutes of Health and U.S. Department of Health, Education, and Welfare, 1958.

Longino, Helen E. *Science as Social Knowledge.* Princeton, NJ: Princeton University Press, 1990.

Longino, Helen E. *The Fate of Knowledge.* Princeton, NJ: Princeton University Press, 2002.

Lunbeck, Elizabeth. *The Psychiatric Persuasion: Knowledge, Gender, and Power in Modern America.* Princeton, NJ: Princeton University Press, 1994.

MacCorquodale, Kenneth, and Paul E. Meehle. "On a Distinction between Hypothetical Constructs and Intervening Variables." *Psychological Reviews* 55 (1948): 95–107.

Macht, David I., N. B. Herman, and C. S. Levy. "A Quantitative Study of the Analgesia Produced by Opium Alkaloids, Individually, and in Combination with Each Other, in Normal Man." *Journal of Pharmacology* 8 (1916): 1–37.

Macklin, Ruth, and Susan Sherwin. "Experimenting on Human Subjects: Philosophical Perspectives." *Case Western Reserve Law Review* 25 (1975): 434–71.

Maclin, Robert. Interview by J. P. Olsen and Luke Walden. Lexington, KY, 2004.

Maddux, James F. "History of the Hospital Treatment Programs, 1935–74." In *Drug Addiction and the U.S. Public Health Service,* ed. William R. Martin and Harris Isbell, 217–50. Rockville, MD: Department of Health, Education, and Welfare, 1978.

Mansky, Peter. Interview by the author. Telephone, January 2006.

Marcuse, Herbert. *One-Dimensional Man.* Boston: Beacon, 1964.

Marja, Fern, and William Duffy. "Drug Addicts, USA." *New York Post,* January 10, 1958, M2.

Marks, Harry M. *The Progress of Experiment: Science and Therapeutic Reform in the United States, 1900–1990.* Cambridge: Cambridge University Press, 1997.

Marks, John. *The Search for the Manchurian Candidate: The CIA and Mind Control.* New York: Times Books, 1979.

Martin, William R., and Harris Isbell, eds. *Drug Addiction and the U.S. Public Health Service.* Rockville, MD: U.S. Department of Health, Education, and Welfare, 1978.

Mason, T. H., and W. B. Hamby. "Frontal Lobotomy in the Treatment of Unbearable Pain." *Archives of Research on Nervous and Mental Disorders* 27 (1947): 715, 1948.

Mason, T. H., and W. B. Hamby. "Relief of Morphine Addiction by Prefrontal Lobotomy." *Journal of the American Medical Association* 136 (1948): 1039.

Masserman, Jules H., and Abraham Wikler. "Effects of Morphine on Learned Adaptive Responses and Experimental Neuroses in Cats." *Archives of Neurology and Psychiatry* 50 (1943): 401–4.

Maurer, David W., and Victor H. Vogel. *Narcotics and Narcotic Addiction.* 3rd ed. Springfield, IL: Charles C. Thomas, 1967.

May, Everette L., and Arthur E. Jacobson. "The Committee on Problems of Drug Dependence: A Legacy of the National Academy of Sciences; An Historical Account." *Drug and Alcohol Dependence* 23 (1989): 183–218.

McFarland, Robert L., and William A. Hall. "A Survey of One Hundred Suspected Drug Addicts." *Journal of Crime, Criminology, and Police Science* 44 (1953–54): 308–19.

McWilliams, John C. *The Protectors: Harry J. Anslinger and the Federal Bureau of Narcotics, 1930–1962.* Newark: University of Delaware Press, 1990.

Mead, George Herbert. *The Philosophy of the Act.* Chicago: University of Chicago Press, 1938/1972.

Meldrum, Marcia. "Departures from Design: The Randomized Clinical Trial in Historical Perspective, 1946–1970." PhD diss., State University of New York at Stony Brook, 1994.

Merchant, Carolyn. *The Death of Nature: Women, Ecology, and the Scientific Revolution.* San Francisco: HarperCollins, 1980.

Meyer, Peter B. *Medical Experimentation on Prisoners: Some Economic Considerations.* Washington, DC: American Bar Association, 1975.

Micale, Mark S., and Roy Porter, eds. *Discovering the History of Psychiatry.* New York: Oxford University Press, 1994.

Mishkin, Barbara. "Factors Enhancing Acceptance of Federal Regulation of Research." In *Responsible Science,* vol. 2, *Background Papers and Resource Documents, Panel on Scientific Responsibility and the Conduct of Research,* 79–89. Washington, DC: National Academies Press, 1993.

Mitford, Jessica. "Experiments behind Bars: Doctors, Drug Companies, and Prisoners." *Atlantic Monthly,* January 1973a, 64–73.

Mitford, Jessica. *Kind and Usual Punishment: The Prison Business.* New York: Alfred A. Knopf, 1973b.

Mol, Annemarie. *The Body Multiple: Ontology in Medical Practice.* Durham, NC: Duke University Press, 2002.

Moreno, Jonathan D. *Undue Risk: Secret State Experiments on Humans.* New York: Routledge, 2001.

Morris, Edward K., and Nathaniel G. Smith. "On the Origin and Preservation of Cumulative Record in Its Struggle for Life as a Favored Term." *Journal of the Experimental Analysis of Behavior* 82.3 (2004): 357–73.

Morris, Norval, and Michael Mills. "Prisoners as Laboratory Animals." *Wall Street Journal,* April 2, 1974.

Morse, William. "An Analysis of Responding in the Presence of a Stimulus Correlated with Periods of Non-reinforcement." PhD diss., Harvard University, 1955.

Mowery, Edward J. "Narco Guards the Squealers: Informers Cringe in Fear of Death from Underworld." *New York World-Telegram and Sun,* November 30, 1951.

Mulkay, Michael J., Nigel Gilbert, and Steve Woolgar. "Problem Areas and Research Networks in Science." *Sociology* 9 (1975): 187–203.

Murphy, Sheigla. Interview by the author. New Orleans, LA, June 2003.

Musto, David. *The American Disease: Origins of Narcotics Control.* 3rd ed. New Haven, CT: Yale University Press, 1973/1999.

Musto, David, and Pamela Korsmeyer. *The Quest for Drug Control: Politics and Federal Policy in a Period of Increasing Substance Abuse, 1963–1981.* New Haven, CT: Yale University Press, 2002.

National Academy of Sciences Committee to Identify Strategies to Raise the Profile of Substance Abuse and Alcoholism Research. *Dispelling the Myths about Addiction.* Washington, DC: National Academy Press, 1997.

National Commission for the Protection of Human Subjects of Biomedical and Behavioral Research. "Report of Site Visit to the Addiction Research Center, Lexington, Kentucky." May 3, 1976a. Collected Papers of Heinz Lehmann, Archives of the American College of Neuropsychopharmacology, Vanderbilt University, Nashville, TN.

National Commission for the Protection of Human Subjects of Biomedical and Behavioral Research. *Research Involving Prisoners: Report and Recommendations.* DHEW Publication (OS) 76-131. Washington, DC: U.S. Government Printing Office, 1976b.

National Commission for the Protection of Human Subjects of Biomedical and Behavioral Research. *The Belmont Report: Ethical Principles and Guidelines for the Protection of Human Subjects.* Washington, DC: U.S. Government Printing Office, 1978.

National Institute of General Medical Sciences. *Status of Research in Pharmacology and Toxicology: Report of the Pharmacology and Toxicology Training Committee of the NIGMS.* Washington, DC: U.S. Government Printing Office, 1966.

National Institute of Mental Health. "Operations Manual, NIMH Clinical Research Center." Lexington, KY: Clinical Research Center, 1971. Located in Record Group 511 ADAMHA Alcohol, Drug Abuse, and Mental Health Administration, Clinical Research Center, Lexington, KY, box 8, folder "Lexington History and Operations," NARA Southeast, Morrow, GA.

Nestler, Eric J., and David Landsman. "Learning about Addiction from the Genome." *Nature,* February 15, 2001.

Nyswander, Marie. *The Drug Addict as Patient.* New York: Grune and Stratton, 1956.

O'Brien, Charles P., Nora Volkow, and Ting-Kai Li. "What's in a Word? Addiction Versus Dependence in DSM-V." *American Journal of Psychiatry* 163.5 (May 2006): 764–65.

O'Brien, Charles P. Interview by Leo Hollister and Thomas Ban. 1998. Archives of the American College of Neuropsychopharmacology, Vanderbilt University, Nashville, TN.

O'Brien, Charles P. Interview by the author. Orlando, FL, June 2005.

O'Donnell, John A. "A Follow-up of Narcotic Addicts: Mortality, Relapse, and Abstinence." *American Journal of Orthopsychiatry* 34.5 (October 1964): 948–54.

Office of Technology Assessment. "The Effectiveness of Drug Abuse Threatment." Washington, DC: Government Printing Office, 1990.

O'Keefe, Charles. Interview by the author. Orlando, FL, June 2005.

Olds, James. "'Reward' from Brain Stimulation in the Rat." *Science* 122 (November 4, 1955): 878.

Olds, James. "Pleasure Center in the Brain." *Scientific American* 195 (1956): 105–16.

Olds, James. "Self-stimulation of the Brain." *Science* 127 (February 14, 1958): 315–24.

Olds, James, and Paul Milner. "Positive Reinforcement Produced by Electrical Stimulation of Septal Area and Other Regions of Rat Brain." *Journal of Comparative Physiology* 47 (1954): 419–27.

Orenstein, Peggy. "Staying Clean." *New York Times Magazine,* February 10, 2002.

Orr, Jackie. *Panic Diaries: A Genealogy of Panic Disorder.* Durham, NC: Duke University Press, 2006.

Oudshoorn, Nelly. *Beyond the Natural Body: An Archeology of Sex Hormones.* New York: Routledge, 1994.

Oudshoorn, Nelly. *The Male Pill: A Biography of a Technology in the Making.* Durham, NC, and London: Duke University Press, 2003.

Patey, Douglas L., ed. *Of Human Bondage: Historical Perspectives on Addiction.* Smith College Studies in History 52. Northampton, MA: Smith College, 2003.

Pavlov, Ivan P. *Conditioned Reflexes.* London: Oxford University Press, 1927.

Pavlov, Ivan P. *Conditioned Reflexes and Psychiatry.* New York: International Publishers, 1941.

Payne, W. J., D. Schreiber, and G. Riley. "Transitions in Counselor Preparation: From Occupational Training Programs to Professional Education." *Journal of Teaching in the Addictions* 3.2 (2004): 19–28.

Pert, Candace. *Molecules of Emotion: The Science behind Mind-Body Medicine.* New York: Scribner, 1997.

Petryna, Adriana. "Globalizing Human Subjects Research." In *Global Pharmaceuticals: Ethics, Markets, and Practices,* ed. Adriana Petryna, Andrew Lakoff, and Arthur Kleinman, 33–60. Durham, NC: Duke University Press, 2006.

Pfeiffer, Carl C. Introduction to part 2 of "Psychotomimetic Agents: Neurophysiological Effects." *Annals of the New York Academy of Science* 66 (1957): 478.

Pickens, Roy. "Behavioral Pharmacology: A Brief History." In *Advances in Behavioral Pharmacology,* vol. 1, ed. Peter B. Dews and Travis Thompson. New York: Academic Press, 1977.

Plummer, Ken. "Continuity and Change in Howard S. Becker's Work: An Interview with Howard S. Becker." *Sociological Perspectives* 46.1 (2003): 21–39.

President's Advisory Commission on Narcotics and Drug Abuse. *Final Report.* Washington, DC: U.S. Government Printing Office, 1963.

Pressman, Jack D. *Last Resort: Psychosurgery and the Limits of Medicine.* Cambridge: Cambridge University Press, 1998.

Rader, Karen A. *Making Mice: Standardizing Animals for American Biomedical Research, 1900–1955.* Princeton, NJ: Princeton University Press, 2004.

Rado, Sandor. "The Psychic Effects of Intoxicants." *International Journal of Psychoanalysis* 7 (1926): 396–413.

Rado, Sandor. "The Psychoanalysis of Pharmacothymia (Drug Addiction)." Trans. B. D. Lewin. *Psychoanalytic Quarterly* 2 (1933): 1–23.

Rado, Sandor. "Narcotic Bondage: A General Theory of the Dependence on Narcotic Drugs." *American Journal of Psychiatry* 114 (1957): 165–70.

Rado, Sandor. "Fighting Narcotic Bondage." *Comprehensive Psychiatry* 4.3 (1963): 160–67.

Rado, Sandor. *Adaptational Psychodynamics: Motivation and Control.* Ed. Jean Jameson and Henriette Klein. New York: Science House, 1969.

Rado, Sandor, and G. E. Daniels, eds. *Changing Concepts of Psychoanalytic Medicine.* New York: Grune and Stratton, 1956.

Rafter, Nicole Hahn. *Creating Born Criminals.* Champaign: University of Illinois Press, 1997.

Rasmussen, Nicolas. "A Prescription for Psychopharmacology." *Social Studies of Science* 33 (2003): 453–61.

Rasor, Robert W., and James F. Maddux. *Institutional Treatment of Narcotic Addiction by the U.S. Public Health Service.* Washington, DC: U.S. Department of Health, Education, and Welfare, 1966.

Reverby, Susan. *Tuskegee's Truths: Rethinking the Tuskegee Syphilis Study.* Chapel Hill: University of North Carolina Press, 2000.

Roberts, Dorothy E. *Killing the Black Body: Race, Reproduction, and the Meaning of Liberty.* New York: Pantheon, 1997.

Roberts, John W. "Work, Education, and Public Safety: A Brief History of Federal Prison Industries." In *Factories with Fences: The History of Federal Prison Industries,* 10–37. Washington, DC: U.S. Government Printing Office, 1996.

Ronald, Lorna. "Empowered to Consume: Direct-to-Consumer Advertising, Free Speech, and Pharmaceutical Governance." PhD diss., Rensselaer Polytechnic Institute, 2006.

Rose, Nikolas. "Becoming Neurochemical Selves." In *Biotechnology between Commerce and Civil Society,* ed. Nico Stehr, 1–43. New Brunswick, NJ: Transaction, 2003.

Rosenfeld, Harold A. *Psychotic States.* London: Hogarth, 1965.

Rothman, David. *Strangers at the Bedside: A History of How Law and Bioethics Transformed Medical Decision Making.* New York: Basic Books, 1994.

Rowan, Andrew N. *Of Mice, Models, and Men: A Critical Evaluation of Animal Research.* Albany: State University of New York Press, 1984.

Rudgley, Richard. *Essential Substances: A Cultural History of Intoxicants in Society.* New York: Kodansha, 1993.

Rudgley, Richard. "The Ethnography of Imaginal States: Archaeology and Altered States." In *Of Human Bondage: Historical Perspectives on Addiction,* ed. Douglas L. Patey, 51–80. Smith College Studies in History 52. Northampton, MA: Smith College, 2003.

Rugaber, Walter. "Prison Drug and Plasma Projects Leave Fatal Trail." *New York Times,* July 29, 1969.

Russell, Roger W. "Drugs as Tools in Behavioral Research." In *Drugs and Behavior,* ed. Leonard Uhr and James G. Miller, 19–40. New York: John Wiley and Sons, 1960.

Rutherford, Alexandra. "Skinner Boxes for Psychotics: Operant Conditioning at Metropolitan State Hospital." *Behavior Analyst* 26 (2003): 267–79.

Salisbury, Karen. "The Junk War." *Newsweek,* September 17, 1951.

Savoy, Robert L. "History and Future Directions of Human Brain Mapping and Functional Neuroimaging." *Acta Psychologica* 107.1–3 (2001): 9–42.

Schram, Sanford F. *Welfare Discipline: Discourse, Governance, and Globalization.* Philadelphia, PA: Temple University Press, 2006.

Schroeder, Kathleen. "A Recommendation to the FDA Concerning Drug Research on Prisoners." *Southern California Law Review* 56 (May 1983): 969–1000.

Schumaker, George A., Helen Goodell, James D. Hardy, and Harold G. Wolff. "Uniformity of the Pain Threshold in Man." *Science* 92 (August 2, 1940): 110–12.

Schuster, Charles R. "Drugs as Reinforcers in Monkey and Man." *Pharmacological Reviews* 27.4 (1976): 511–21.

Schuster, Charles R. Interview by the author. San Juan, PR, June 2004.

Scull, Andrew. *Social Order/Mental Disorder: Anglo-American Psychiatry in Historical Perspective.* Berkeley: University of California Press, 1989.

Sedgwick, Eve Kosofky. *Tendencies.* Durham, NC: Duke University Press, 1993.

Seevers, Maurice H. "Acute and Chronic Narcotic Drug Poisoning." PhD diss., University of Chicago, 1930.

Seevers, Maurice H. "Opiate Addiction in the Monkey: Dilaudid in Comparison with Morphine, Heroine and Codeine." *Journal of Pharmacology and Experimental Therapeutics* 56.2 (1936a): 157.

Seevers, Maurice H. "Opiate Addiction in the Monkey: Methods of Study." *Journal of Pharmacology and Experimental Therapeutics* 56.2 (1936b): 147.

Seevers, Maurice H. "Drug Addiction Problems." *Sigma Xi Quarterly* 27 (June 1939): 91–102.

Seevers, Maurice H. "Test Planning." Proceedings of the Annual Research and Development Conference of the Proprietary Association, 4–12. New York, Biltmore Hotel, December 8, 1960.

Seevers, Maurice H. "Drugs, Monkeys, and Men." *Michigan Quarterly Review* 8.1 (January 1969a): 3–14.

Seevers, Maurice H. Chapter 3, "Publications," and Chapter 8, "Projection to the Future." In *The American Society for Pharmacology and Experimental Therapeutics: The First Sixty Years,* ed. K. K. Chen, 123–36, 207–20. Washington, DC: Judd and Detweiler, 1969b.

Seevers, Maurice H. "Science and Medicine: Puppets in International Drug Abuse Control." Paper presented at the annual meeting of the Committee on Problems of Drug Dependence, Ann Arbor, MI, 1972.

Seiden, Lewis S., and Robert L. Balster, eds. *Behavioral Pharmacology: The Current Status.* New York: Alan R. Liss, 1985.

Senechal, Marjorie. "Narco Brat." In *Of Human Bondage: Historical Perspectives on Addiction,* ed. Douglas L. Patey, 173–200. Smith College Studies in History 52. Northampton, MA: Smith College, 2003.

Senechal, Marjorie. Interview by the author. Northampton, MA, 2004.

Shah, Sonia. *The Body Hunters: How the Drug Industry Tests Its Products on the World's Poorest Patients.* New York: New Press, 2006.

Shapiro, Arthur K., and Elaine Shapiro. "The Placebo: Is It Much Ado about Nothing?"

In *The Placebo Effect: An Interdisciplinary Exploration*, ed. Anne Harrington, 12–36. Cambridge, MA: Harvard University Press, 1997.

Shaw, Susan J., and Nancy D. Campbell. "The Incitement to Discourse: The Historical Travels of Harm Reduction in Drug Ethnography." *Cultural Anthropology* 22.3 (forthcoming).

Shubin, Seymour. "Prisoner Research." Rochester, NY: Center for the Study of Drug Development, 1980.

Siegel, Ronald K. *Intoxication: Life in Pursuit of Artificial Paradise.* New York: E. P. Dutton, 1989.

Siegel, Ronald K., and Louis J. West, eds. *Hallucinations: Behavior, Experience, and Theory.* London: John Wiley and Sons, 1975.

Smith, Barbara Herrnstein. *Scandalous Knowledge: Science, Truth, and the Human.* Durham, NC: Duke University Press, 2005.

Smith, Mickey C. *A Social History of the Minor Tranquilizers: The Quest for Small Comfort in the Age of Anxiety.* London: Haworth Press, 1991.

Snyder, Solomon H. *Brainstorming: The Science and Politics of Opiate Research.* Cambridge, MA: Harvard University Press, 1989.

Spiegel, Rene. *Psychopharmacology: An Introduction.* Trans. David Oliver. New York: John Wiley and Sons, 1989.

Spragg, S. D. S. "Morphine Addiction in Chimpanzees." *Comparative Psychology Monographs* 15 (1940): 1–132.

Starr, Paul. *The Social Transformation of American Medicine.* New York: Basic Books, 1982.

Stepan, Nancy. *The Idea of Race in Science.* Hamden, CT: Archon, 1982.

Stephens, Trent, and Rock Brynner. *Dark Remedy: The Impact of Thalidomide and Its Revival as a Vital Medicine.* Cambridge, MA: Perseus, 2001.

Straus, Erwin, ed. *Phenomenology: Pure and Applied.* Pittsburgh, PA: University of Pittsburgh Press, 1964.

Su, Tsung-Ping. Interview by the author. San Juan, PR, June 14, 2004.

Substance Abuse and Mental Health Services Administration. "Practice Improvement Collaboratives: Bridging the Gap," *SAMHSA News* 9.3 (Summer 2001): 1–4.

Swain, Henry. *One Hundred Years of Pharmacology, 1891–1991.* Ann Arbor, MI: Department of Pharmacology, 1991.

Swann, John P. *Academic Scientists and the Pharmaceutical Industry: Cooperative Research in Twentieth-Century America.* Baltimore: Johns Hopkins University Press, 1988.

Swinburn, Woods C. "Medical Research and Experimentation and Pharmaceutical Testing: A Protocol." Research and Development Division, Texas Department of Corrections, Huntsville, 1974.

Tabenanika, Candace. "Ethical Issues of Human Experimentation with Emphasis on Experiments Conducted at the Texas Prison System." Master's thesis, College of Criminal Justice, Sam Houston State University, 2002.

Tatum, Arthur L., K. H. Collins, and Maurice H. Seevers. "Further Observations in Experimental Chronic Morphinism." *Journal of Pharmacology and Experimental Therapeutics* 31.3 (1927): 213.

Tatum, Arthur L., K. H. Collins, and Maurice H. Seevers. "Morphine Addiction and Its Physiological Interpretation Based on Experimental Evidences." *Journal of Pharmacology and Experimental Therapeutics* 36.3 (1929): 447–75.

Tatum, Arthur L., and Maurice H. Seevers. "Experimental Cocaine Addiction." *Journal of Pharmacology and Experimental Therapeutics* 36.3 (1929): 401–10.

Terry, Charles E., and Mildred Pellens. *The Opium Problem.* Montclair, NJ: Patterson Smith, 1928/1970.

Terry, Jennifer. *An American Obsession: Science, Medicine, and Homosexuality in Modern Society.* Chicago: University of Chicago Press, 1999.

Thompson, Paul. "Oral History and the History of Medicine: A Review." *Social History of Medicine* 4 (1991): 371–83.

Thompson, Travis, and Charles R. Schuster. *Behavioral Pharmacology.* Englewood Cliffs, NJ: Prentice Hall, 1968.

Tomes, Nancy. *The Art of Asylum-Keeping: Thomas Story Kirkbride and the Origins of American Psychiatry.* Philadelphia: University of Pennsylvania Press, 1994.

Tone, Andrea. *The Age of Anxiety: Tranquilizers and Psychiatry in Modern America.* New York: Basic Books, forthcoming.

Tousignant, Noemi. "Pain and the Pursuit of Objectivity: Pain-Measuring Technologies in the United States, c. 1890–1975." PhD diss., McGill University, 2006.

Tracy, Sarah, and Caroline J. Acker, eds. *Altering American Consciousness: The History of Alcohol and Drug Use in the United States, 1800–2000.* Boston: University of Massachusetts Press, 2004.

Traweek, Sharon. *Beamtimes and Lifetimes: The World of High Energy Physics.* Cambridge, MA: Harvard University Press, 1988.

Treadway, Walter L. "Medical Service in Federal Prisons." *Public Health Reports* 45 (1930): 2–8.

Tuana, Nancy. *Feminism and Science.* Bloomington: Indiana University Press, 1989.

Tuana, Nancy. *The Less Noble Sex: Scientific, Religious, and Philosophical Conceptions of Woman's Nature.* Bloomington: Indiana University Press, 1993.

Ubel, Peter A., Brian J. Zikmund-Fisher, Brianna Sarr, and Angelina Fagerlin. "A Matter of Perspective: Choosing for Others Differs from Choosing for Yourself in Medical Treatment Decisions." *Journal of General Internal Medicine* 21.6 (June 2006): 618–22.

Uhl, George. Interview by the author. Baltimore, MD. May 2003.

Urbina, Ian. "Panel Suggests Using Inmates in Drug Trials." *New York Times,* August 13, 2006.

U.S. Congress. Senate Committee on the Judiciary, Subcommittee on Improvements to the Criminal Code. *The Illicit Narcotics Traffic.* 84th Cong., 1st sess., 1955.

U.S. Congress. Senate Select Committee on Small Business, Subcommittee on Monopoly. *Competitive Problems in the Drug Industry: Present Status of Competition in the Pharmaceutical Industry.* 91st Cong., 1st sess., part 14, June 19, August 7, and August 12, 1969.

U.S. Congress. Senate Committee on Labor and Public Welfare, Subcommittee on Health. *Quality of Health Care—Human Experimentation.* 93d Cong., 1st sess., March 7 and June 28, 1973.

U.S. Congress. House Committee on the Judiciary, Subcommittee on Courts, Civil Liberties, and the Administration of Justice. On HR 3603. 94th Cong., 1st sess., September 29 and October 1, 1975.

U.S. Congress. Senate Committee on Human Resources, Subcommittee on Health and Scientific Research. *Human Drug Testing by the CIA.* On S 1893. 95th Cong., 1st sess., September 20–21, 1977a.

U.S. Congress. Senate Committee on Human Resources, Subcommittee on Health and Scientific Research, and Select Committee on Intelligence. *Project MKULTRA, the CIA's Program of Research in Behavioral Modification.* 95th Cong., 1st sess., August 3, 1977b.

U.S. Department of Health, Education, and Welfare. *Rehabilitating the Narcotic Addict.* Rockville, MD: Department of Health, Education, and Welfare, 1967.

U.S. Department of Health, Education, and Welfare. "Report of the President's Biomedical Research Panel." [OS] 76-500. Rockville, MD: Department of Health, Education, and Welfare, 1976.

U.S. Department of Health, Education, and Welfare. *Annotated Bibliography of Papers from the Addiction Research Center, 1935 to 1975.* [ADM] 77-435. Rockville, MD: Department of Health, Education, and Welfare, 1978.

Valverde, Mariana. *Diseases of the Will: Alcohol and the Dilemmas of Freedom.* Cambridge: Cambridge University Press, 1998.

Van Winkle, Walton, Jr. "Report to the Council." *Journal of the American Medical Association* 141 (1949): 1051.

Vocci, Frank. Interview by the author. Orlando, FL, June 2005.

Volkow, Nora. "Drug Addiction: Neurobiology of Disrupted Free Will." Bethesda, MD: National Institutes of Health, 2006.

Volkow, Nora, and Ting-Kai Li. "Drug Addiction: The Neurobiology of Behavior Gone Awry." *Nature Reviews Neuroscience* 12 (December 2004): 963–70.

Volkow, Nora, and Ting-Kai Li. "The Neuroscience of Addiction." *Nature Neuroscience* 8 (2005): 1429–30.

Von Felsinger, John M., Louis Lasagna, and Henry K. Beecher. "Drug-Induced Mood Changes in Man." Part 2, "Personality and Reactions to Drugs." *Journal of the American Medical Association* 157 (1955): 1113–19.

Wailoo, Keith. *Drawing Blood: Technology and Disease Identity in Twentieth-Century America.* Baltimore: Johns Hopkins University Press, 1997.

Walsh, John. "Addiction Research Center: Pioneers Still on the Frontier." *Science* 182 (December 21, 1973a): 1229–31.

Walsh, John. "Lexington Narcotics Hospital: A Special Sort of Alma Mater." *Science* 182 (December 7, 1973b): 1004–5, 1007–8.

Weeks, James R. "Self-Maintained Morphine 'Addiction': A Method for Chronic, Programmed Intravenous Injection in Unrestricted Rats." *Federation Proceedings* 20 (1961): 397.

Weeks, James R. "Experimental Morphine Addiction: Methods for Automatic Intravenous Injections in Unrestrained Rats." *Science* 138 (October 12, 1962): 143–144.

Weil, Andrew. *The Natural Mind.* Boston: Houghton Mifflin, 1972.

Weiss, Bernard, Victor Laties, and F. L. Blanton. "Amphetamine Toxicity in Rats and

Mice Subjected to Stress." *Journal of Pharmacology and Experimental Therapeutics* 132.3 (1961): 366.

Wells, Stephen H., Patricia M. Kennedy, John Kenny, Marvin Reznikoff, and Michael H. Sheard. *Pharmacological Testing in a Correctional Institution.* Springfield, IL: Charles C. Thomas, 1975.

White, William L. *Slaying the Dragon: A History of Addiction Treatment in America.* Bloomington, IN: Chestnut Health Systems/Lighthouse Institute, 1998.

White, William L. "The Lesson of Language: Historical Perspectives on the Language of Addiction." In *Altering American Consciousness: The History of Alcohol and Drug Use in the United States, 1800–2000,* ed. Sarah W. Tracy and Caroline Jean Acker, 33–60. Amherst, MA: University of Massachusetts Press, 2004.

Wikler, Abraham. "Organic Factors in the Etiology of Mental Disorders." *Kentucky Medical Journal* 40 (1942): 399–404.

Wikler, Abraham. "Conferences on Therapy: Treatment of Drug Addiction." *New York State Journal of Medicine,* October 1, 1944, 1–8.

Wikler, Abraham. "Discussion of the Paper by Maurice H. Seevers, 'Animal Experimentation in Studying Addiction to the Newer Synthetic Analgesics.'" *Annals of the New York Academy of Science* 51 (1948a): 98–107.

Wikler, Abraham. "Recent Progress in Research on the Neurophysiologic Basis of Morphine Addiction." *American Journal of Psychiatry* 105 (November 1948b): 329–38.

Wikler, Abraham. "Sites and Mechanisms of Action of Morphine and Related Drugs in the Central Nervous System." Part 2. *Journal of Pharmacology and Experimental Therapeutics* 100.4 (1950): 436–506.

Wikler, Abraham. "Clinical Aspects of Diagnosis and Treatment of Addictions." *Bulletin of the Menninger Clinic* 15.1 (September 1951): 157–66.

Wikler, Abraham. "A Critical Analysis of Some Current Concepts in Psychiatry." *Psychosomatic Medicine* 14 (1952a): 10–17.

Wikler, Abraham. "Discussion of Experimental Pharmacology and the Measurement of the Subjective Response." *Biometrics* 8 (1952b): 227–29.

Wikler, Abraham. "Fundamentals of Scientific Research in Psychiatry." *Neuropsychiatry* 2.3 (Fall 1952c): 87–98.

Wikler, Abraham. "A Psychodynamic Study of a Patient during Experimental Self-regulated Readdiction to Morphine." *Psychiatric Quarterly* 26 (1952d): 279–93.

Wikler, Abraham. *Opiate Addiction: Psychological and Neurophysiological Aspects in Relation to Clinical Problems.* Springfield, IL: Charles C. Thomas, 1953.

Wikler, Abraham. "Clinical and Electroencephalographic Studies on the Effects of Mescaline, N-allylnormorphine and Morphine in Man." *Journal of Nervous and Mental Diseases* 120 (1954): 157–75.

Wikler, Abraham. *The Relation of Psychiatry to Pharmacology.* Baltimore: Williams and Wilkins, 1957.

Wikler, Abraham. "Research Program of NIMH Addiction Research Center: Past Development and Future Prospects." Report to Congress, 1960.

Wikler, Abraham. "Comments." In *Phenomenology: Pure and Applied,* ed. Erwin Straus, 185–88. Pittsburgh, PA: University of Pittsburgh Press, 1964.

Wikler, Abraham. "Conditioning Factors in Opiate Addiction and Relapse," *Narcotics,* eds. Daniel M. Wilner and Gene G. Kassebaum, 86–100. New York: McGraw-Hill, 1965.

Wikler, Abraham. "Review of the NIMH Intramural Research Program on Drugs of Abuse: Behavioral and Psychosocial Studies." Bethesda, MD: National Institute on Mental Health, 1972.

Wikler, Abraham. "The Search for the Psyche in Drug Dependence." Nathan B. Eddy Memorial Award Lecture, College on Problems of Drug Dependence, 1974.

Wikler, Abraham. "The Search for the Psyche in Drug Dependence: A 35-Year Retrospective Study." *Journal of Nervous and Mental Disease* 165.1 (1977): 29–40.

Wikler, Abraham. "Neurophysiological and Neuropsychiatric Aspects of Opioid Dependence." In *Drug Addiction and the U.S. Public Health Service*, ed. William R. Martin and Harris Isbell, 63–88. Rockville, MD: U.S. Department of Health, Education, and Welfare, 1978.

Wikler, Abraham, and R. L. Carter. "Effects of Single Doses of N-allylnormorphine on Hindlimb Reflexes of Chronic Spinal Dogs during Cycles of Morphine Addiction." *Journal of Pharmacology and Experimental Therapeutics* 109.1 (1953): 92–101.

Wikler, Abraham, H. Franklin Fraser, and Harris Isbell. "N-Allylnormorphine: Effects of Single Doses and Precipitation of Acute 'Abstinence Syndromes' during Addiction to Morphine, Methadone, or Heroin in Man (Post-addicts)." *Journal of Pharmacology and Experimental Therapeutics* 109.1 (1953): 8–20.

Wikler, Abraham, Helen Goodell, and Harold G. Wolff. "Studies on Pain: The Effects of Analgesic Agents on Sensations other than Pain." *Journal of Pharmacology and Experimental Therapeutics* 83.4 (1945): 294–99.

Wikler, Abraham, and J. H. Linson. "A Study of the Horner Syndrome with Presentation of Five Cases." *Hospital News* 6 (1939): 1–14.

Wikler, Abraham, Michael J. Pescor, Elmore P. Kalbaugh, and Ralph J. Angelucci. "Effects of Frontal Lobotomy on the Morphine Abstinence Syndrome in Man: An Experimental Study." *Archives of Neurology and Psychiatry* 67 (1952): 510–21.

Wikler, Abraham, Edwin G. Williams, and Carl Weisel. "Monilemia Associated with Toxic Purpura." *Archives of Neurology and Psychiatry* 50 (1943): 661–68.

Wilner, Daniel M., and Gene G. Kassebaum, eds. *Narcotics*. New York: McGraw-Hill, 1965.

Wilson, Elizabeth. *Psychosomatic: Feminism and the Neurological Body*. Durham, NC: Duke University Press, 2004.

Woods, James. Interview by the author. San Juan, PR, June 2004.

Woods, James. Interview by the author. Ann Arbor, MI, March 2005.

World Health Organization. Expert Committee on Drugs Liable to Produce Addiction. Technical Report Series 21. 1950.

Xie, Xuemei. "Brain, Gender, Culture, and the Neurosciences in the United States and China." PhD diss., Rensselaer Polytechnic Institute, 1999.

Yalisove, Daniel L., ed. *Essential Papers on Addiction*. New York: New York University Press, 1997.

Index

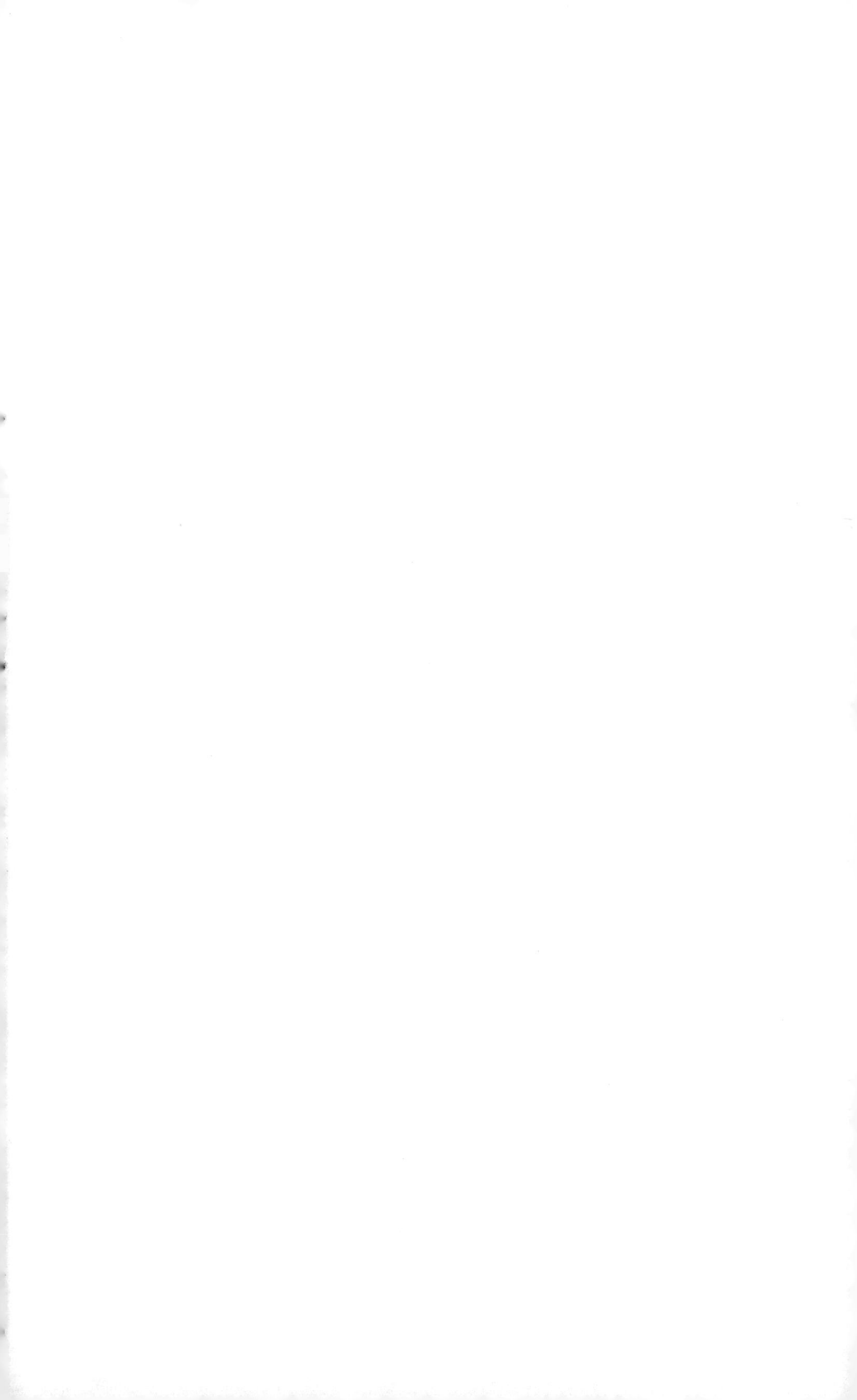